Bone Marrow

Interpretation

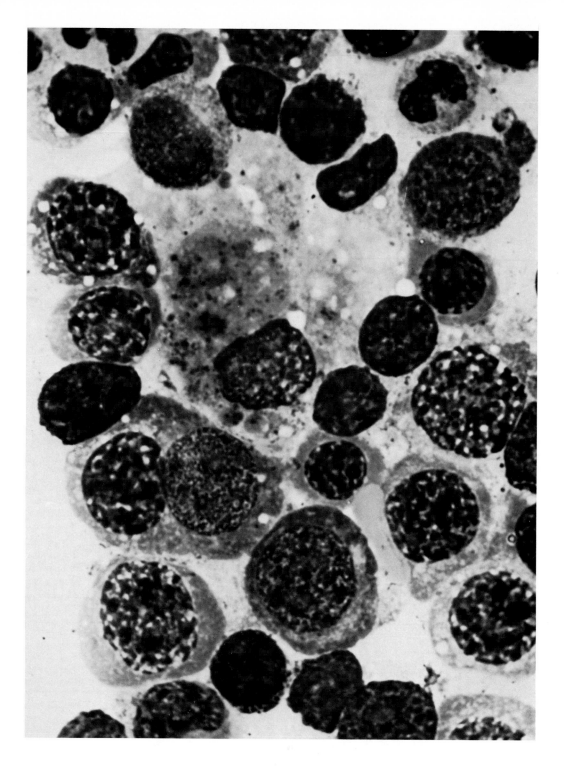

J. B. Lippincott Company Philadelphia

London   Mexico City   New York   St. Louis   São Paulo   Sydney

Lawrence Kass M.D.

Professor of Medicine, Pathology, and Hematopathology,
Case Western Reserve University School of Medicine,
Cleveland, Ohio

BONE MARROW

INTERPRETATION

Second Edition

Acquisitions Editor: Micaela Palumbo
Sponsoring Editor: Richard Winters
Manuscript Editor: Linda Fitzpatrick
Art Director and Designer: Tracy Baldwin
Production Supervisor: J. Corey Gray
Production Coordinator: Barney Fernandes
Compositor: Ruttle, Shaw & Wetherill
Printer/Binder: Halliday Lithograph

Frontispiece. Macrophage and megaloblastoid intermediate macronormoblasts in chronic erythemic myelosis.

The author and publisher have exerted every effort to ensure that drug selection and dosage set forth in this text are in accord with current recommendations and practice at the time of publication. However, in view of ongoing research, changes in government regulations, and the constant flow of information relating to drug therapy and drug reactions, the reader is urged to check the package insert for each drug for any change in indications and dosage and for added warnings and precautions. This is particularly important when the recommended agent is a new or infrequently employed drug.

6 5 4 3 2 1

Library of Congress Cataloging in Publication Data

Kass, Lawrence, DATE
    Bone marrow interpretation.

    Bibliography: p.
    Includes index.
    1. Marrow—Examination. 2. Diagnosis, Cytologic.
I. Title. [DNLM: 1. Bone Marrow—pathology. 2. Bone Marrow Examination. 3. Hematologic Diseases—pathology. WH 380 K19b]
RB55.2.K37 1985   616.1'507583   84-23537
ISBN 0-397-50701-1

For my wife, Sara Fran

Preface

Since the publication of the original edition of *Bone Marrow Interpretation* in 1973, the value and importance of bone marrow interpretation as a diagnostic tool have increased dramatically. Particularly over the past decade, bone marrow aspirations and biopsies have been essential in the continuing observation of evolutionary patterns in leukemias and lymphomas. With parallel advances in immunology, cytogenetics, and cytochemistry, it is now possible to identify preleukemic disorders with greater assurance than before and to categorize them according to their proliferative potential and likelihood of leukemic evolution. Likewise, the advent of the FAB (French-American-British) classification of the acute leukemias has provided a sound basis for the cytological diagnosis of the various types of leukemic blasts.

Of ever-increasing value in the staging of solid tumors is the use of bone marrow aspirates and biopsies to detect bone marrow involvement, and subsequently to formulate appropriate treatment. With the development of immunoperoxidase techniques using monoclonal antibodies, interpretation of bone marrow aspirates and biopsies in the staging of malignant lymphomas and Hodgkin's disease has attained new sophistication. In bone marrow specimens, it is now possible to identify small numbers of lymphoma cells on the basis of their monoclonality, and thereby determine the extent of disease.

As bone marrow transplantation has become more widespread in the treatment of aplastic anemia and acute leukemia, examination of serial bone marrow specimens has been of critical importance in assessing whether or not a transplant has been successful. Of course, bone marrow interpretation retains a time-honored place in the diagnosis of obscure anemias and pancytopenias and in the investigation of peripheral blood abnormalities such as neutropenia, monocytosis, lymphocytosis, eosinophilia, basophilia, thrombocytosis, and thrombocytopenia. As in the past, the only certain way to diagnose a disorder of the formed elements of the blood is to examine a patient's bone marrow.

This edition of *Bone Marrow Interpretation* has several important additions. First, 178 new black-and-white photomicrographs have been added. These include panoptically stained bone marrow aspirates, H&E stained sections of bone marrow biopsies, and cytochemical stains. Second, 16 new plates in full color have been included; these display representative disorders of erythropoiesis, diseases of megakaryocytes, unusual forms of leukemia, and typical cytochemical reactions. Third, the sections on lymphocytosis and acute non-lymphoblastic leukemia have been rewritten and revised to bring these areas into line with present-day observations and concepts. Fourth, selected classical and contemporary references have been added at the end of the text.

Current trends in cytology indicate that many of the dramatic developments in cytogenetics and in flow cytometry are being applied to the study of bone marrow cells in health and disease. With greater awareness of these developments and their integration into hematopathology, morphologic abnormalities will be regarded as visible expressions of more fundamental biochemical and biophysical aberrations occurring within the cells. As new cytochemical and immunocytochemical stains become available, identification of cell types and their progenitors will become precise and accurate. With these applications of advances in morphology, cytochemistry, and immunology, it is likely that bone marrow interpretation will continue to grow in importance and in significance in the years to come.

Lawrence Kass, M.D.

Preface to the First Edition

This is a book about bone marrow interpretation. It has been written for hematologists, oncologists, pathologists, and medical laboratory technologists.

Unlike many traditional bone marrow atlases, this book proposes that most hematologic disorders are characterized by an increase of one or more cell lines (hyperplasia) accompanied by a relative decrease of one or another cell line (hypoplasia). Within this framework of hyperplasia and hypoplasia, cells may show distinctive morphologic and cytochemical abnormalities.

Recognition of abnormalities in composition, appearance, and cytochemistry of marrow cells is an initial step in the complex cognitive process of interpretation. These abnormalities are visible manifestations of important biochemical and biophysical aberrations. Some of these have been identified. Others are as yet unknown.

With an understanding of disease processes and their effects upon blood-forming tissues, the significance of cytologic and cytochemical abnormalities can be elucidated. Only then does bone marrow interpretation approach what it ought to be: a meaningful statement of pathophysiology occurring in the patient's marrow at a given moment in time.

Lawrence Kass, M.D.

Contents

Bone Marrow

Interpretation

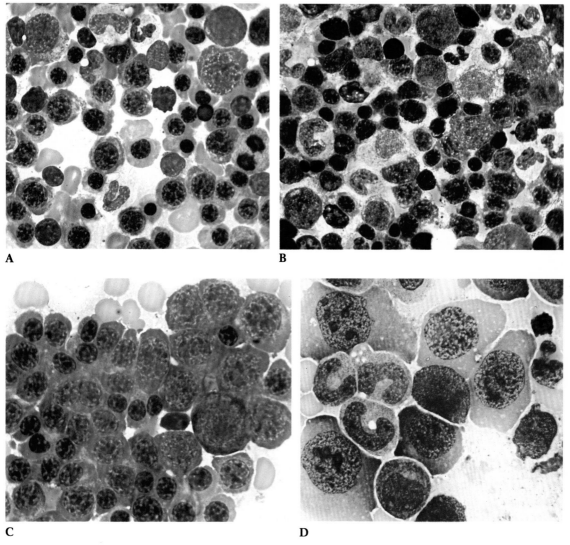

Plate 1   *Disorders of erythropoiesis. (A) Autoimmune hemolytic anemia. (B) Iron deficiency anemia. (C) Chronic erythremic myelosis. (D) Pernicious anemia.*

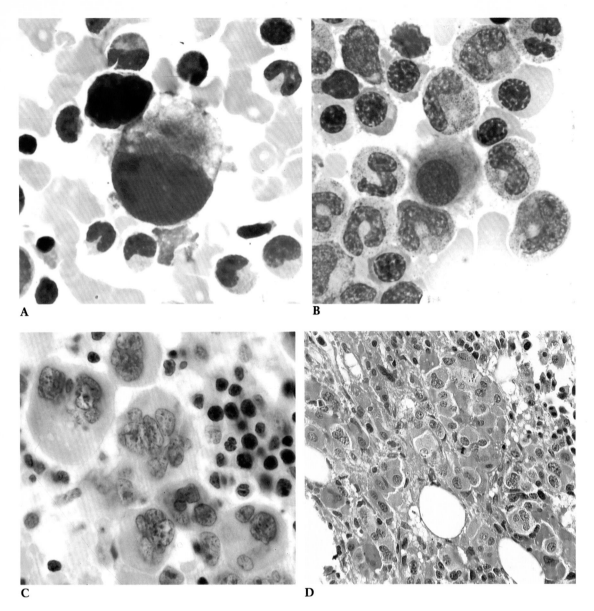

Plate 2   *Disorders of megakaryocytes. (A) Idiopathic thrombocytopenic purpura.*
(B) Micromegakaryocyte in preleukemia. (C) Essential thrombocythemia.
(D) Acute megakaryocytic myelosis.

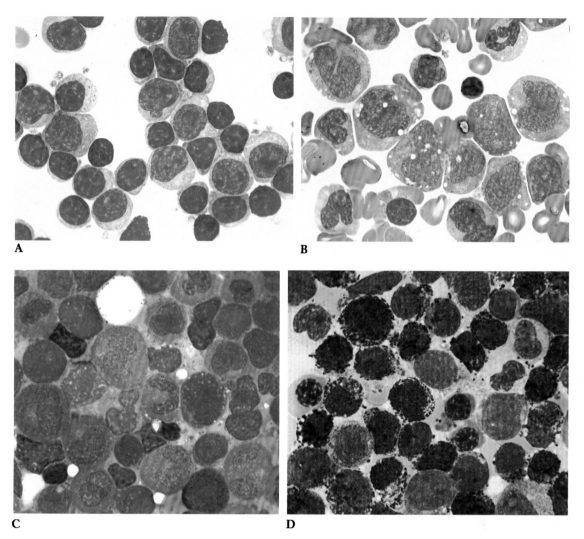

Plate 3   *Unusual forms of leukemia. (A) Prolymphocytic leukemia.*
(B) Microgranular promyelocytic leukemia. (C) Acute myelomonocytic
leukemia (M4) with increased eosinophils. (D) Basophilic leukemia.

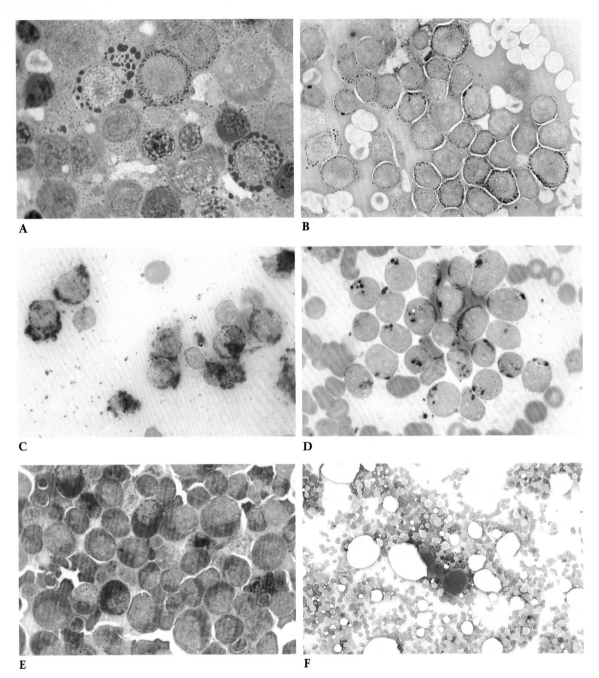

Plate 4   *Cytochemical stains for bone marrow cells. (A) PAS-positive erythroblasts in erythroleukemia. (B) PAS positivity in leukemic lymphoblasts. (C) Tartrate-resistant acid phosphatase in hairy cells, hairy cell leukemia. (D) Focal, unipolar acid phosphatase in T-cell convoluted leukemic lymphoblasts. (E) Eosinophils (dark blue granules) and neutrophilic granulocytic cells (violet granules), acid blue 1 stain. (F) Megakaryocytes, rhodanile blue stain after ribonuclease digestion.*

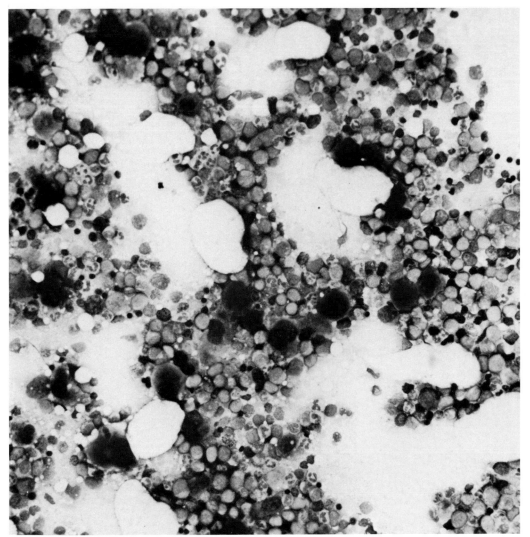

Normocellular bone marrow.

1   *Cellularity*

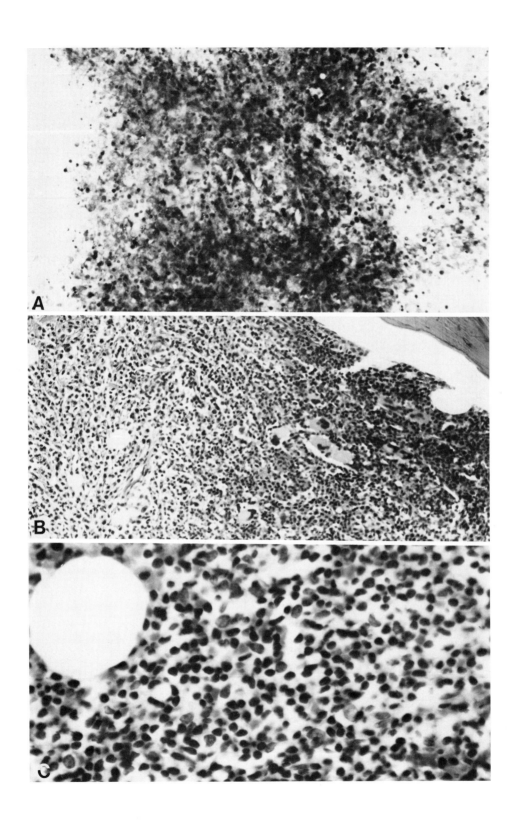

Assessment of the cellularity of the marrow is an important initial step in the evaluation and interpretation of a marrow aspirate and biopsy.

Hypercellular marrows show few or no fat spaces. These marrows are composed largely of cellular elements (Fig. 1–1).

Normocellular marrows contain occasional fat spaces of varying sizes (Fig. 1–2). In aspirates of normal bone marrow, different cell types at various stages of maturation are found (Fig. 1–3). On hematoxylin-eosin (H and E) stained sections of normal bone marrow, proerythroblasts appear as pale vesicular nuclei that have prominent chromatin aggregates and well-demarcated nuclear membranes (Fig. 1–4A, *inset*). Intermediate normoblasts have darkly stained nuclei that have a checkerboard nuclear chromatin pattern. Cytoplasm of these cells is deeply eosinophilic because of their increased hemoglobin content (Fig. 1–4A).

Granulocytic precursors have round to oval nuclei with finely dispersed aggregates of chromatin and a few particles of chromatin adhering to the nuclear membrane. Cytoplasm of immature granulocytes stains lightly eosinophilic, and specific granules may be visualized poorly (Fig. 1–4B). Plasma cells have eccentric nuclei that show a radial chromatin pattern. Cytoplasm is deeply eosinophilic because of increased ribosomal ribonucleic acid (RNA).

Hypocellular marrows contain numerous fat spaces (Fig. 1–5). Fibroblasts are numerous, as are strands of collagen. Mast cells, lymphocytes, and plasma cells are often increased in number. Other marrow cells are decreased in number.

Hypocellularity of the marrow can occur after exposure to a specific toxin, such as an organic solvent or drug, and may result in pancytopenia. Hypocellularity of the marrow is often found after exposure to therapeutic doses of ionizing radiation and after chemotherapy. Hypocellularity can also represent a preleukemic state, as found in some cases of idiopathic acquired aplastic anemia, Fanconi's hypoplastic anemia, and paroxysmal nocturnal hemoglobinuria.

(Text continued on page 8)

Figure 1–1
(opposite)

Hypercellular marrow, showing low-power view of aspirate (A), low-power view of H and E section of biopsy (B), and higher-power view of biopsy section (C).

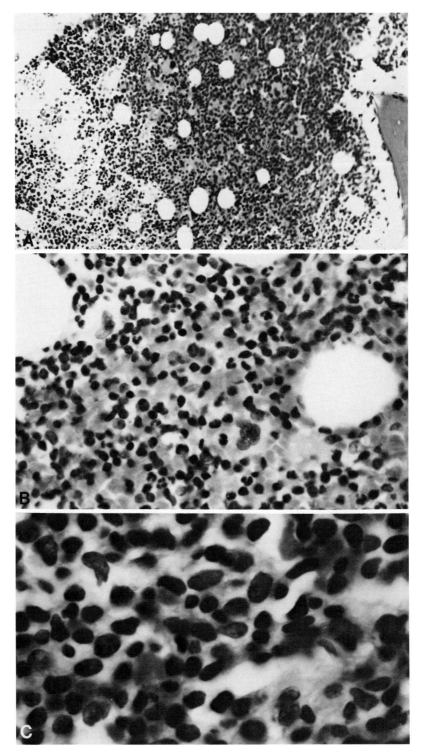

Figure 1–2   *Normocellular marrow, depicting Wright-stained aspirate under low magnification (A), low-power view of bone marrow biopsy showing megakaryocytes and fat spaces (B), and higher-power view of biopsy section (C).*

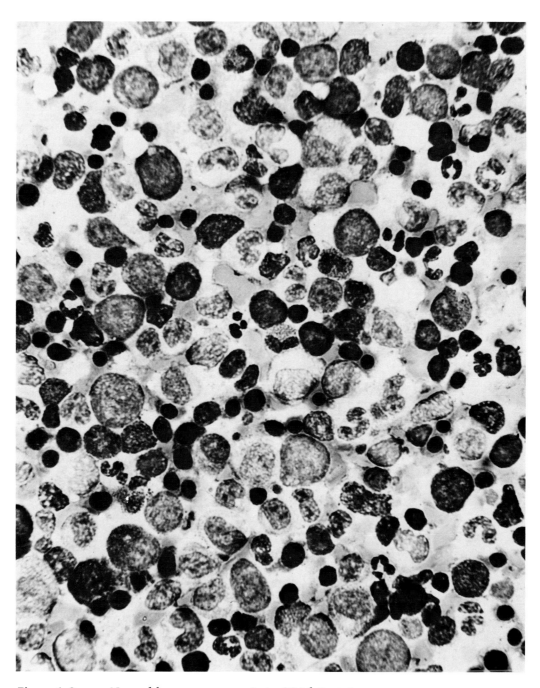

Figure 1–3   *Normal bone marrow aspirate, Wright's stain.*

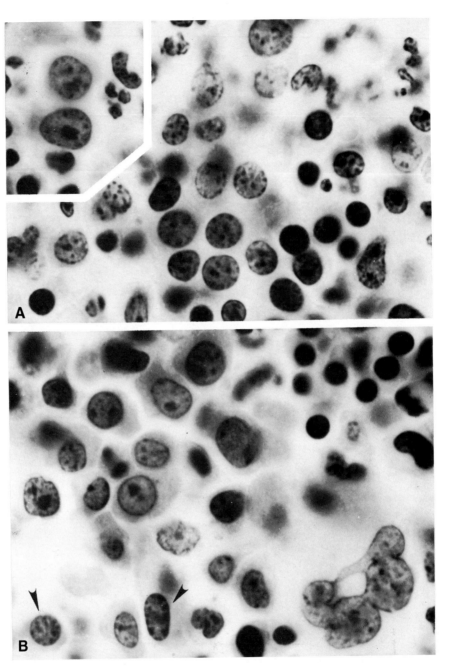

Figure 1–4   (A) *H and E section of normal marrow, showing predominantly intermediate normoblasts with darkly staining nuclei containing a checkerboard chromatin pattern. Inset shows large pale-staining nuclei with prominent nuclear membranes that are characteristic of proerythroblasts.* (B) *H and E section of normal marrow, showing megakaryocyte and nuclei of immature granulocytic cells, most likely myelocytes and promyelocytes. Nuclear chromatin in these cells appears punctate and tenuous with few aggregates of chromatin. Cells at lower left and at bottom (arrows) are normal plasma cells with eccentric nuclei that contain prominent aggregates of chromatin and deeply eosinophilic-staining cytoplasm.*

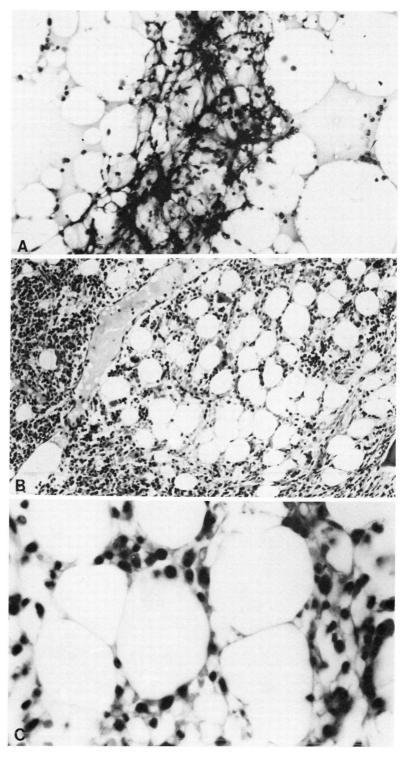

Figure 1–5   *Hypocellular marrow seen in low-power view of marrow aspirate* (A), *marrow biopsy* (B), *and higher-power view of biopsy* (C).

In other instances, hypocellular marrows can be comprised of 10% to 20% myeloblasts and represent instances of refractory anemia with excess blasts (RAEB) or smoldering acute leukemia. When the number of myeloblasts exceeds 40% of the differential cell count in these hypocellular marrows, the diagnosis of acute myeloblastic leukemia is made. Rarely some cases of agnogenic myeloid metaplasia in a proliferative phase demonstrate areas of hypercellularity alternating with areas of hypocellularity. In the hypocellular as well as hypercellular areas, focal proliferation of erythroblasts can be detected within marrow sinusoids.

In addition to judging the cellularity of the marrow, assessment of the marrow specimen under the low-power objective lens of a microscope permits the identification of abnormal clusters of malignant nonhematopoietic cells, which are seen in carcinomatosis of the marrow.

Figure 1–6   *Low-power view of normal marrow biopsy section stained with H and E, showing megakaryocytes of various sizes. Normoblasts have darkly stained nuclei.*

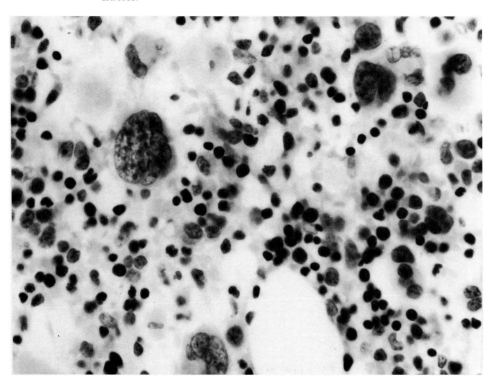

Using the low-power objective lens, the following abnormalities can be detected in an H and E section of bone marrow biopsy: granulomas found in sarcoidosis and myobacterial infections; foci of necrosis found in hemoglobinopathies such as sickle cell anemia (hemoglobin SS disease) and osteomyelitis; areas of lymphomatous involvement found in Hodgkin's disease and non-Hodgkin's lymphomas; areas of focal or diffuse fibrosis found in agnogenic myeloid metaplasia, Hodgkin's disease, or angioimmunoblastic lymphadenopathy; areas in which there are increased numbers of eosinophils, as found in myeloproliferative disorders, Hodgkin's disease, and angioimmunoblastic lymphadenopathy; areas of diffuse or focal accumulations of large, primitive-appearing cells found in acute leukemia; and areas of proliferation of storage cells seen in Gaucher's disease and Niemann-Pick disease. With this lens, the number and size of megakaryocytes (Fig. 1–6) and lymphoid follicles or aggregates in the bone marrow can also be detected.

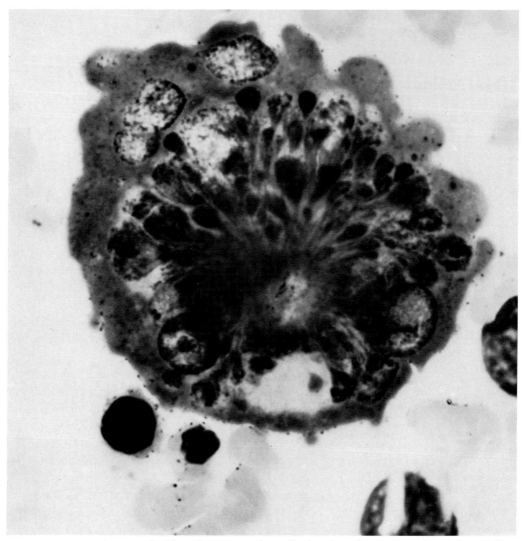

Giant erythroblast showing accelerated pyknosis and coarse cytoplasmic basophilic stippling from a patient with erythroleukemia.

2   *Erythroblastosis*

Maturation of Erythroblasts

In normal marrows, erythroblasts usually constitute between 25% and 30% of the marrow cells in a differential cell count.

Stages of the maturation of erythroblasts have been given arbitrary designations. Actually, erythroblastic maturation reflects a continuum in the process of increasing cytoplasmic hemoglobinization and decreasing size and eventual expulsion of the nucleus.

Proerythroblast is the earliest recognizable erythroid precursor. Nuclear chromatin is delicate with few aggregates. One or two small nucleoli may be present. Cytoplasm is deeply basophilic because of increased amounts of ribosomal RNA and may appear radially striated (Fig. 2–1). Binuclear proerythroblasts are found in normal marrows (Fig. 2–2) and are increased in number in marrows from patients with disorders of erythropoiesis.

Increased numbers of proerythroblasts can be found in disorders like autoimmune hemolytic anemia that are characterized by accelerated destruction of erythrocytes, striking erythroblastic proliferation of the marrow, and marked reticulocytosis as a reflection of marrow erythropoietic activity. Presumably, increased numbers of proerythroblasts in these examples of "effective erythropoiesis" represent generations of erythroid precursors that eventually develop into mature erythrocytes (Fig. 2–3A). Increased numbers of proerythroblasts can also occur in marrows that show evidence of erythroblastic regeneration, as in recovery from drug-induced marrow hypoplasis following treatment of acute leukemia or after toxic exposure to an organic solvent or drug.

Figure 2–1   *Proerythroblast, normal marrow.*

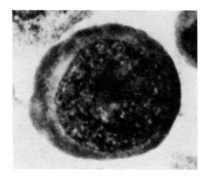

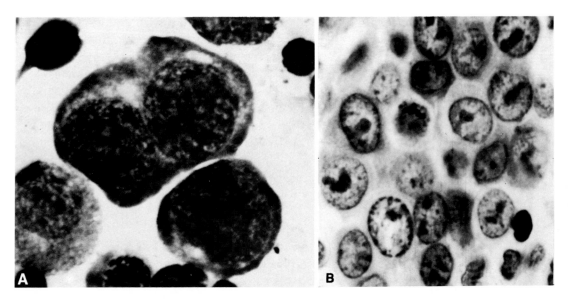

Figure 2–2 (A) *Binuclear proerythroblasts, normal marrow. (B) H and E section of normal bone marrow, showing increased numbers of proerythroblasts occurring in a cluster. These cells have a prominent nuclear membrane with an irregularly shaped nucleolus and small darkly stained aggregates of chromatin adherent to the inner aspect of the membrane. Nucleoli are prominent and sometimes extend from the center of the nucleus to the nuclear membrane.*

Figure 2–3 *Increased numbers of proerythroblasts in thrombotic thrombocytopenic purpura (A) and in chronic erythremic myelosis (B).*

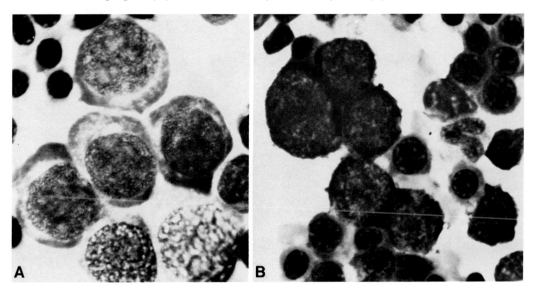

Increased numbers of proerythroblasts are also found in disorders in which erythropoiesis is "ineffective." In these disorders, such as pernicious anemia, folate deficiency, acute erythremic myelosis, chronic erythremic myelosis, erythroleukemia, preleukemic disorders like smoldering acute leukemia, and, in rare cases, pyridoxine-responsive sideroblastic anemia, accelerated destruction of erythroblasts and mature erythrocytes occurs predominantly in the bone marrow. This intramedullary cell death is accompanied by low numbers of reticulocytes in the blood and by anemia. Accumulation of increased numbers of proerythroblasts in these disorders may be due in part to impediment to their maturation beyond this stage of development (Fig. 2–3*B*).

Early intermediate normoblast, or polychromatophilic erythroblast, has nuclear chromatin that appears more aggregated than in the proerythroblast. Compared to the proerythroblast, the nucleus of the

Figure 2–4   *Early intermediate normoblasts, normal marrow.*

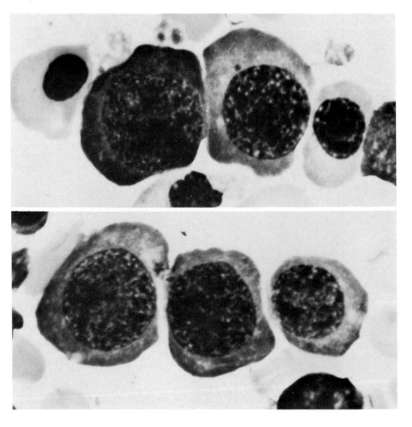

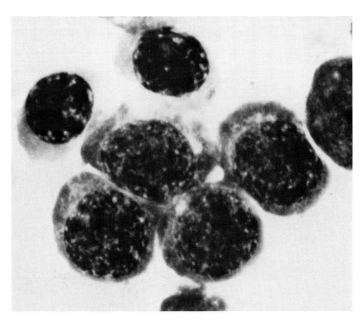

Figure 2–5   *Early intermediate normoblasts, normal marrow.*

early intermediate normoblast is smaller and lacks nucleoli. Nuclear chromatin strands are connected to adjacent aggregates and strands by coarse connections of chromatin. With panoptic stains like Wright's or Giemsa's, the cytoplasm of these cells stains purple to orange, depending on the amount of hemoglobin (Figs. 2–4 and 2–5).

Late intermediate normoblasts demonstrate progressive hemoglobinization of the cytoplasm by staining orange or orange green. Nuclear chromatin is dense and often homogeneous (Fig. 2–6). One or two Howell-Jolly bodies may be present. Sometimes the normoblast is binuclear (Fig. 2–7).

Intermediate stages of erythroblastic maturation are those in which distinctions between megaloblastic, megaloblastoid, and normoblastic chromatin patterns become apparent.

In disorders of erythropoiesis, nuclear and cytoplasmic abnormalities are found in erythroblasts at varying stages of maturation. In some instances, an individual erythroblast may demonstrate both nuclear and cytoplasmic abnormalities in the same cell.

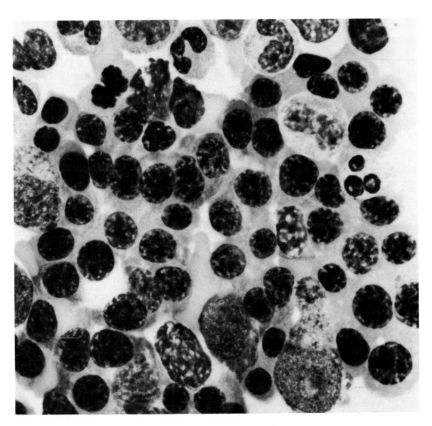

Figure 2–6   *Late intermediate normoblasts showing prominent darkly-stained aggregates of nuclear chromatin and well-hemoglobinized cytoplasm.*

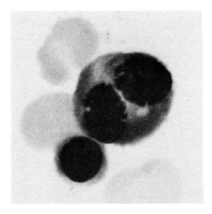

Figure 2–7   *Binuclear normoblast, normal marrow.*

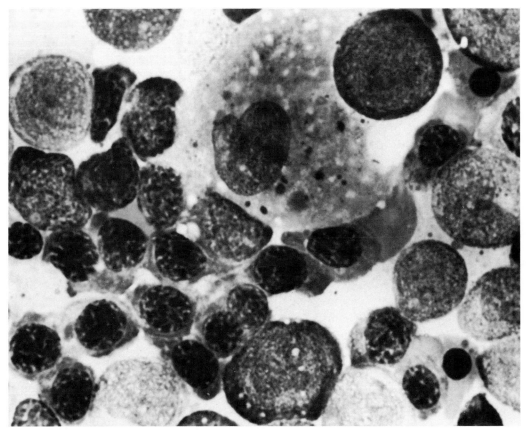

Figure 2–8   *Erythroid island, normal marrow. A large macrophage (top) contains abundant cytoplasmic debris, including hemosiderin. Surrounding the macrophage are erythroblasts in various stages of maturation, including a proerythroblast at the top and numerous intermediate normoblasts at the lower margins of the macrophage.*

Erythroid islands are cellular composites that include histiocytes containing ferritin and erythroblasts in varying stages of maturation; these surround the histiocytes (Fig. 2–8). It is thought that erythroblasts acquire iron from the histiocytes by a process called rhopheocytosis. Increased numbers of erythroid islands are found in hemolytic anemias, particularly thrombotic thrombocytopenic purpura, and in primary acquired refractory sideroblastic anemias (Di Guglielmo syndrome).

Nuclear Abnormalities

Nuclei of abnormal erythroblasts can demonstrate abnormalities of size, configuration, and nuclear chromatin.

Asynchronous Nuclei. In conditions in which there is a deficiency of vitamin B_{12} or folate and in erythroleukemia, some multinuclear erythroblasts show abnormalities of individual nuclei within a single cell (Fig. 2–9). Nuclear chromatin patterns in the small nucleus or nuclei often appear different from those in the large nucleus. In some erythroblasts, the larger nucleus shows megaloblastoid nuclear chromatin patterns, and one or more small nuclei exhibit a fine or coarse reticular chromatin pattern. In other erythroblasts, the larger nucleus demonstrates a reticular chromatin pattern, whereas the smaller nucleus in the same cell exhibits marked megaloblastoid chromatin features. Finally, in other erythroblasts, the larger nucleus appears intact and may demonstrate megaloblastic or megaloblastoid nuclear chromatin (Fig. 2–10), whereas one or more small nuclei in the erythroblast demonstrate pyknosis and degeneration.

In some of these instances, the nuclei vary considerably in size. Some may show chromosomal polarization as though the nucleus were in mitosis. Other nuclei are in the process of nuclear division, and adjacent nuclei in the same cell appear quiescent. These abnormalities reflect aberrations in cellular replication and cellular division.

Figure 2–9   *Nuclear asynchronism in erythroblasts from patients with acute and chronic erythremic myelosis and erythroleukemia. Nuclei at arrows are smaller than larger nucleus in the same cell and often show a different type of chromatin pattern than found in the larger nucleus.*

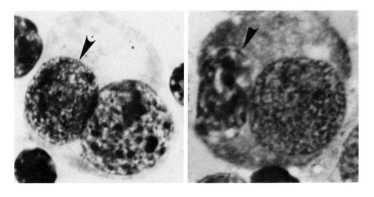

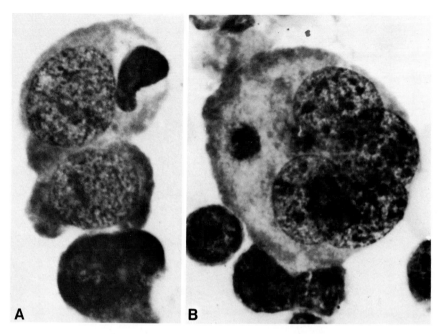

Figure 2–10   *Erythroblasts in pernicious anemia (A) and erythroleukemia (B). Both show degenerating nuclei within multinuclear erythroblasts. These degenerating nuclei are smaller than adjacent nuclei and stain darkly.*

"Fried-Egg" Nucleus. In megaloblasts from patients with untreated erythroleukemia, the nucleus often occupies a central position within the cell, giving it a "fried-egg" appearance (Fig. 2–11). The significance of this abnormality is uncertain.

Multinuclearity. Some proerythroblasts and early intermediate normoblasts contain more than one nucleus (Fig. 2–12). Abnormalities of this type are found frequently when there is a deficiency of vitamin B_{12} or folate and in neoplastic disorders such as erythroleukemia. They are also found in disorders that precede the development of leukemia, such as preleukemia, smoldering acute leukemia, and acute and chronic erythremic myelosis. Often multinuclearity is observed in unusually large erythroblasts or gigantoblasts (Fig. 2–13). Multinuclearity signifies abnormalities in cellular replication and cellular division.

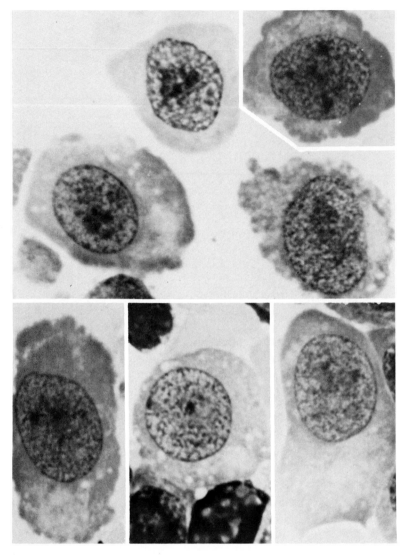

Figure 2–11   *Megaloblasts in erythroleukemia. These cells have unusually attenuated nuclear chromatin, with few chromatin aggregates. The nucleus often occupies a central position in the cell.*

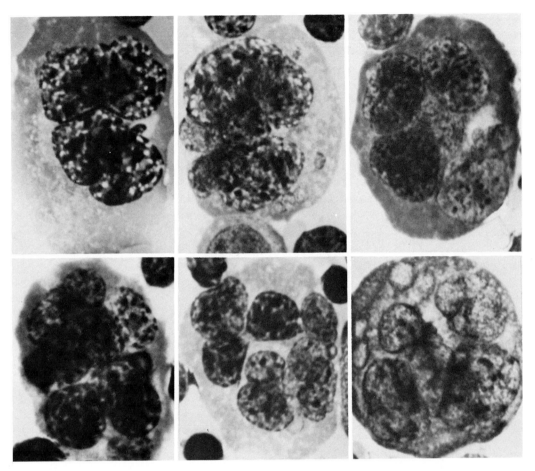

Figure 2–12   *Giant multinuclear and multilobular erythroblasts in erythroleukemia.*

Multiple Nuclear Lobulations. In conditions in which there is a deficiency of vitamin B_{12} or folate or in erythroleukemia, nuclei of erythroblasts often show one or more lobulations. These look like outpouchings of various sizes that seem to emanate from the nuclear membrane and contain nucleoplasm (Figs. 2–14 and 2–15).

Nuclear Foldings. In some patients with erythroleukemia, the nuclei of erythroblasts show delicate foldings, such as those found in cells of monocytic origin (Fig. 2–16).

(Text continued on page 24)

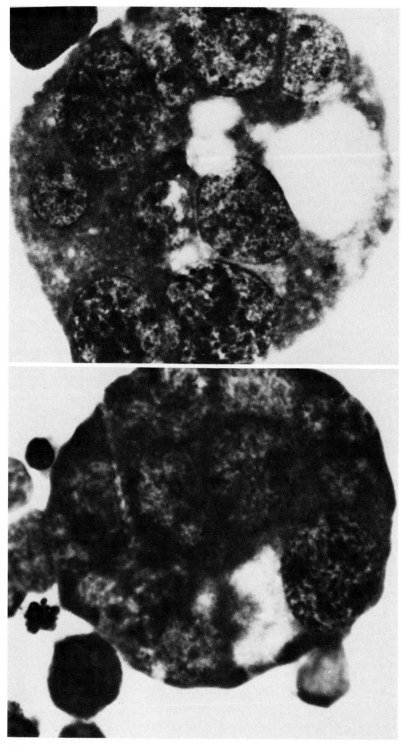

Figure 2–13   *Giant, bizarre-appearing multinuclear erythroblasts, acute erythremic myelosis.*

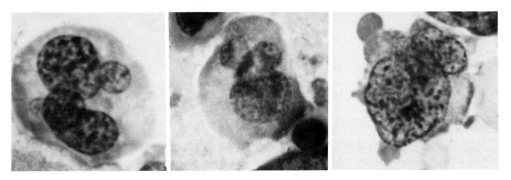

Figure 2–14   Erythroblasts in erythroleukemia, showing multiple small nuclear lobulations.

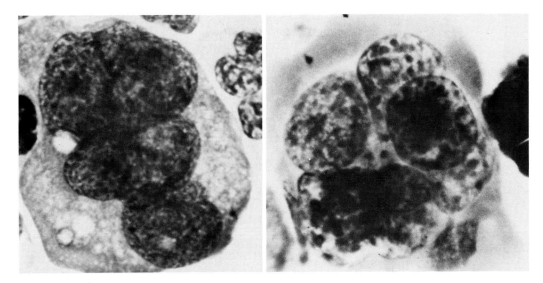

Figure 2–15   Giant erythroblasts with large nuclear lobulations.

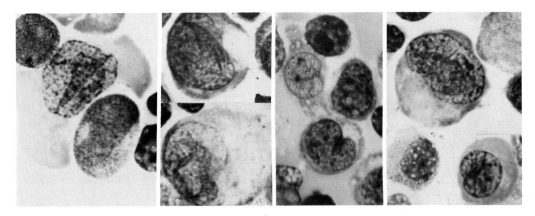

Figure 2–16   Monocytoid-type nuclear foldings in erythroleukemia erythroblasts.

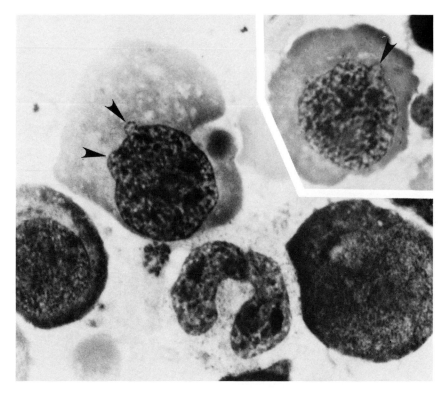

Figure 2–17   *Arrows point to nuclear blebs in pernicious anemia megaloblasts.*

Nuclear Bleb. Nuclei from erythroblasts where there is a deficiency of vitamin B_{12} or folate may frequently contain small outpouchings from the nuclear membrane in the form of "blebs" (Fig. 2–17). In phase-contrast studies of living megaloblasts, blebs of this type have been observed as they detach from the nuclear membrane. They become free floating in the cytoplasm and appear as either Howell-Jolly bodies or tiny accessory nuclei (Fig. 2–18).

Nuclear Bubble. In megaloblasts from patients with untreated pernicious anemia or folate deficiency, progressive enlargement of the nuclear bleb leads to the formation of nuclear protrusions containing nucleoplasm. Possibly these protrusions or bubbles enlarge progressively and become attached to the main nucleus by tenuous connections which then sever; this leads to the formation of multiple nuclei and/or Howell-Jolly bodies (Fig. 2–19).

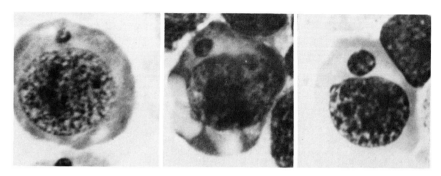

Figure 2–18   *Single, large accessory nucleus, pernicious anemia megaloblasts.*

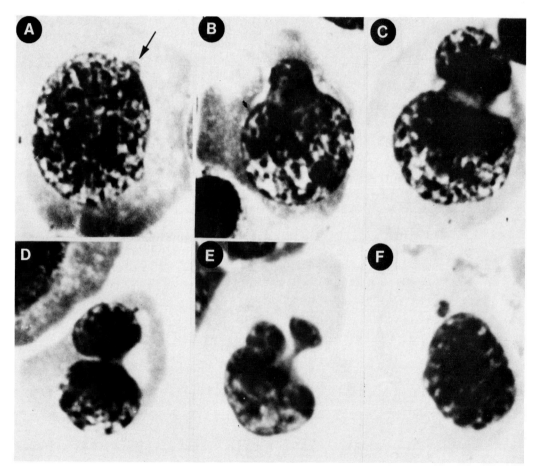

Figure 2–19   *Proposed sequence of Howell-Jolly body formation (A through F) from nuclear blebs and bubbles. Arrow in A points to a nuclear bleb. (Kass L: Pernicious Anemia. Philadelphia, WB Saunders, 1976)*

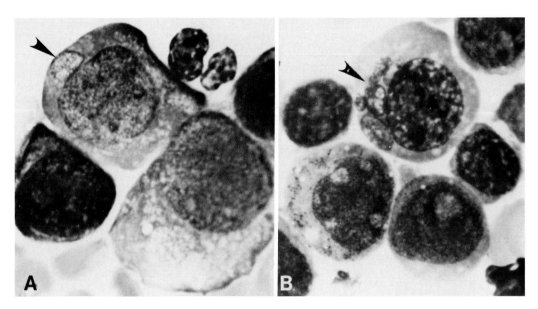

Figure 2–20   *Multiple small nuclear lobulations and accessory nuclei* (arrows) *in erythroblasts from patients with acute erythremic myelosis* (A) *and from patients with refractory anemia with excess blasts* (B).

Small Accessory Nuclei. These small nuclei result from bleb or bubble formation (see above). They can also form as a result of asynchronous nuclear divisions (Fig. 2–20).

Multiple Howell-Jolly Bodies. Multiple Howell-Jolly bodies often appear in erythroblasts from patients with a deficiency of vitamin B_{12} or folate and in erythroblasts from patients with other disorders of erythropoiesis such as primary acquired sideroblastic anemias (Di Guglielmo syndrome) and erythroleukemia. Although as many as two small Howell-Jolly bodies may be found in normal erythroblasts, more than two Howell-Jolly bodies of varying sizes occur in pathologic erythroblasts (Fig. 2–21). In some instances, Howell-Jolly bodies are connected to the main nucleus by a delicate stalk of chromatin. This abnormality is particularly frequent in untreated pernicious anemia and folate deficiency.

Orange Nuclear Deposits. Some erythroblasts from patients with Di Guglielmo syndrome and preleukemic disorders such as "preleukemia" contain small orange-staining deposits within the interstices of nuclear chromatin (Fig. 2–22). These deposits vary in size and shape and can be globular and confluent or punctate. Although they are

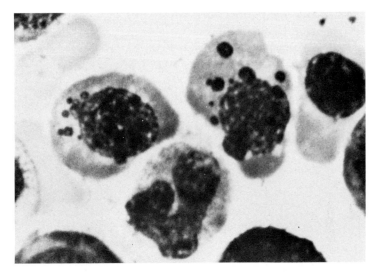

Figure 2–21   *Multiple Howell-Jolly bodies of varying sizes, pernicious anemia megaloblasts.*

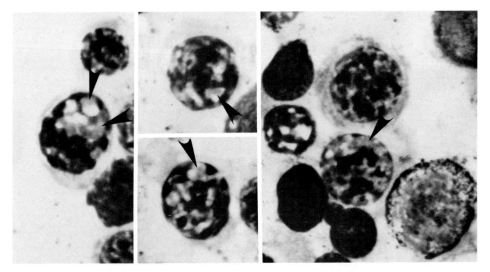

Figure 2–22   *The arrows denote areas of orange-colored deposits in nuclei of megaloblastoid intermediate macronormoblasts, chronic erythremic myelosis. Nuclear membranes of these erythroblasts show multiple discontinuities that may represent "pores."*

usually located between chromatin strands, in some instances they seem to be continuous with chromatin strands, as though the material in these areas possessed staining properties that differed from adjacent deoxyribonucleic acid (DNA). On cytochemical examination, these orange-staining deposits do not contain either hemoglobin or DNA, and as yet their composition is unknown. Erythroblasts containing the orange nuclear deposits also have multiple areas of discontinuity of the nuclear membranes that appear as "pores." Both nuclear abnormalities may serve as useful markers of erythroblasts in disorders that precede the emergence of acute leukemia.

Figure 2–23   *Normoblast (A), showing circularity of nuclear chromatin. Megaloblastoid intermediate macronormoblast (B) and megaloblast (C), showing the loss of circularity of chromatin and disarrangement of chromatin.*

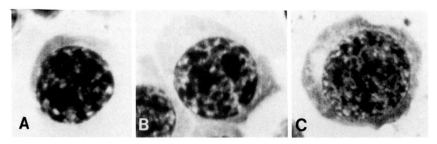

Figure 2–24   *Megaloblasts, pernicious anemia (A), and large megaloblast, refractory anemia with excess blasts (B).*

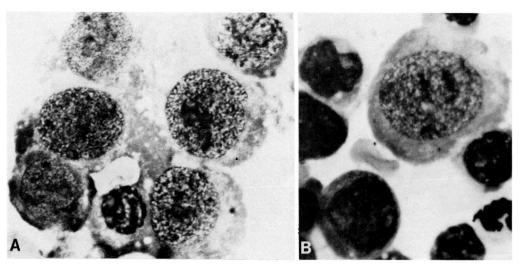

Disarrangement of Nuclear Circularity. In early intermediate normoblasts the pattern of nuclear chromatin is often circular, with strands of nuclear chromatin arranged in concentric fashion (Fig. 2–23*A*). In megaloblastoid erythropoiesis (Fig. 2–23*B*) and in megaloblastic erythropoiesis (Fig. 2–23*C*), this circular pattern is not apparent and the nuclear chromatin pattern appears disorganized.

Loss of Nuclear Chromatin Aggregates. In erythroblasts from patients with untreated deficiency of vitamin B_{12} or folate and in other pathologic erythroblasts, the number and size of chromatin aggregates are often reduced compared to normal erythroblasts. Loss of size and number of chromatin aggregates is an early morphologic manifestation of megaloblastosis due to deficiency of vitamin B_{12} or folate. These abnormalities may be caused in part by aberrations in the biosynthesis of DNA and histones (Fig. 2–24).

Clockface Chromatin Pattern. In nuclei of megaloblasts from patients with untreated deficiency of vitamin B_{12} or folate, small masses of chromatin surround the nuclear membrane in a "clockface" configuration (Fig. 2–25). Often these masses of chromatin

Figure 2–25   *Clockface chromatin configuration in megaloblast, pernicious anemia. Arrows point to aggregates of chromatin that adhere to the inner surface of the nuclear membrane in a circumferential pattern.*

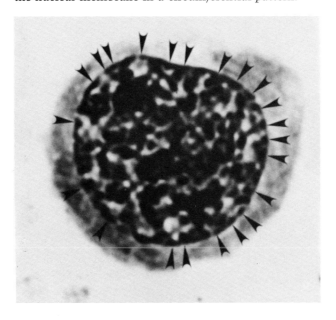

appear to be unconnected to other masses of chromatin in the nucleus. This abnormality may be due in part to aberrations in the biosynthesis of DNA and histones in megaloblasts. The clockface chromatin pattern is usually not observed in erythroblasts having megaloblastoid nuclear chromatin patterns.

Vacuous Nuclear Chromatin. Loss of chromatin strands is found in megaloblasts and megaloblastoid cells that may be degenerating (Fig. 2–26). In these cells, portions of the nucleus appear vacuous

Figure 2–26   *Megaloblasts, pernicious anemia, showing unusually vacuous-appearing nuclear chromatin. This probably represents a degenerative change.*

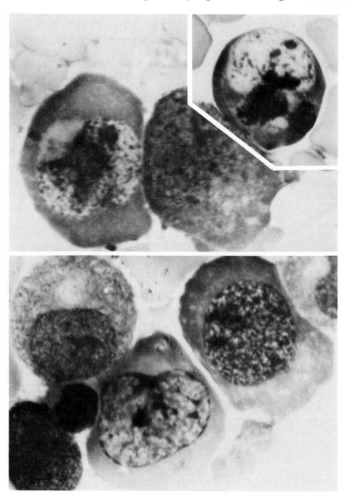

because of loss of nuclear chromatin strands and aggregates. Remaining chromatin strands in these cells often form delicate reticular patterns resembling those found in fully developed megaloblasts. Erythroblasts with vacuous nuclear chromatin also demonstrate loss of cytoplasmic details, leading to a ragged appearance of the cytoplasm. Presumably, these cytoplasmic abnormalities are also manifestations of cellular degeneration.

Extreme Chromatin Attenuation. Nuclei of some erythroblasts from patients with untreated erythroleukemia or untreated deficiency of vitamin B_{12} or folate demonstrate marked attenuation of nuclear chromatin. At times, it is difficult to visualize individual chromatin strands, and the chromatin strands themselves may show reduced affinity for panoptic stains (Fig. 2–27). Chromatin aggregates appear punctate and are greatly reduced in number compared to those in normal erythroblasts.

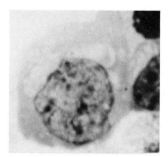

Figure 2–27   *Unusually attenuated nuclear chromatin in an erythroleukemia erythroblast.*

"Pince-Nez" Chromatin Configuration. In patients with severe untreated pernicious anemia, mitotic figures in some megaloblasts are connected by a thin arc-shaped filament of chromatin (Fig. 2–28). It has been suggested that this filament is the precursor of Cabot's ring (Figs. 2–29 and 2–30). Similar-appearing connections between nuclei of erythroblasts have been called nuclear "bridging" and are found in marrows of patients with hereditary erythroblastic multinuclearity.

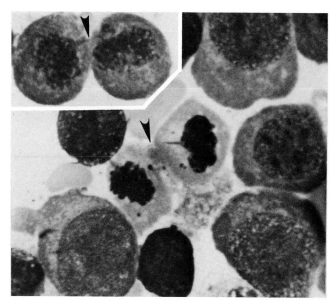

Figure 2–28   *Arrows point to the "pince-nez" configuration of a nuclear chromatin strand in a pernicious anemia megaloblast. This thin strand may be the precursor of Cabot's ring. Nuclear "bridging" of this type is also found in erythroblasts from patients with hereditary erythroblastic multinuclearity.*

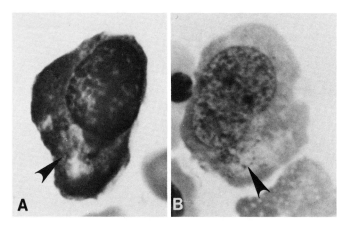

Figure 2–29   *Arrows denote Cabot's rings in pernicious anemia megaloblast (A) and in erythroleukemia erythroblast (B).*

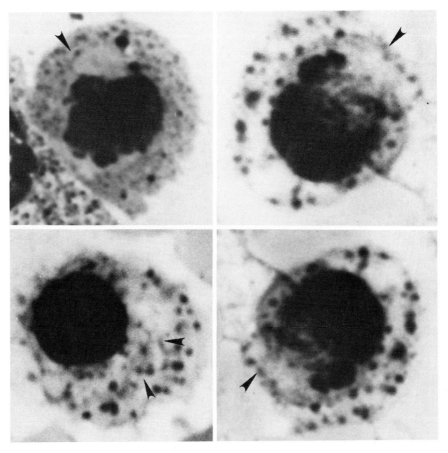

Figure 2–30   *Arrows point to the precursors of or actual Cabot's rings in pernicious anemia megaloblasts that have unusually coarse basophilic stippling.*

Elongated chromosomes are found in erythroblasts from patients with a deficiency of vitamin B_{12} and/or folate. It is thought that elongation of chromosomes in these disorders is due to abnormalities of biosynthesis of DNA and histones (Fig. 2–31).

Multipolar Mitotic Figures. Abnormal gigantoblasts from patients with acute erythremic myelosis or erythroleukemia may show multipolar mitoses (Fig. 2–32). These represent disturbances in cellular division.

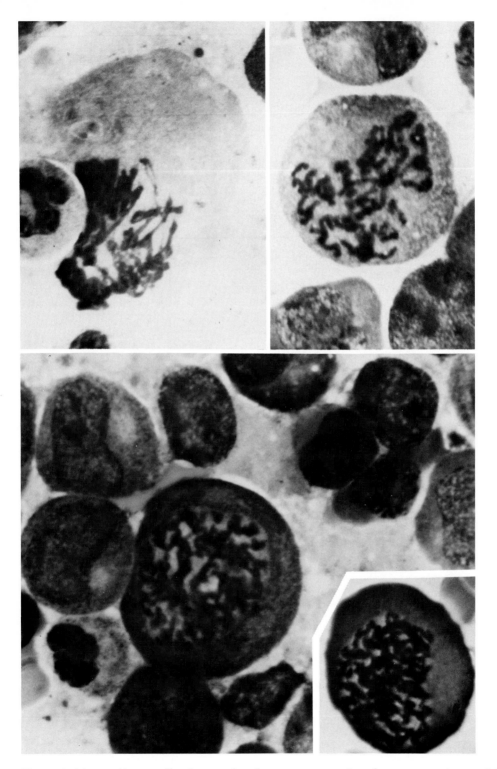

Figure 2–31   *Abnormally elongated and tenuous-appearing chromosomes in pernicious anemia megaloblasts.*

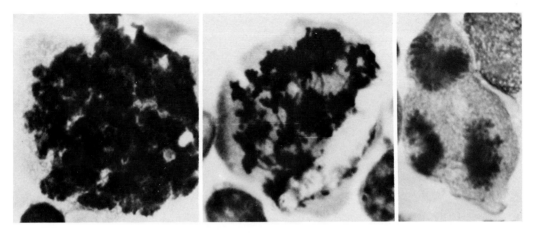

Figure 2–32   *Aberrant-appearing multipolar mitotic figures in erythroblasts from a patient with acute erythremic myelosis.*

Abnormal Karyorrhexis. In erythroblasts from patients with untreated deficiency of vitamin B_{12} or folate, erythroleukemia, or preleukemic disorders, small fragments of chromosomes fail to unite with chromosome during the process of nuclear division. These chromosomal fragments may become free in the cytoplasm and appear as Howell-Jolly bodies (Fig. 2–33).

Accelerated Pyknosis. In pathologic erythroblasts such as those found in deficiency of vitamin B_{12} or folate, erythroleukemia, preleukemic disorders of erythropoiesis, and acute nonlymphoblastic leukemia, processes of nuclear condensation prior to nuclear expulsion seem to be accelerated. This acceleration of pyknosis leads to the formation of multiple aggregates of dense chromatin connected to the main nucleus. These aggregates detach and appear in the cytoplasm as Howell-Jolly bodies (Figs. 2–34*A* through *D* and 2–35). Accelerated pyknosis can also be found in normoblasts from patients with chronic heavy metal intoxication, as in arsenic poisoning (Fig. 2–34*C* and *D*).

(Text continued on page 38)

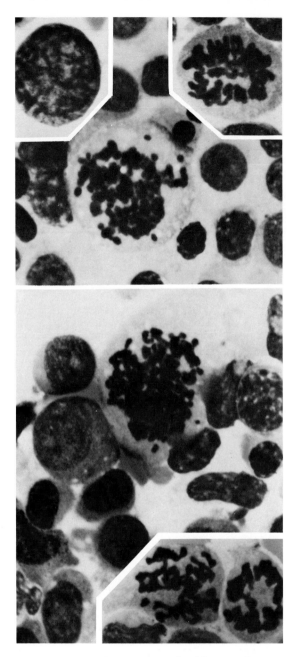

Figure 2–33   *Bizarre mitotic figures in erythroblasts, refractory anemia with excess blasts, demonstrating abnormal karyorrhexis.*

Figure 2–34
(opposite)   *Accelerated pyknosis in megaloblasts from patients with pernicious anemia (A) and in erythroblasts from patients with acute erythremic myelosis (B). Nuclear lobulations in these cells have a teardrop configuration and seem to be connected to a central portion by thin filaments of chromatin. Normoblasts from a patient with chronic arsenic poisoning, showing accelerated pyknosis (C) along with cloverleaf-shaped nuclei and coarse cytoplasmic basophilic stippling (D).*

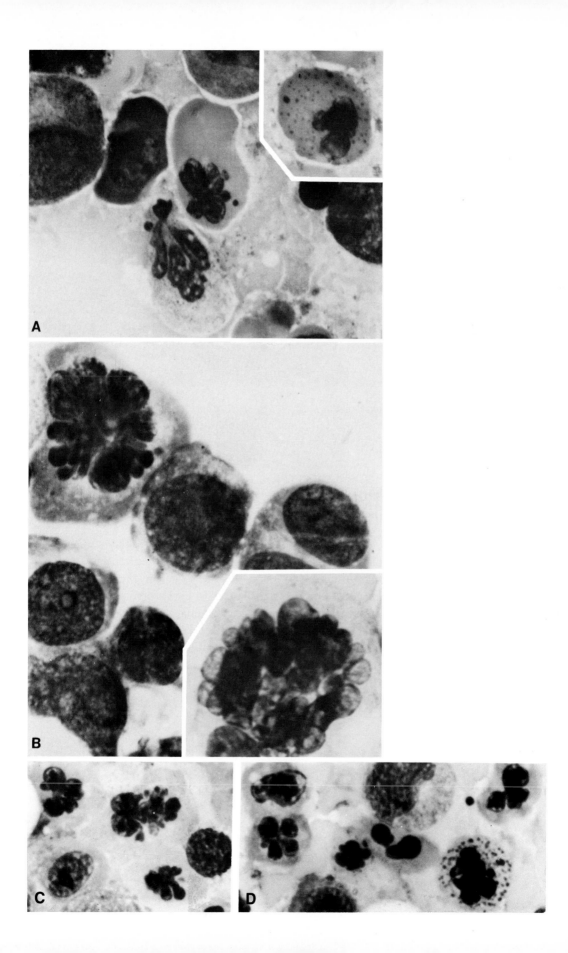

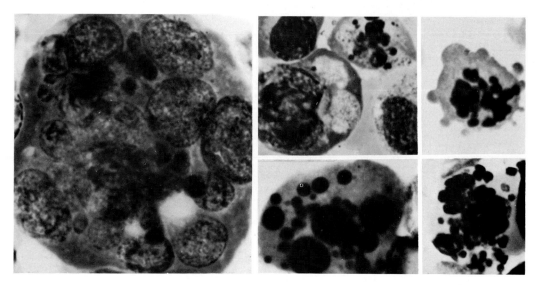

Figure 2–35   *Abnormal, accelerated pyknosis in erythroblasts from patients with acute erythremic myelosis (left), pernicious anemia (top, right), and erythroleukemia (bottom, right).*

Cytoplasmic Abnormalities

Gigantism. A marked increase in the size of erythroblasts is seen in deficiency of vitamin B_{12} or folate and in erythroleukemia (Fig. 2–36). The increase in size is also observed in preleukemic disorders. Gigantism is found in all stages of erythroblastic maturation but is seen most frequently in proerythroblast and early intermediate normoblast stages. Gigantism is often associated with abnormalities of the nucleus such as multilobularity and multinuclearity (Fig. 2–37).

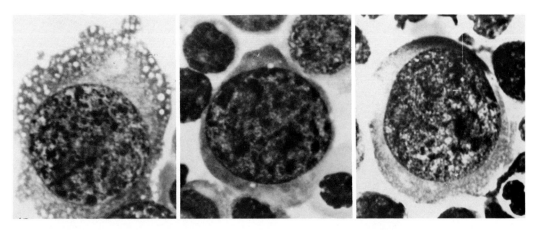

Figure 2–36   *Giant bizarre-appearing erythroblasts from patients with acute erythremic myelosis (right) and acute myeloblastic leukemia (center and left).*

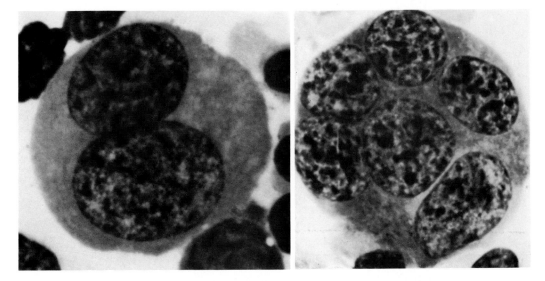

Figure 2–37   *Giant multinuclear erythroblasts, acute myeloblastic leukemia. The erythroblast on the right shows a prominent megaloblastoid-type chromatin pattern with large blocklike aggregates of nuclear chromatin connected to adjacent aggregates by coarse-appearing strands.*

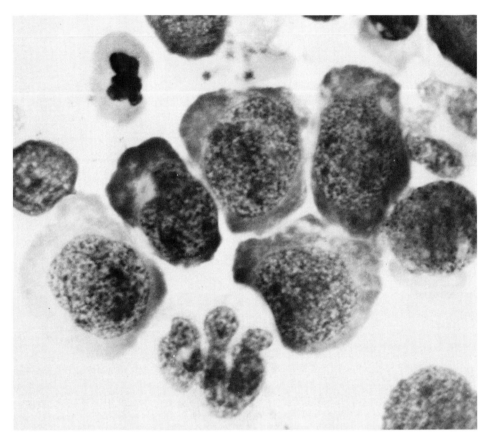

Figure 2–38   *Intermediate megaloblasts, pernicious anemia, showing nucleocytoplasmic asynchronism.*

Nucleocytoplasmic Asynchronism. Erythroblasts from patients with deficiency of vitamin B_{12} or folate and from patients with erythroleukemia or preleukemic disorders of erythropoiesis often show discrepancies between development and maturation of the nucleus and cytoplasm. In these cells, typically megaloblasts in untreated pernicious anemia, the nucleus contains unusually attenuated nuclear chromatin typical of immature erythroblasts, whereas the cytoplasm shows advanced hemoglobinization as found in more mature erythroblasts (Fig. 2–38). Asynchronous maturation of the nucleus and the cytoplasm is found in disorders in which abnormalities of DNA and histone biosynthesis have been demonstrated.

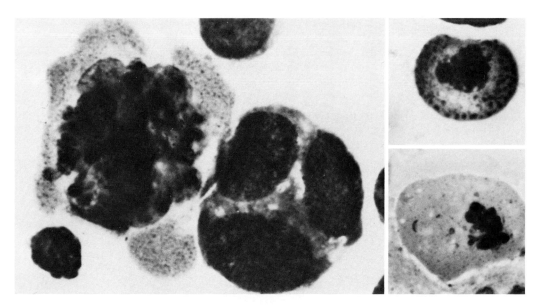

Figure 2–39   *Coarse basophilic stippling in a large erythroblast from a patient with acute erythremic myelosis and in megaloblasts from patients with untreated pernicious anemia* (right insets).

Coarse Basophilic Stippling. Unusually coarse basophilic stippling occurs in erythroblasts from patients who have disorders in which the incorporation of iron into hemoglobin is abnormal (Fig. 2–39). These disorders include hemoglobinopathies, primary acquired sideroblastic anemias, erythroleukemia, heavy metal intoxication, and deficiency of vitamin B_{12} or folate. Stippling is seen most frequently in later stages of erythroblastic maturation and in pernicious anemia may be associated with Cabot's ring formation.

Cytoplasmic Vacuoles. Vacuolation of the cytoplasm represents toxic or degenerative changes. Vacuolation is often prominent in the proerythroblast stage of maturation. Multiple vacuoles may occur. Vacuoles are observed in proerythroblasts from patients with acute erythremic myelosis and erythroleukemia, and in patients after exposure to alcohol. They are also seen in preleukemic disorders of erythropoiesis, phenylalanine deficiency, and phenylketonuria. Cytoplasmic vacuoles in proerythroblasts are often observed in patients treated with chloramphenicol, but these usually disappear after discontinuation of the drug (Fig. 2–40).

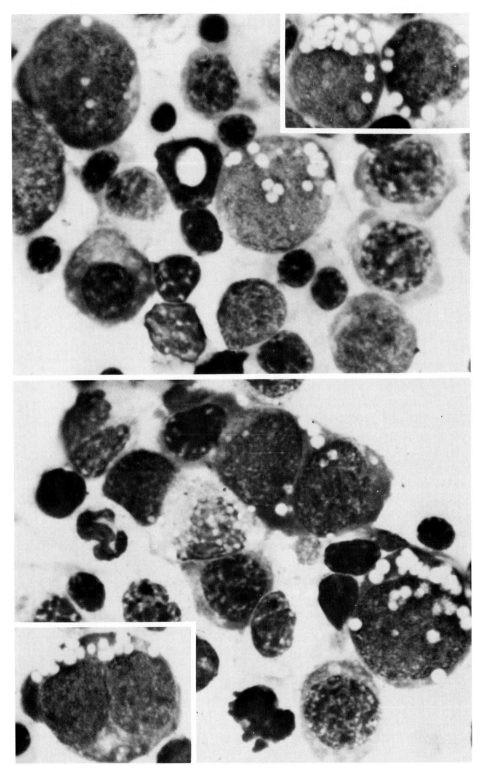

Figure 2–40   *Multiple cytoplasmic vacuoles in proerythroblasts from patients with erythroleukemia. (Kass L: Preleukemic Disorders. Springfield, IL, Charles C Thomas, 1979)*

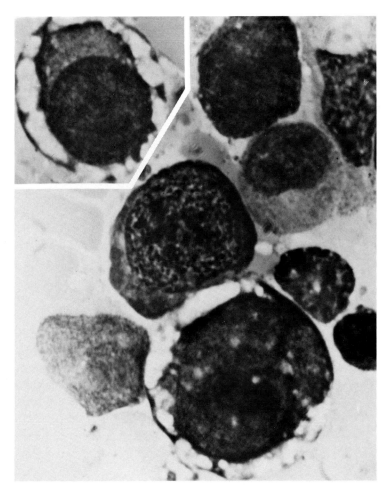

Figure 2–41   *Unusually large cytoplasmic vacuoles in erythroblasts, acute erythremic myelosis.*

Unusually Large Cytoplasmic Vacuoles. Particularly in proerythroblasts from patients with acute erythremic myelosis or erythroleukemia, especially large vacuoles can be found in the cytoplasm (Fig. 2–41). These vacuoles probably represent degenerative changes in the erythroblasts. They often contain abundant deposits of glycogen.

Cytoplasmic Vacuoles Containing Debris. In some megaloblasts, vacuoles contain finely granular acidophilic-staining material (Fig. 2–42). It is uncertain whether these represent phagocytic vacuoles or whether the acidophilic-staining material is degenerated nuclear chromatin.

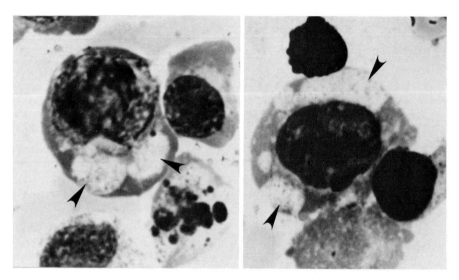

Figure 2–42   *Cytoplasmic vacuoles* (arrows) *containing debris, pernicious anemia megaloblasts.*

Hemoglobin Lakes. Some erythroblasts from patients with untreated deficiency of vitamin B_{12} or folate, chronic erythremic myelosis, or erythroleukemia show sequestrations of hemoglobin within the cytoplasm (Figs. 2–43 and 2–44). These hemoglobinized areas appear to be demarcated by adjacent polychromatophilic cytoplasm of the erythroblast. Hemoglobin lakes are usually oval or triangular. They represent uneven hemoglobinization of the cytoplasm.

Degenerative Changes in Cytoplasm. In pernicious anemia and folate deficiency, the cytoplasm of some megaloblasts may appear ragged and lacking in detail (Fig. 2–45). These cells usually have nuclei that also lack detail and consequently may be degenerating cells. They constitute cytologic evidence of intramedullary cell death and ineffective erythropoiesis in these disorders.

Erythrocytophagy by Erythroblasts. In patients with untreated pernicious anemia and in acute erythremic myelosis (Di Guglielmo disease), some erythroblasts show phagocytosis of erythrocytes and/or other degenerating erythroblasts (Fig. 2–46). The significance of the apparent "cannibalism" is unknown.

(Text continued on page 48)

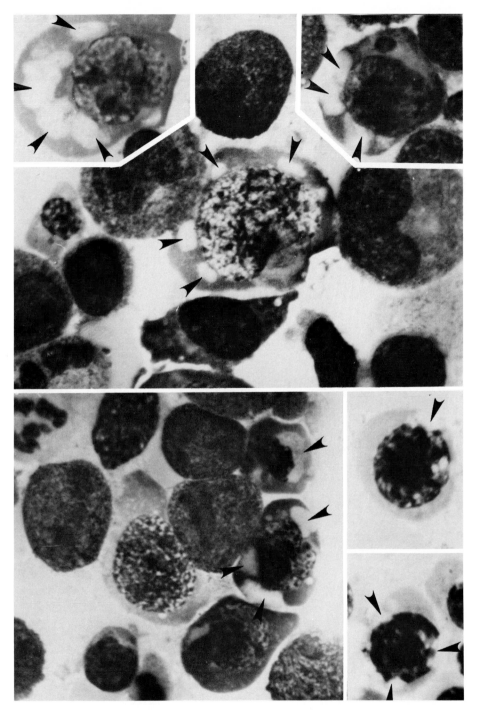

Figure 2–43   *Hemoglobin lakes (arrows) in pernicious anemia megaloblasts and in megaloblastoid intermediate macronormoblasts from patients with chronic erythremic myelosis (bottom, right insets).*

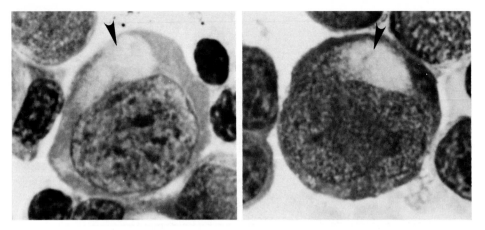

Figure 2–44 Hemoglobin lakes (arrows) in erythroleukemia erythroblasts. (Kass L: Preleukemic Disorders, Springfield, IL, Charles C Thomas, 1979)

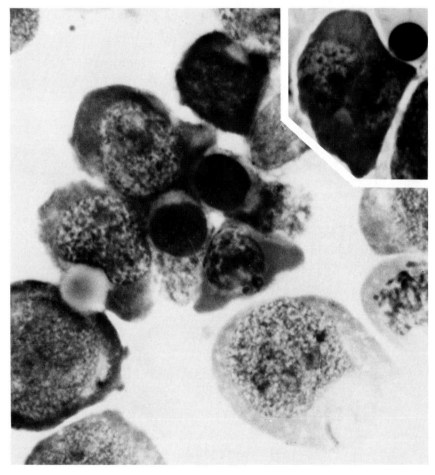

Figure 2–45 Degenerating megaloblasts with indistinct nuclear and cytoplasmic details. Nuclei appear dense and darkly stained.

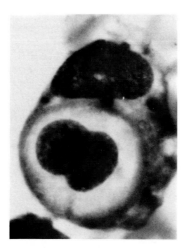

Figure 2–46   *Erythrocytophagy of an erythroblast by another erythroblast.*

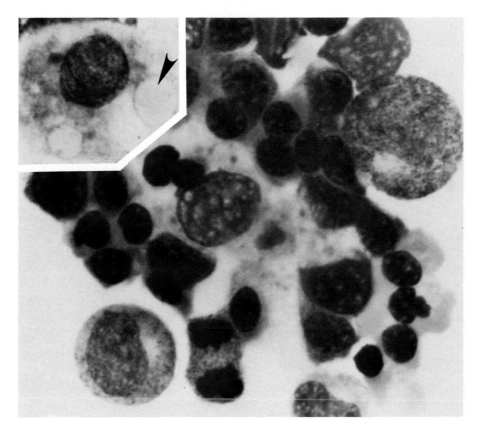

Figure 2–47   *Erythroid island. Inset shows erythrocytophagy by macrophage. Arrow designates an erythrocyte within the cell.*

Erythrocytophagy by Macrophages. Erythrocytophagy may be found in a variety of disorders, including malignant histiocytosis, monocytic leukemia, autoimmune hemolytic anemia, untreated pernicious anemia, folate deficiency, chronic erythremic myelosis, septicemia, erythroleukemia, and thrombotic thrombocytopenic purpura (Fig. 2–47). In some instances, macrophages contain both mature erythrocytes and degenerating late intermediate erythroblasts. Erythrocytophagy provides cytologic evidence of ineffective erythropoiesis.

Normoblastic Erythroid Hyperplasia. Increased numbers of normoblasts, particularly intermediate and late normoblasts, are found in a variety of disorders, including autoimmune hemolytic anemia (Fig. 2–48 and Plate 1*A*), thrombotic thrombocytopenic purpura, hemolytic anemia due to artificial heart valve prosthesis, and hemoglobinopathies. Normoblastic erythroid hyperplasia is also found in hereditary spherocytosis and polycythemia vera (Fig. 2–49).

Figure 2–48   *Increased numbers of intermediate normoblasts in autoimmune hemolytic anemia (A). H and E section of biopsy of intermediate normoblasts, showing darkly stained nuclei with checkerboard chromatin pattern typical of erythroblasts (B).*

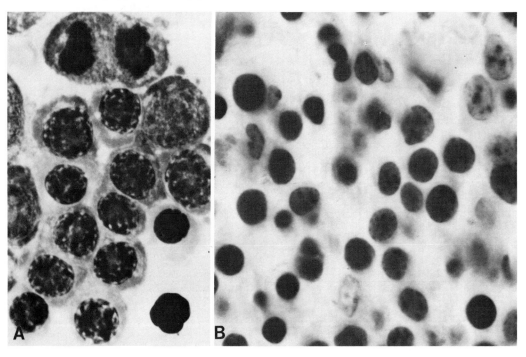

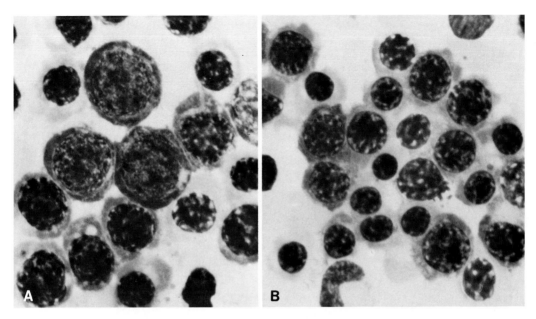

Figure 2–49   *Increased numbers of intermediate normoblasts in (A) hereditary spherocytosis and (B) polycythemia vera.*

In thrombotic thrombocytopenic purpura, marrows show marked hyperplasia of normoblasts (Fig. 2–50), numerous erythroid islands, and megakaryocytic abnormalities (Chap. 7). If capillaries are included in the marrow biopsies, they often show typical hyaline thrombotic lesions.

In untreated iron deficiency anemia, normoblasts are smaller than normal and show indistinct cytoplasmic details with frayed, ragged-appearing cytoplasmic borders (Fig. 2–51 and Plate 1*B*). In these erythroblasts, polychromasia persists into the late stages of erythroid maturation. Delayed hemoglobinization of erythroblasts is a characteristic finding in severe untreated iron deficiency anemia.

Marrows from patients with hemoglobinopathies usually do not show distinctive features other than normoblastic erythroid hyperplasia. In some patients with sickle cell anemia, hemoglobin SC disease, or hemoglobin S–thalassemia, megaloblastic changes occur in the marrow presumably as the result of folate deficiency due to increased utilization of folate.

Normoblastic erythroid hyperplasia can also occur in chronic lymphocytic leukemia or lymphocytic lymphoma in which there is concomitant hemolytic anemia. It is also found in hemolytic anemias due to accelerated destruction of erythrocytes by an enlarged spleen (hypersplenism).

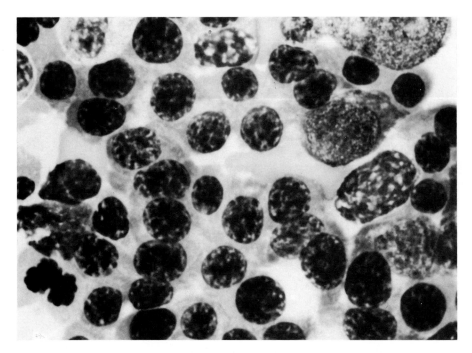

Figure 2–50   *Increased numbers of late intermediate macronormoblasts in thrombotic thrombocytopenic purpura.*

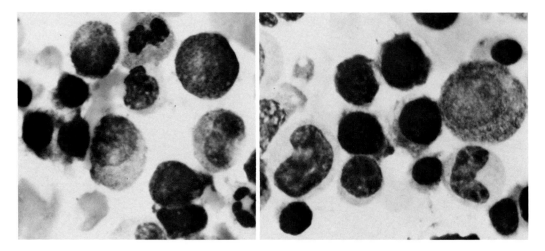

Figure 2–51   *Iron deficiency anemia, showing erythroblasts that are smaller than normal, with ragged-appearing cytoplasm and the persistence of basophilia as a reflection of delayed hemoglobinization.*

Di Guglielmo Syndrome

Di Guglielmo syndrome is a spectrum of erythroblastic disorders that includes acute erythremic myelosis (Di Guglielmo disease), chronic erythremic myelosis, and erythroleukemia. Probably, some cases of refractory anemia and refractory anemia with ringed sideroblasts (both of which have been included in the current designation, "myelodysplastic syndrome") fit within the concept of Di Guglielmo syndrome. In some instances, patients with acute erythremic myelosis and chronic erythremic myelosis have developed erythroleukemia and/or acute myeloblastic or myelomonocytic leukemia. In other instances, obvious leukemic evolution does not seem to occur within the patient's lifetime.

Megaloblastoid-type nuclear chromatin patterns are often found in erythroblasts from patients with Di Guglielmo syndrome. Megaloblastoid erythropoiesis is first noticeable in early intermediate macronormoblasts. Megaloblastoid erythroblasts are larger than normoblasts. Nuclear chromatin shows disarrangement of the usual normoblastic circularity and also demonstrates large blocklike aggregates of chromatin, irregular in size and shape, that are connected to adjacent aggregates of chromatin and chromatin strands by coarse filaments of nuclear chromatin (Fig. 2–52A and B).

Nucleocytoplasmic asynchronism usually occurs. In some megaloblastoid cells, portions of the nucleus show a megaloblastoid nuclear chromatin pattern, whereas other areas of the nucleus demonstrate more finely attenuated nuclear chromatin and reduction of number and size of aggregates typical of megaloblastic maturation. Orange nuclear deposits may be found. These are usually punctate and located in the interstices between chromatin strands, but may also be globular and large.

Under the light microscope, megaloblastoid maturation can usually be distinguished from megaloblastic maturation. In megaloblastoid maturation, nuclear chromatin strands appear coarser than in megaloblastic maturation and nuclear chromatin aggregates are considerably larger and more numerous. In both types of chromatin patterns, aggregates and chromatin strands are widely separated, imparting an open appearance to the cell. In both instances, normal erythroid chromatin circularity is lost and is replaced by a disorganized-appearing chromatin pattern. Although most instances are typical, sometimes it may be difficult to distinguish earliest megaloblastic changes from megaloblastoid patterns.

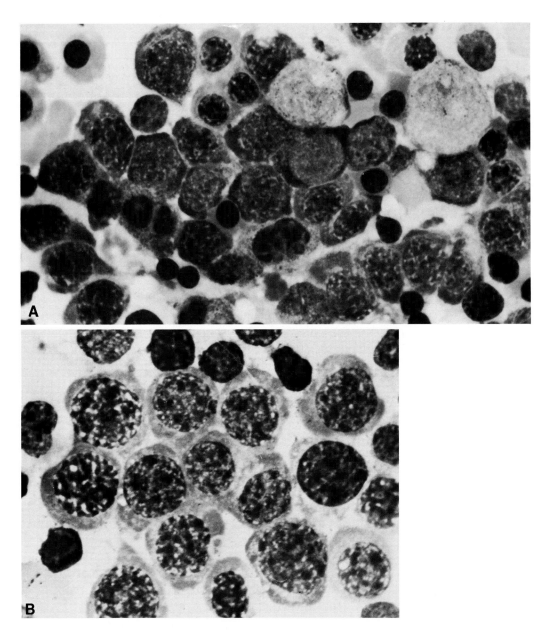

Figure 2–52   (A) *Low-power view of cluster of proerythroblasts and megaloblastoid intermediate macronormoblasts, chronic erythremic myelosis.* (B) *Higher-power view of megaloblastoid intermediate macronormoblasts, chronic erythremic myelosis. Aggregates of nuclear chromatin are prominent and blocklike and are connected to adjacent aggregates by coarse-appearing strands of chromatin.*

Pathogenesis of the megaloblastoid nuclear chromatin pattern is not fully understood. Abnormalities in the biosynthesis of DNA probably contribute to the morphologic lesion of megaloblastoid nuclear chromatin. Abnormalities in type and composition of histones also contribute to the pathogenesis of megaloblastoid erythropoiesis. Megaloblastoid erythroid precursors have increased amounts of arginine-rich histone arranged in an abnormal spatial distribution in the nucleus and localized in areas of heterochromatin or metabolically repressed DNA. Megaloblastoid erythroblasts also have increased nuclear deposits of methylated arginine-rich histone that may arise in part as a result of increased activity of S-adenosyl-methionine-dependent arginine methyltransferase. Perhaps as a result of the abnormalities in DNA biosynthesis, arginine-rich histone, and methylated arginine-rich histone, chromatin strands assume the blocklike configurations typical of megaloblastoid erythropoiesis.

Megaloblastoid maturation occurs in Di Guglielmo syndrome and in acute myeloblastic and myelomonocytic leukemia. Megaloblastoid maturation can also be seen after exposure to various agents such as organic phosphorous and a variety of antibiotics. Megaloblastoid and megaloblastic nuclear chromatin patterns occur after administration of antineoplastic agents such as fluorouracil, cyclophosphamide, and 6-mercaptopurine.

Acute Erythremic Myelosis

Acute erythremic myelosis is a rare disorder characterized by the proliferation of atypical erythroblasts in the marrow and visceral organs. Erythroblastic hyperplasia is intense (Figs. 2–53 and 2–54), and many erythroblasts are bizarre-appearing, gigantic, and multinuclear (Figs. 2–55 through 2–57). Some of them have large cytoplasmic vacuoles (Fig. 2–58). Occasionally, multinuclear histiocytic cells are found (Fig. 2–59). Giant, bizarre-appearing mitotic figures may occur.

(Text continued on page 60)

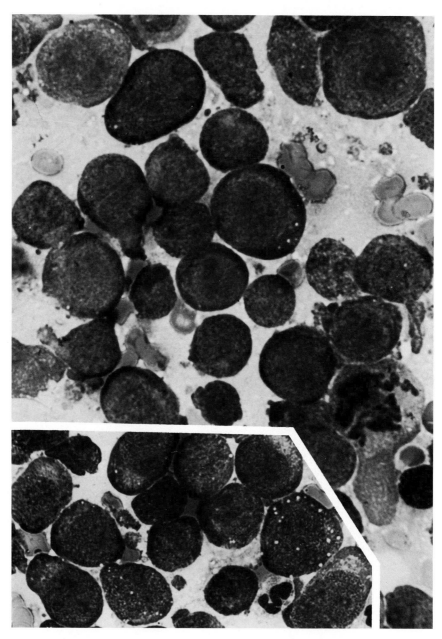

Figure 2–53   *Acute erythremic myelosis, showing hypercellular marrow composed largely of proerythroblasts and aberrant-appearing mitotic figures.*

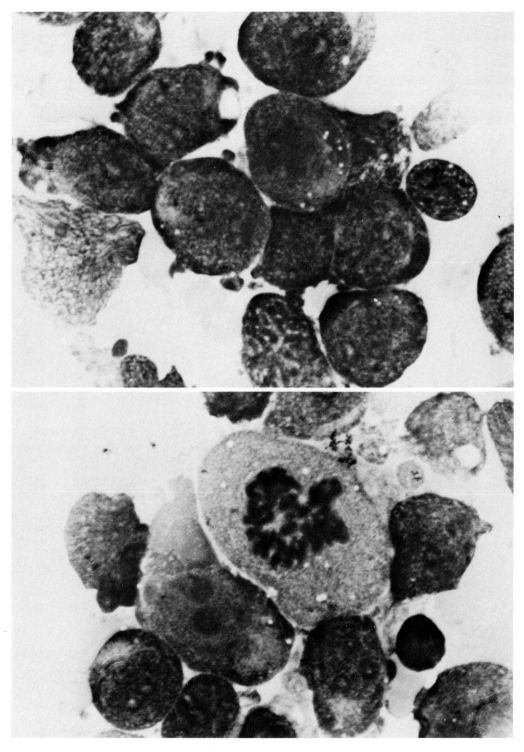

Figure 2–54   *Acute erythremic myelosis, showing increased numbers of proerythroblasts and aberrant-appearing mitotic figures.*

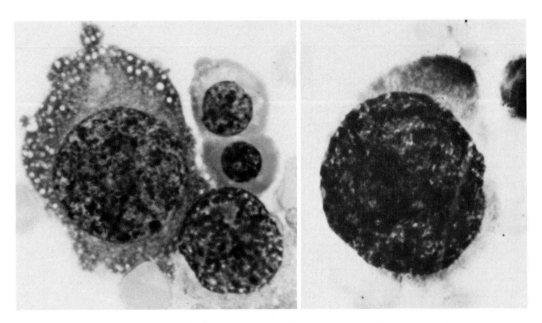

Figure 2–55   *Giant intermediate macronormoblasts, acute erythremic myelosis.*

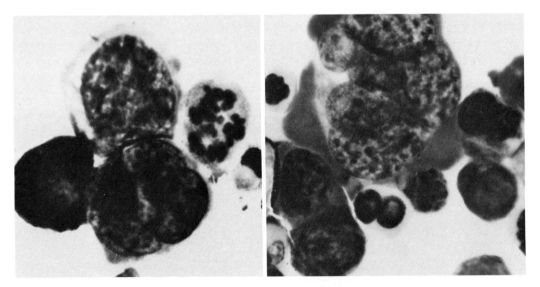

Figure 2–56   *Bizarre-appearing multinuclear erythroblasts and aberrant mitotic figures in acute erythremic myelosis.*

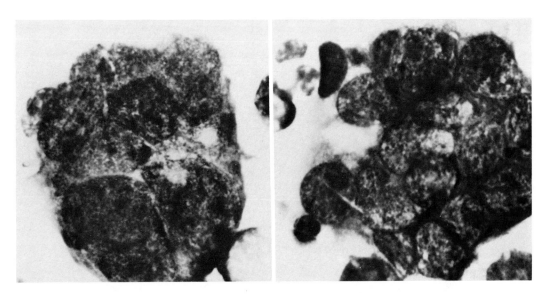

Figure 2–57   Bizarre multinuclear giant erythroblasts, acute erythremic myelosis.

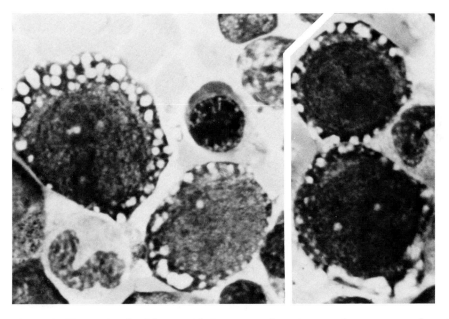

Figure 2–58   Erythroblasts with large cytoplasmic vacuoles, acute erythremic myelosis.

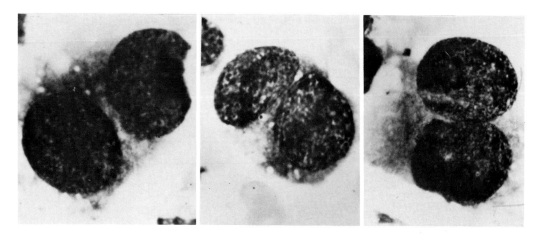

Figure 2–59   *Bizarre-appearing histiocytoid cells, acute erythremic myelosis.*

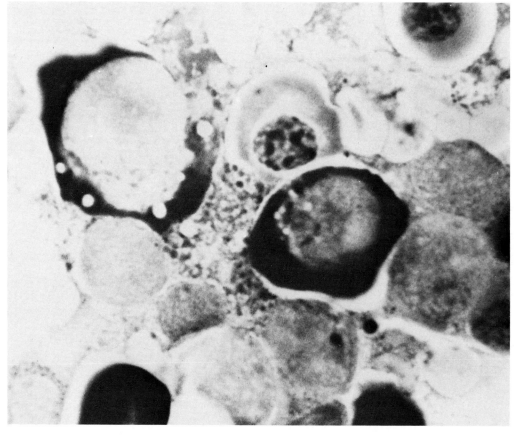

Figure 2–60   *Intense PAS-positive material in erythroblasts, acute erythremic myelosis.*

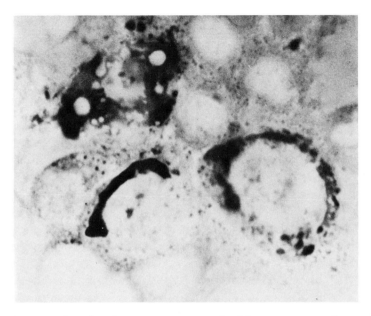

Figure 2–61   *Intense phosphorylase activity in erythroblasts, acute erythremic myelosis.*

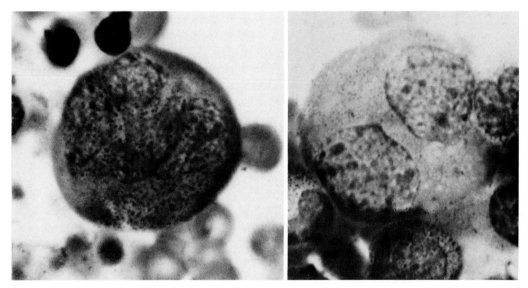

Figure 2–62   *Black punctate-appearing specific esterase activity and gray-appearing nonspecific esterase activity in erythroblasts from patients with acute erythremic myelosis. Specific esterase activity is demonstrated with naphthol ASD-chloroacetate and fast blue BBN, and nonspecific esterase activity is detected with alpha naphthyl acetate and hexazotized pararosaniline.*

Possibly, all patients with acute nonlymphoblastic leukemia pass through an erythremic phase. Only those patients who sustain consequences of pancytopenia come to medical attention. According to this view, acute erythremic myelosis may be the initial and erythroid expression of a disorder that is basically myeloblastic.

Cytochemically, erythroblasts from patients with acute erythremic myelosis demonstrate a number of abnormalities. Using the *PAS* (periodic acid–Schiff) *reagent* for glycogen, the cytoplasm of erythroblasts stains intensely. PAS-positive material is usually diffuse in distribution and often seems to extrude from the cellular margins (Fig. 2–60). *Phosphorylase activity* is also intense in these cells (Fig. 2–61).

Prussian blue stain for ferric iron demonstrates numerous siderotic granules in the cytoplasm, representing deposition of hemosiderin within mitochondria.

Nonspecific esterase activity using alpha naphthyl acetate as a substrate is intense in erythroblasts. *Specific esterase activity* utilizing naphthol ASD-chloroacetate as a substrate also occurs in the cytoplasm of the abnormal erythroblasts (Fig. 2–62). The presence of specific esterase activity reflects granulocytic properties of these cells and indicates disturbances of cellular differentiation in erythroblasts that exhibit both erythroid and granulocytic properties. Accordingly, the presence of specific esterase activity in these pathologic erythroblasts is consistent with the concept of Di Guglielmo syndrome in which a preleukemic disorder of erythropoiesis may be the initial manifestation of myeloblastic leukemia and may precede the emergence of this leukemia by varying periods of time.

Chronic Erythremic Myelosis

Chronic erythremic myelosis is the most commonly encountered form of Di Guglielmo syndrome. It is characterized by refractory macrocytic anemia, monocytosis, and pancytopenia. Often, pseudo-Pelger-Huët anomaly is found in polymorphonuclear leukocytes in the blood and marrow. The presence of this abnormality is believed to represent a greater likelihood of leukemic transformation in a particular patient than if the abnormality were not present. Enlargements of the liver and the spleen are often found.

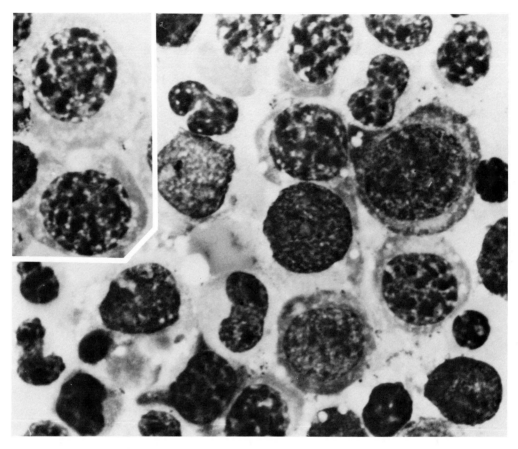

Figure 2–63   *Megaloblastoid intermediate macronormoblasts, chronic erythremic myelosis.*

Marrows from patients with chronic erythremic myelosis are markedly hypercellular. Erythroblastic hyperplasia is intense, and megaloblastoid erythropoiesis is found (Figs. 2–63, through 2–65 and Plate 1C). Increased numbers of proerythroblasts and early intermediate macronormoblasts are observed (Fig. 2–66). Some show nuclear abnormalities in the form of multinuclearity. Most of the erythroblastic hyperplasia is due to increased numbers of megaloblastoid intermediate macronormoblasts. At this stage of erythroblastic maturation, these cells are believed to be unusually susceptible to intramedullary cell death. Late normoblasts show multiple Howell-Jolly bodies and coarse basophilic stippling.

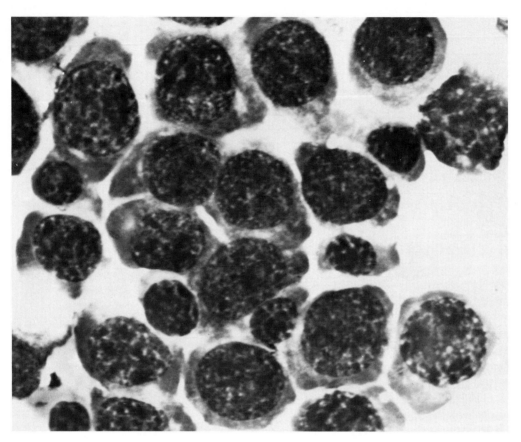

Figure 2–64   *Megaloblastoid intermediate macronormoblasts, chronic erythremic myelosis, showing blocklike aggregates of nuclear chromatin connected by delicate strands of chromatin.*

Other nuclear abnormalities include deposits of orange-staining material in the nucleus (Fig. 2–67) and, in some instances, megaloblastic-type erythropoiesis (Fig. 2–68). Cytoplasmic abnormalities such as the presence of hemoglobin lakes indicate defective hemoglobinization. Nucleocytoplasmic asynchronism can also be found. Aberrant-appearing mitotic figures are prominent (Fig. 2–69).

Granulocytopoiesis is usually left shifted with increased numbers of myelocytes and promyelocytes. Megakaryocytes show numerous abnormalities, and micromegakaryocytes with heavily vacuolated cytoplasm are found frequently. Numerous macrophages showing erythrocytophagy of mature erythrocytes and degenerating

(Text continued on page 66)

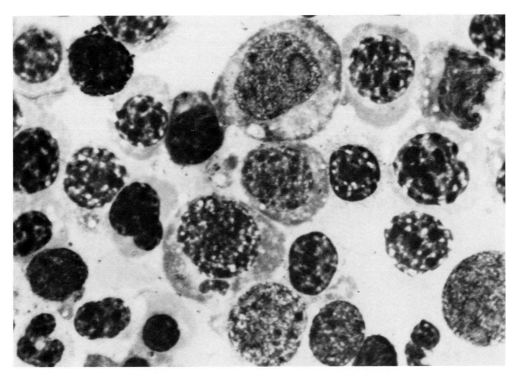

Figure 2–65   *Megaloblastoid intermediate macronormoblasts, chronic erythremic myelosis, depicting accessory nucleus (center) and prominent nucleolus in proerythroblast (top).*

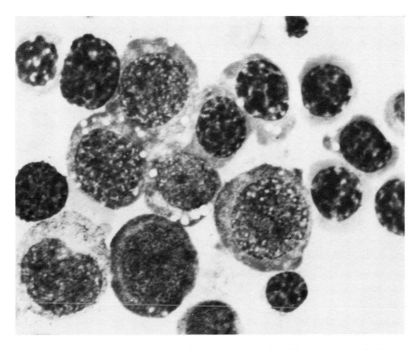

Figure 2–66   *Increased numbers of proerythroblasts and early intermediate macronormoblasts, chronic erythremic myelosis.*

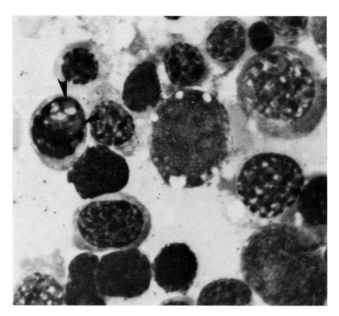

Figure 2–67   *Orange-staining intranuclear deposits (arrows) in erythroblast from patient with chronic erythremic myelosis. Vacuolated proerythroblasts and megaloblastoid intermediate macronormoblasts also are shown.*

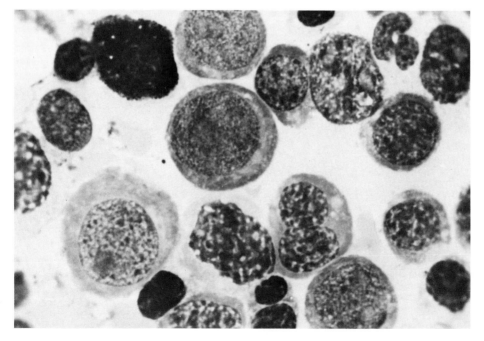

Figure 2–68   *Megaloblasts, megaloblastoid intermediate macronormoblasts, and mast cell (upper left) in marrow of patient with chronic erythremic myelosis.*

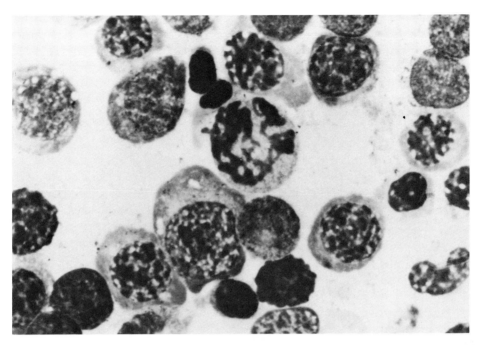

Figure 2–69   *Chronic erythremic myelosis, showing large megaloblastoid intermediate macronormoblasts and aberrant mitotic figure in erythroblast (center).*

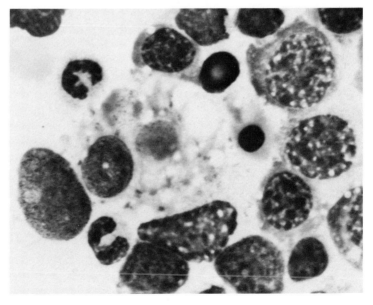

Figure 2–70   *Erythrocytophagy of mature erythroblasts and erythrocytes by macrophage, chronic erythremic myelosis.*

erythroblasts constitute cytologic evidence of ineffective erythropoiesis (Fig. 2–70). Macrophages containing cellular debris are also present in increased numbers (Fig. 2–71). Mast cells are increased in number. In typical cases, myeloblasts are less than 1%.

Biopsies of marrows from patients with chronic erythremic myelosis show markedly increased numbers of erythroblasts, particularly proerythroblasts and early intermediate normoblasts (Fig. 2–72). On routine H and E sections, proerythroblasts have a pale vesicular nucleus with a random pattern of nuclear chromatin particles, and the nuclear membrane is usually distinct and uniform appearing. Later stages of erythroblastic maturation show darkly staining nuclei with checkerboard nuclear chromatin patterns. Aberrant-appearing mitotic figures may also occur.

Figure 2–71   *Large macrophage containing cytoplasmic debris, chronic erythremic myelosis.*

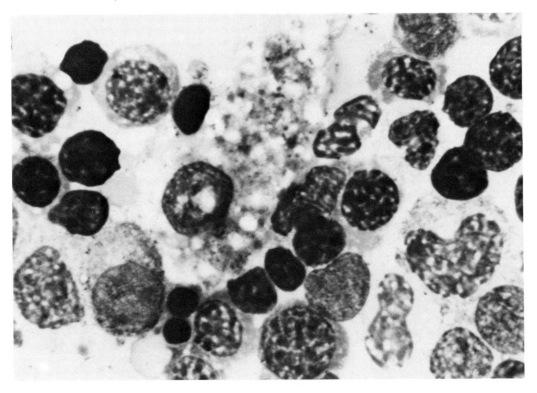

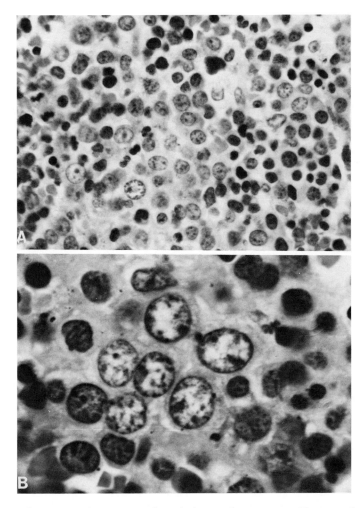

Figure 2–72   *Chronic erythremic myelosis (A) H and E section of biopsy, showing hypercellularity and increased numbers of erythroblasts. (B) Higher magnification, showing pale vesicular nuclei of proerythroblasts and darker-staining nuclei of more mature erythroblasts.*

Cytochemical Abnormalities in Chronic Erythremic Myelosis

A number of cytochemical abnormalities of nuclear constituents have been observed in erythroblasts from patients with chronic erythremic myelosis. Using the *ammoniacal silver* stain, nuclei of erythroblasts from patients with this disorder have abundant arginine-rich

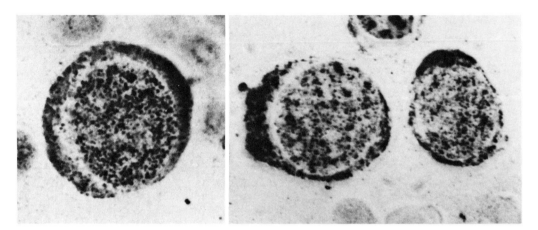

Figure 2–73   *Ammoniacal silver stain, chronic erythremic myelosis. Punctate black- to brown-staining areas in the nuclei represent sites of arginine-rich histone.*

histone arranged in a granular or speckled pattern (Fig. 2–73). Abnormalities in the distribution of this histone have been observed in ultrastructural studies in which the histone has been found to be localized predominantly in areas of metabolically repressed DNA or heterochromatin. Localization of arginine-rich histone in these areas of metabolically inactive DNA may contribute by means as yet unknown to the cellular abnormalities leading to the evolution of acute leukemia.

With the blue thiazine dye *azure A,* nuclei of erythroblasts from patients with chronic erythremic myelosis stain a metachromatic pink color after removal of nucleic acids by acid digestion (Fig. 2–74). This pink metachromasia is believed to be due to the high content of methylated arginine present in basic nucleoprotein (histone) of these erythroblasts. Nuclear metachromasia with azure A may be a distinctive abnormality for erythroblasts in chronic erythremic myelosis and reflects aberrations in type and composition of basic nuclear proteins.

With the use of *gold chloride,* punctate deposits of metallic (colloidal) gold have been observed in nuclei of erythroblasts from patients with chronic erythremic myelosis (Fig. 2–75). The ability of nuclei to reduce gold chloride to colloidal or elemental gold may reflect the presence of reducing substance(s), perhaps enzymatic, in the nuclei of these pathologic erythroblasts.

Abnormalities of cytoplasmic constituents have also been described in erythroblasts from patients with chronic erythremic myelosis. Aberrations of iron storage and metabolism can be

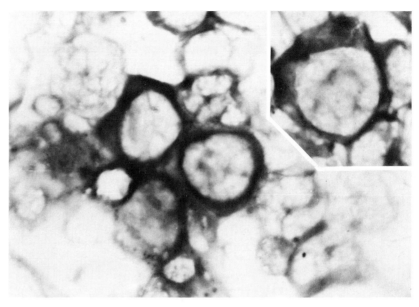

Figure 2–74 *Azure A stain, chronic erythremic myelosis, demonstrating pink metachromatic staining of the nuclei in erythroblasts.*

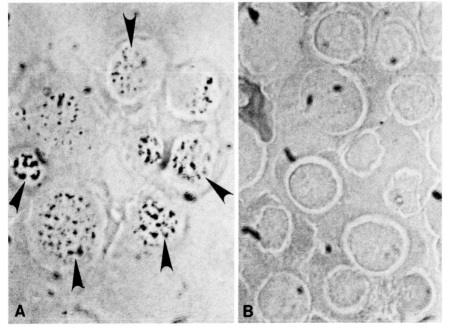

Figure 2–75 *Gold chloride stain. (A) Erythroblasts in chronic erythremic myelosis, showing black punctate nuclear staining, as delineated by arrows. (B) Lack of staining in normal erythroblasts.*

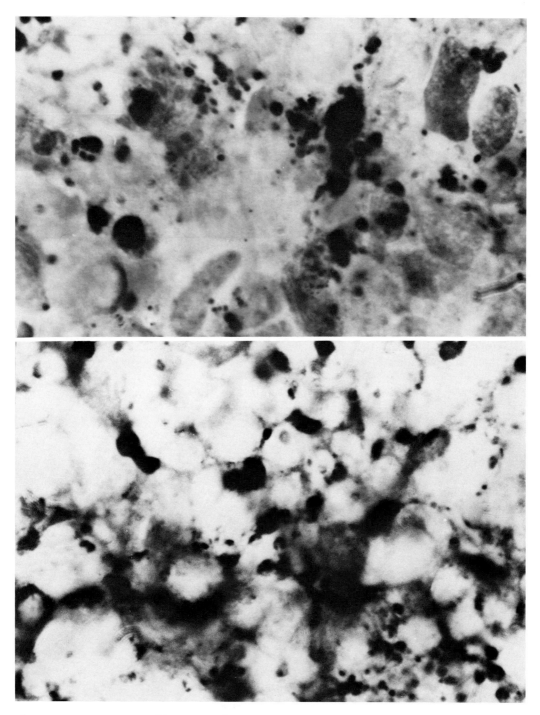

Figure 2–76   *Prussian blue stain, chronic erythremic myelosis, demonstrating large agglomerates of hemosiderin that are typical of disorders in which the turnover of iron is slow, such as refractory anemias.*

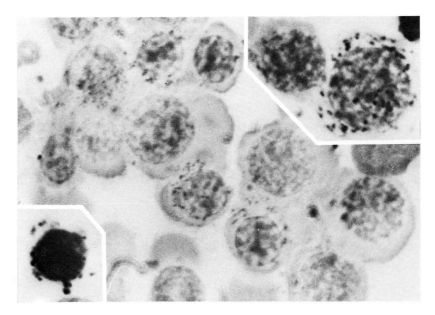

Figure 2–77 *Prussian blue stain, chronic erythremic myelosis, depicting ringed sideroblasts.*

detected with a variety of cytochemical stains. *Prussian blue* demonstrates hemosiderin iron in which iron is in the form of ferric hydroxide. Using the *Prussian blue* stain, abnormalities in the distribution and content of hemosiderin have been detected. In chronic erythremic myelosis, large blocklike deposits of hemosiderin are observed in the marrow (Fig. 2–76). Some of this iron is within the cytoplasm of macrophages. Other hemosiderin appears to be extracellular.

This type of pattern of hemosiderin deposition is seen in anemias in which there is slow turnover of iron, such as in the refractory anemias. By contrast, in anemias characterized by rapid iron turnover, such as hemolytic anemias, the iron-particle pattern is small and punctate.

Within the cytoplasm of erythroblasts, iron can be demonstrated within the lamellae and cristae of mitochondria. In chronic erythremic myelosis and other types of anemias characterized by abnormalities of iron metabolism and faulty incorporation of iron into hemoglobin, mitochondria containing iron surround the nucleus in a ringed fashion, leading to the designation "ringed sideroblast" (Fig. 2–77). Ringed sideroblasts are seen first in those stages of erythroblastic maturation in which hemoglobin synthesis becomes apparent (i.e., early intermediate macronormoblasts). In some sideroblasts, Prussian blue–positive material occurs in a circumferential fashion surrounding the nucleus. In other erythroblasts, siderotic granules occur in a cluster in one area of the cytoplasm, indicating that iron-laden mitochondria have accumulated in a discrete area. Rarely, sideroblasts show diffuse, pale blue staining of the cytoplasm, representing dispersal of iron-containing substances throughout the cell.

Pathologic siderotic granules are usually multiple and coarse appearing, in contrast to normal siderotic granules, which are small and usually do not number more than two to four in a normal erythroblast. In some instances, pathologic siderocytes (mature erythrocytes containing siderotic granules) contain siderotic granules that seem to be arranged in a weblike or netlike configuration.

Figure 2–78   *Alizarin red S stain, demonstrating purple-staining coccoid structures and purple perinuclear halos in ringed sideroblasts. These purple-staining areas represent sites of iron deposition in mitochondria.*

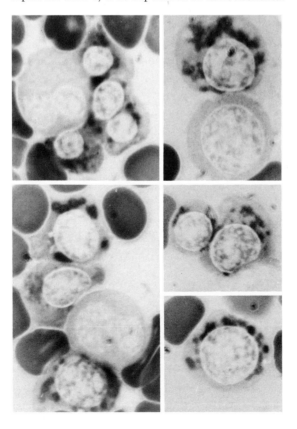

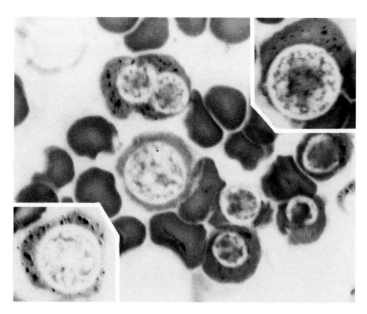

Figure 2–79 *Bromochlorophenol blue stain, chronic erythremic myelosis, demonstrating punctate black-staining areas that represent iron in mitochondria in ringed sideroblasts.*

Alizarin red S is an anthraquinone dye capable of forming colored, insoluble dye lakes or precipitates with various heavy metal salts. With ferric iron, alizarin red S forms a purple or black precipitate. In sideroblasts from patients with chronic erythremic myelosis and other types of sideroblastic anemias, exposure to alizarin red S leads to the visualization of a purple perinuclear halo and violaceous-appearing coccoid structures, probably representing mitochondria containing iron (Fig. 2–78).

Using the dye indicator *bromochlorophenol blue,* ferric salts form an insoluble black precipitate composed of the dye and the heavy metal. After staining pathologic sideroblasts with bromochlorophenol blue, punctate black-staining structures can be seen surrounding the nucleus (Fig. 2–79). Apparently, bromochlorophenol blue reacts with iron in mitochondria to produce the punctate black staining.

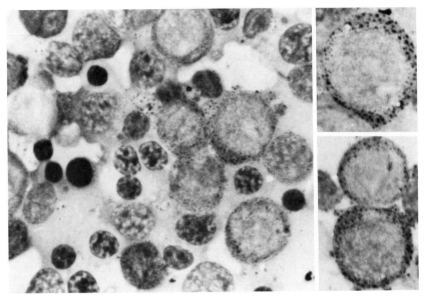

Figure 2–80   *PAS positivity of erythroblasts in chronic erythremic myelosis. In late intermediate macronormoblasts, PAS-positive material can be diffuse or punctate. In early intermediate macronormoblasts and in proerythroblasts (right insets), PAS-positive material is often punctate.*

Periodic acid–Schiff (PAS) reaction for glycogen is often positive in erythroblasts from patients with chronic erythremic myelosis (Fig. 2–80). In proerythroblasts, the PAS reaction is usually finely punctate, although some diffuse staining may also be found. In later intermediate erythroblasts, PAS positivity is usually diffuse. Generally, in chronic erythremic myelosis, PAS positivity of erythroblasts is less intense than in acute erythremic myelosis or erythroleukemia. In some instances, PAS positivity of erythroblasts and/or ringed sideroblasts does not occur. Absence of these abnormalities does not constitute evidence against the diagnosis of chronic erythremic myelosis, since these abnormalities show some variability.

Phosphorylase activity is also increased in erythroblasts (Fig. 2–81). The reasons for increased phosphorylase activity are unclear. Increased activity usually occurs in cells that show abundant glycogen as demonstrated by the PAS reagent, suggesting that increased phosphorylase activity is induced by increased amounts of glycogen as a compensatory mechanism for glycogen breakdown.

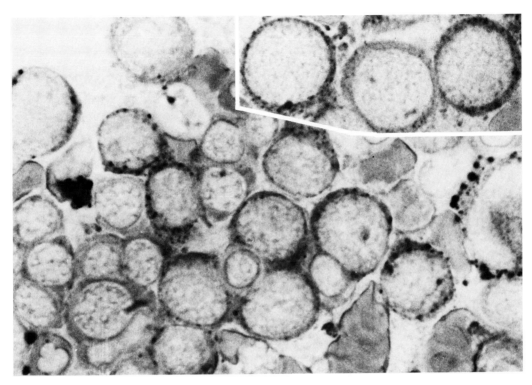

Figure 2–81   *Increased phosphorylase activity in megaloblastoid intermediate macronormoblasts, chronic erythremic myelosis.*

Alternatively, phosphorylase may act in a reverse direction in pathologic erythroblasts to facilitate biosynthesis rather than breakdown of glycogen.

Nonspecific esterase activity using alpha naphthyl acetate as the substrate is usually intense in erythroblasts from patients with chronic erythremic myelosis. The reasons for increased activity of this enzyme are unclear. By isoenzymatic analysis in polyacrylamide gel, nonspecific esterase derived predominantly from erythroblasts in chronic erythremic myelosis does not show a distinctive pattern compared to other types of predominantly erythroid esterases. *Specific esterase activity* is not detectable in erythroblasts from patients with chronic erythremic myelosis.

Refractory Anemia With Excess Blasts (RAEB)

Refractory anemia with excess blasts is known by a wide variety of other designations including smoldering acute leukemia, oligoblastic leukemia, aregenerative anemia, and partial myeloblastosis. Along with refractory anemia, refractory anemia with ringed sideroblasts

Figure 2–82   *Refractory anemia with excess blasts, showing increased numbers of small myeloblasts and megaloblastoid intermediate macronormoblasts* (main figure *and* inset).

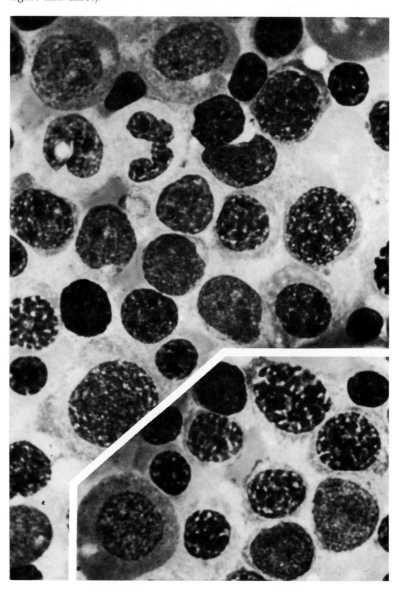

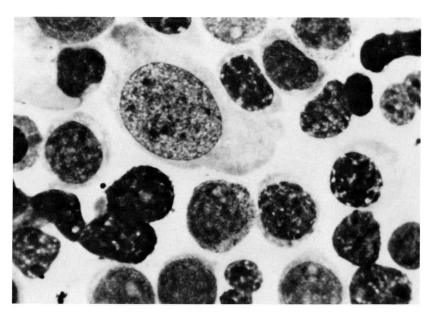

Figure 2–83   *Refractory anemia with excess blasts, illustrating a large bizarre erythroblast at the top and increased numbers of small myeloblasts with a delicate nuclear chromatin pattern and prominent nucleoli with perinucleolar chromatin condensation.*

(acquired idiopathic sideroblastic anemia), and chronic myelomonocytic leukemia (CMML), refractory anemia with excess blasts is currently included under the broad descriptive term, "myelodysplastic syndrome." Refractory anemia with excess blasts is a disorder characterized by pancytopenia, a variable clinical course, and frequent evolution into acute leukemia. Marrows are hypercellular with increased numbers of megaloblastoid intermediate macronormoblasts, proerythroblasts, and increased numbers of myeloblasts (Figs. 2–82 and 2–83). Myeloblasts usually do not exceed 20% of the marrow cells in a differential cell count. They do not contain Auer rods. Mitotic figures are numerous and appear bizarre (Fig. 2–84A).

Myeloblastic proliferation is usually indolent, and the percentage of myeloblasts in the marrow increases over a prolonged period of time in most patients. In others, myeloblastic proliferation is more rapid and the tempo of leukemic evolution is accelerated, leading to replacement of the marrow by leukemic blasts within weeks or months. When myeloblasts exceed 20% to 30% in the bone marrow

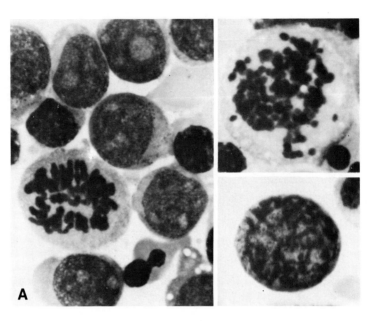

Figure 2–84 *(above and opposite)* (A) *Myeloblasts and aberrant-appearing mitotic figures in refractory anemia with excess blasts.* (B) (Top): *Increased numbers of eosinophil myelocytes and basophils along with increased numbers of small myeloblasts, megaloblastoid intermediate macronormoblasts, and micromegakaryocytes* (inset). (Bottom): *Eosinophils and atypical-appearing megakaryocytes. Refractory anemia with excess blasts.*

and Auer rods can be detected in granulocytic precursors, the disorder can be called "refractory anemia with excess blasts in transformation." In most cases of refractory anemia with excess blasts, myeloblasts are small, in contrast to acute myeloblastic leukemia, in which many of the myeloblasts are large. Small myeloblasts are believed to be resting or dormant and may reflect the smoldering or indolent behavior of refractory anemia with excess blasts. In contrast, large myeloblasts as found in acute myeloblastic leukemia are metabolically active and rapidly proliferative.

Increased numbers of eosinophil myelocytes and plasma cells may also be seen, and in some instances increased numbers of basophils occurs (Fig. 2–84B). Macrophages demonstrating erythrocytophagy constitute cytologic evidence of intramedullary cell death.

Megakaryocytes show numerous although nonspecific nuclear and cytoplasmic abnormalities. In many instances, micromegakaryocytes such as those seen in acute myeloblastic or myelomonocytic leukemia and in the cellular phase of agnogenic myeloid metaplasia are found (Figs. 2–84B and 2–85).

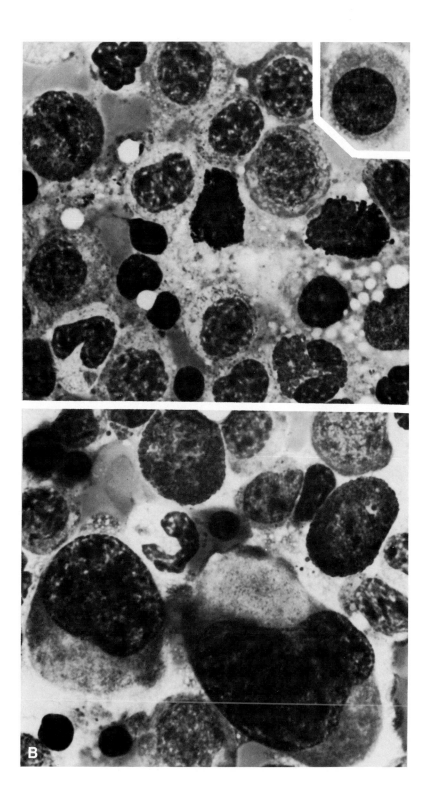

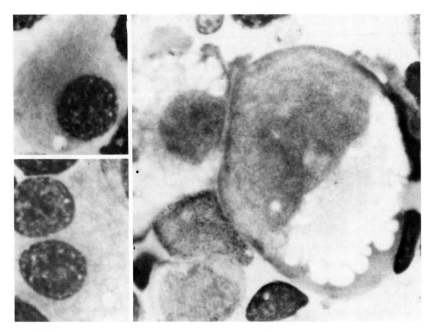

Figure 2–85   *Megakaryocytes, refractory anemia with excess blasts. Most of the megakaryocytes are micromegakaryocytes.*

On H and E sections, nuclei of erythroblasts appear as large vesicular structures containing one or more nucleoli in the immature erythroblasts. In more mature erythroblasts, nuclear chromatin forms a checkerboard pattern and the nucleus stains diffusely dark. Numerous mitotic figures are seen (Fig. 2–86).

Nuclei of immature granulocytic precursors have a nuclear membrane that is less uniform in caliber and more irregular in shape than in early erythroblasts (Fig. 2–87). In these granulocytic cells, nuclear chromatin is unusually diffuse and sometimes shows small punctate aggregates. In contrast to the nuclear chromatin of granulocytic cells, the chromatin of erythroblasts usually shows prominent, darkly staining aggregates. Megakaryocytes may also be increased in number.

Cytochemically, abnormalities in refractory anemia with excess blasts are nonspecific and include occasional PAS-positive erythroblasts and ringed sideroblasts.

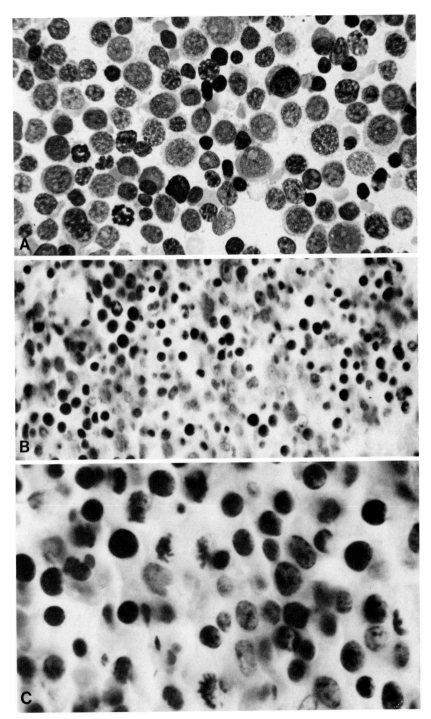

Figure 2–86 *Refractory anemia with excess blasts. (A) Hypercellular marrow with increased myeloblasts, promyelocytes, and erythroblasts. (B) Low-power view of marrow biopsy. (C) Higher magnification of marrow biopsy, showing darkly stained nuclei of erythroblasts and numerous mitotic figures.*

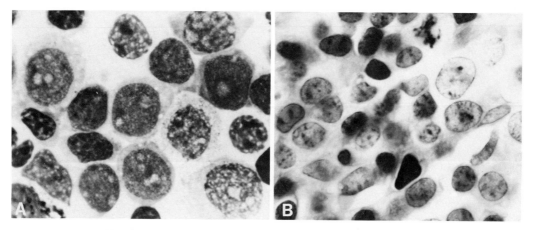

Figure 2–87   *Refractory anemia with excess blasts. (A) Increased numbers of myeloblasts and promyelocytes. (B) H and E section of biopsy, showing nuclei of promyelocytes and darkly staining nuclei of erythroblasts.*

Erythroleukemia

Erythroleukemia is a fatal disorder characterized by pancytopenia, infrequent occurrences of erythroblasts and myeloblasts in the peripheral blood, and erythroblastosis and myeloblastosis of the bone marrow and visceral organs. Marrows from patients with erythroleukemia can be hypercellular, normocellular, or hypocellular and show considerable variability from case to case. According to the FAB (French-American-British) classification of the acute leukemias, erythroleukemia has been designated M6.

In all instances, marrows show a more or less even admixture of erythroblasts and myeloblasts. When the proportion of myeloblasts exceeds 50%, it may be more accurate to interpret the marrow sample as showing acute myeloblastic leukemia based on cytologic and clinical considerations.

Currently, erythroleukemia is believed to be a transitory stage in the evolution of acute myeloblastic or myelomonocytic leukemia. Perhaps all patients with acute myeloblastic or myelomonocytic leukemia pass through an erythroleukemic phase that may be clinically inapparent in most instances. Evolution of erythroleukemia into acute myeloblastic or myelomonocytic leukemia occurs with marked rapidity in some individuals and more slowly in others.

In marrows from most patients with erythroleukemia, erythroblastic abnormalities are striking. Increased numbers of proerythroblasts occur, and many of them are binuclear, multinuclear, and bizarre appearing (Figs. 2–88 and 2–89). Gigantism of erythroblasts is observed frequently. Some erythroblasts have nuclear lobulations of

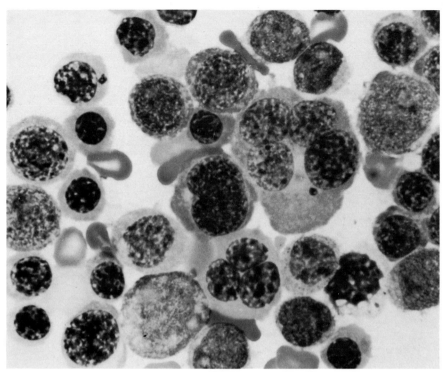

Figure 2–88   *Gigantic multinuclear erythroblasts, showing nucleocytoplasmic asynchronism and increased numbers of myeloblasts in erythroleukemia.*

Figure 2–89   *Erythroleukemia, showing bizarre erythroblasts and myeloblasts. (Kass L: Enzymatic abnormalities in megakaryocytes. Acta Haematol 59:302, 1978)*

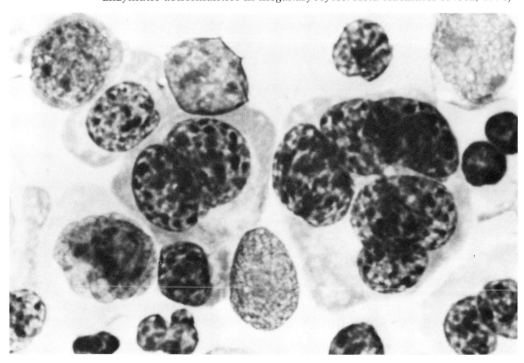

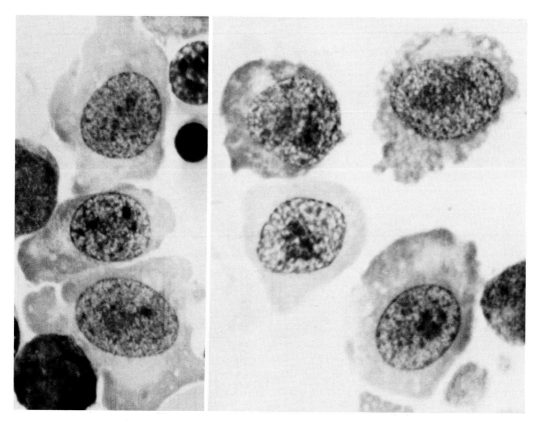

Figure 2–90   *Megaloblasts in erythroleukemia.*

various sizes within the same nucleus. Others show nuclear protrusions, accelerated pyknosis, and abnormal karyorrhexis. Multiple Howell-Jolly bodies and coarse basophlic stippling also occur.

Nuclear chromatin patterns in erythroblasts are usually megaloblastoid. In erythroblasts with multiple nuclei, some nuclei show a megaloblastoid nuclear chromatin pattern whereas others in the same cell exhibit a megaloblastic nuclear chromatin pattern. Some nuclei are pyknotic and degenerating whereas others in the same cell are in mitosis.

In other erythroblasts, megaloblastic nuclear chromatin patterns are found (Fig. 2–90). In these megaloblasts in erythroleukemia, the caliber of strands is markedly decreased, as are the number and size of chromatin aggregates. In some megaloblasts the nuclear chromatin strands are barely visible with the light microscope. Nuclei of megaloblasts in erythroleukemia are often centrally located, imparting a "fried-egg" appearance to the cell. Cytoplasm of these megaloblasts has a stellate configuration and appears elongated.

Hemoglobin lakes as well as apparent sequestrations of hemoglobin in the nucleus are also seen in megaloblasts and megaloblastoid intermediate macronormoblasts in erythroleukemia (Fig. 2–91).

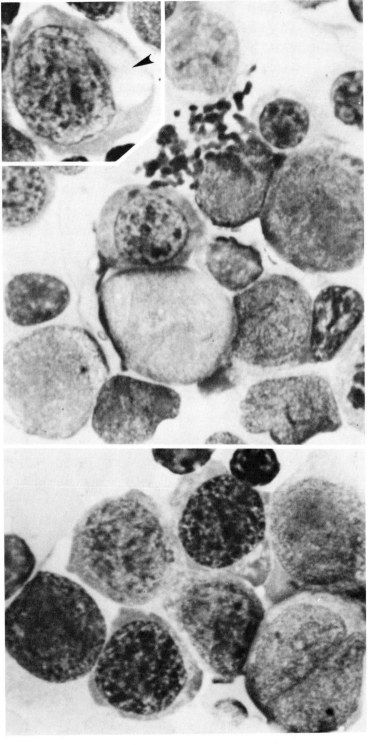

Figure 2–91   *Erythroleukemia, showing myeloblasts and erythroblasts. One erythroblast* (inset) *has a prominent hemoglobin lake* (arrow).

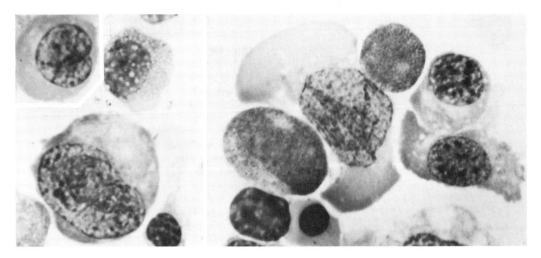

Figure 2–92   *Monocytoid-type foldings and lobulations of nuclei of erythroblasts in
erythroleukemia.*

Figure 2–93   (A) *Erythroleukemia, showing increased numbers of promyelocytes,*
(below and   *myeloblasts, and multinuclear bizarre-appearing erythroblasts (figure and*
opposite)   *inset). (B) Atypical promyelocytes, erythroleukemia, demonstrating*
           simultaneous eosinophilic and basophilic granules.

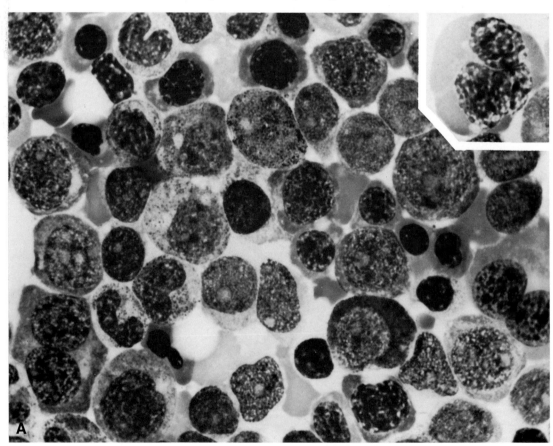

Hemoglobin lakes represent defective hemoglobinization of these cells. In other erythroleukemia megaloblasts, nuclear folding occurs, resembling that seen in cells of monocytic origin (Fig. 2–92). Nucleocytoplasmic asynchronism is also found. Bizarre-appearing and often multipolar mitotic figures in erythroblasts have been noted.

Granulocytic abnormalities include increased numbers of pro-myelocytes and myelocytes as well as increased numbers of myelo-blasts (Figs. 2–91 and 2–93*A*). Atypical promyelocytes containing both eosinophilic and basophilic granules in the same cell can be detected (Fig. 2–93*B*). Some myeloblasts contain Auer rods. The

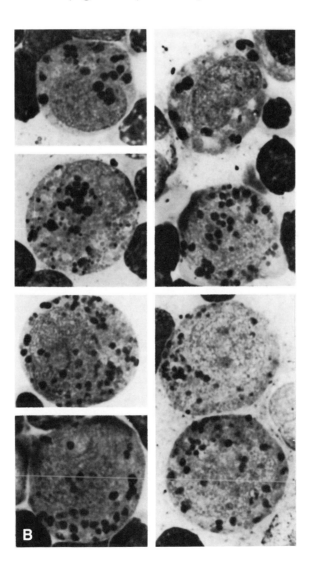

number of mature polymorphonuclear leukocytes is reduced. Evolution of erythroleukemia into acute leukemia can be rapid in some patients and protracted in others (Fig. 2–94).

On routine H and E sections, unusual-appearing gigantic erythroblasts and abnormal mitotic figures are seen (Fig. 2–95). Other nuclei appear pale and vesicular and may represent nuclei of myeloblasts and other primitive granulocytic cells.

Although erythropoiesis in erythroleukemia is morphologically bizarre appearing, as yet it is uncertain whether the bizarre erythropoiesis is actually a manifestation of neoplastic processes involving erythroblasts or whether erythropoiesis is abnormal because it is in the microenvironment of myeloblastic leukemia. Supporting the contention that erythropoiesis is physiologic in erythroleukemia, studies have shown that red cell development is under the control of erythropoietin. In contrast, cytochemical studies have indicated dual paths of differentiation in erythroleukemia erythroblasts, suggesting that they may have profound disturbances in cellular development as found in neoplastic cells. As yet, these issues are unresolved.

Figure 2–94
(opposite)   (A) *Erythroleukemia, showing erythroblasts with cytoplasmic vacuoles.* (B) *Acute leukemia that developed in the patient whose marrow is shown above* (A) *2 days after the original marrow showed erythroleukemia.*

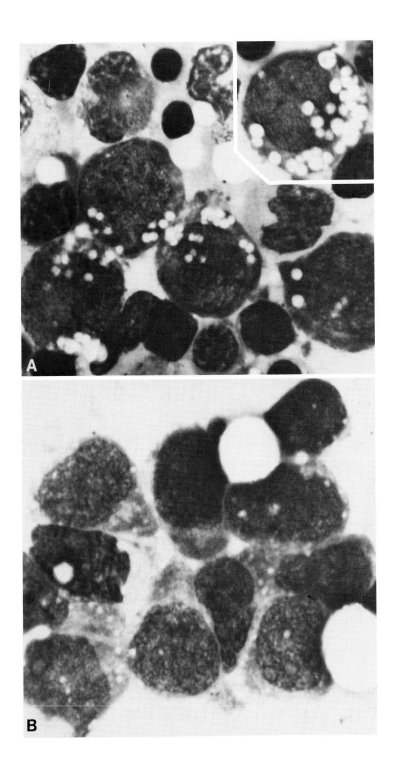

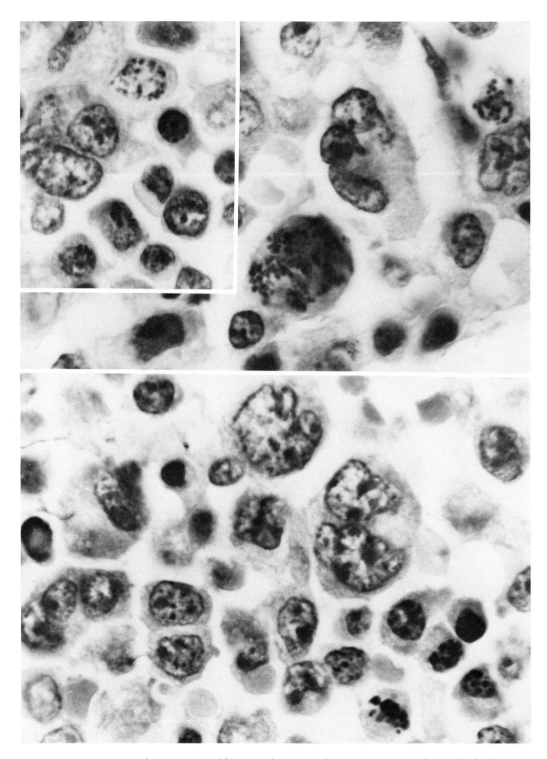

Figure 2–95   *H and E sections of biopsy of marrow from a patient with erythroleukemia, showing increased numbers of bizarre-appearing multinuclear erythroblasts and mitotic figures.*

Cytochemistry of Erythroleukemia

Ammoniacal silver reagent visualizes coarse deposits of arginine-rich histone in the nuclei of erythroblasts, similar to those in chronic erythremic myelosis (Fig. 2–96).

Prussian blue reagent visualizes coarse multiple siderotic granules in erythroblasts from patients with erythroleukemia. In those erythroblasts that are most bizarre appearing, such as gigantoblasts with multiple nuclear lobulations or multiple nuclei, the number and size of siderotic granules are often increased compared to more normal-appearing erythroblasts (Fig. 2–97).

Using the *PAS* reagent, erythroblasts in erythroleukemia usually show intensely positive reactions (Fig. 2–98). They are of several types. Large chunklike aggregates of PAS-positive material are often found (Fig. 2–98 and Plate 4*A*). More punctate types of positivity are also observed but less frequently than the prominent deposits. In

Figure 2–96 *Ammoniacal silver stain visualizes arginine-rich histone (black punctate) in erythroleukemia erythroblasts.*

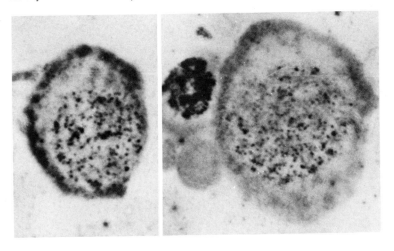

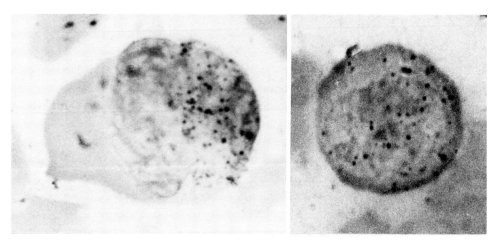

Figure 2–97   Siderotic granules in erythroleukemia erythroblasts visualized by Prussian blue reagent. (Kass L: Preleukemic Disorders. Springfield IL, Charles C Thomas, 1979)

Figure 2–98   Intense PAS-positive material in erythroleukemia erythroblasts. In some of these cells, both diffuse and blocklike positive material can be detected.

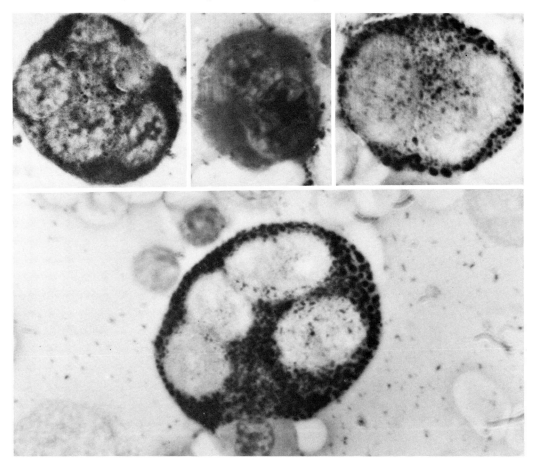

those cells that appear most bizarre, such as multinuclear gigantoblasts, PAS positivity is often most intense and blocklike in configuration. In other erythroblasts, diffuse PAS positivity is seen. This diffuse staining may be intense and in some instances is associated with coarse chunklike positivity.

Phosphorylase activity is unusually intense in erythroleukemia erythroblasts and may have pathophysiologic significance similar to that in chronic erythremic myelosis (Fig. 2–99).

Studies of *esterases* have provided insight into metabolic abnormalities of erythroblasts in erythroleukemia and may indicate profound disturbances of cellular differentiation. Using alpha naphthyl acetate as the substrate, erythroblasts from patients with erythroleukemia show strong nonspecific esterase activity. As in cells of granulocytic origin, the activity of this enzyme in erythroleukemia erythroblasts is only minimally inhibited by sodium fluoride. Using naphthol ASD-chloroacetate as a substrate to demonstrate the granulocytic properties of cells, erythroblasts from patients with erythro-

Figure 2–99   *Intense phosphorylase activity in erythroleukemia erythroblast. (Kass L: Enzymatic abnormalities in erythroleukemia. Acta Haematol 59:302, 1978)*

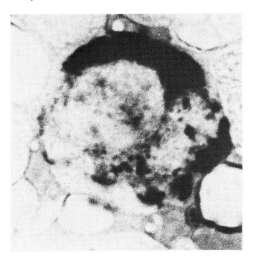

leukemia contain specific esterase activity (Fig. 2–100). Similar evidence of the granulocytic properties of erythroblasts in erythroleukemia is found in the presence of peroxidase activity, utilizing either benzidine or O-tolidine (Fig. 2–101).

Finding lysosomal enzymes typical of granulocytic cells in these erythroleukemia erythroblasts is consistent with the interpretation that these cells not only are morphologically erythroid and capable of synthesizing hemoglobin but also contain properties of cells of granulocytic origin. Accordingly, they seem to have differentiated along two cell lines, erythroid and granulocytic. Presumably, disturbances of differentiation of this type are seen in neoplastic cells. Activities of glycolytic enzymes like lactic dehydrogenase are increased in erythroleukemia erythroblasts (Fig. 2–102).

In some patients, evolution of erythroleukemia into acute myeloblastic or myelomonocytic leukemia does not occur. Possibly they die of the consequences of pancytopenia and/or treatment before obvious leukemic evolution. With the emergence of acute leukemia, the marked erythroblastic abnormalities present in the erythroleukemic phase disappear and only a few erythroblasts remain in the myeloblastic marrow. Whether the erythroblasts actually transform into myeloblasts or whether, more likely, they undergo intramedullary cell death as myeloblastic proliferation intensifies is unknown.

Figure 2–100   *Specific esterase activity (arrows) in erythroleukemia erythroblasts, naphthol ASD-chloroacetate and fast blue BBN. (Kass L: Esterase activity in erythroleukemia. Am J Clin Pathol 67:368, 1977)*

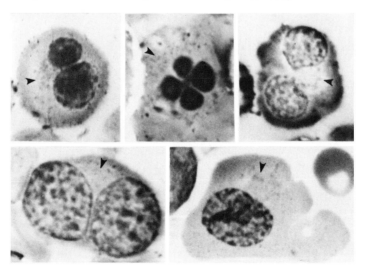

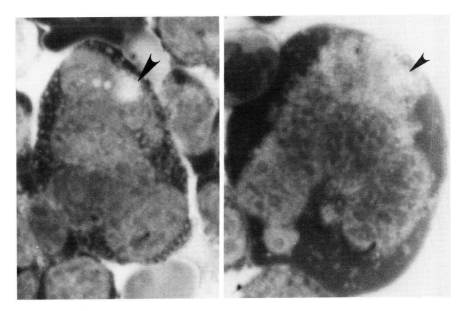

Figure 2–101   Peroxidase activity (arrows) in erythroleukemia erythroblasts, O-tolidine.

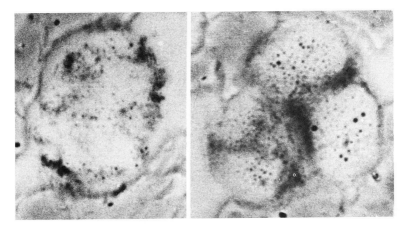

Figure 2–102   Increased activity of lactic dehydrogenase (black punctate) in erythroleukemia erythroblasts. (Kass L: Enzymatic abnormalities in erythroleukemia. Acta Haematol 59:302, 1978)

Megaloblastic Anemia

Megaloblastic anemia is a broad descriptive term indicating an anemia associated with megaloblasts in the bone marrow. In fact, anemia does not usually occur until megaloblasts are identifiable as such in the marrow. In most instances, the anemia is macrocytic, and the mean corpuscular volume of erythrocytes is usually greater than 105 cubic microns. Most cases of megaloblastic anemia are caused by deficiency of vitamin B_{12}, folate, or both. Deficiency of vitamin B_{12} may be heredofamilial (as in cases of pernicious anemia) or acquired (as in cases of intestinal malabsorption). Most instances of folate deficiency are attributable to dietary deficiency of the vitamin. However, drugs such as methotrexate can induce folate deficiency and megaloblastic anemia. Other chemotherapeutic drugs such as cytoxan and 6-mercaptopurine can also be associated with megaloblastic anemia. In rare instances, megaloblastic anemia can occur in patients with erythroleukemia. In all instances of megaloblastic anemia, abnormalities in the biosynthesis of DNA and perhaps histones are important factors that contribute to the pathogenesis of the megaloblastic lesion.

Morphologically, the earliest manifestations of megaloblastosis include a modest increase in the number of proerythroblasts and nuclear abnormalities of metamyelocytes such as gigantism and nuclear clubbing. Nuclei of bands may show twisting (Fig. 2–103). Hypersegmentation of the nucleus of polymorphonuclear leukocytes also occurs, and mild eosinophilia and plasmacytosis are often seen (Fig. 2–104).

Several morphologic features are among the earliest to indicate megaloblastic maturation in erythroblasts. In the clockface chromatin pattern, "hillocks" and "lumps" of chromatin are arranged in a circumferential fashion around the nuclear membrane, imparting a clockface appearance to it. These masses of chromatin are usually unconnected to other masses or strands of nuclear chromatin.

Another early morphologic manifestation of megaloblastosis is reduction in the number and size of chromatin aggregates. Similarly, there is reduction in the caliber of chromatin strands, leading to attenuation of chromatin strands. In some megaloblasts, these changes may be localized in one sector of the nucleus, imparting the appearance of focal attenuation of chromatin strands of the nucleus (Fig. 2–105). As a result of these alterations, among the earliest changes to occur in the nuclear chromatin of erythroblasts in mega-

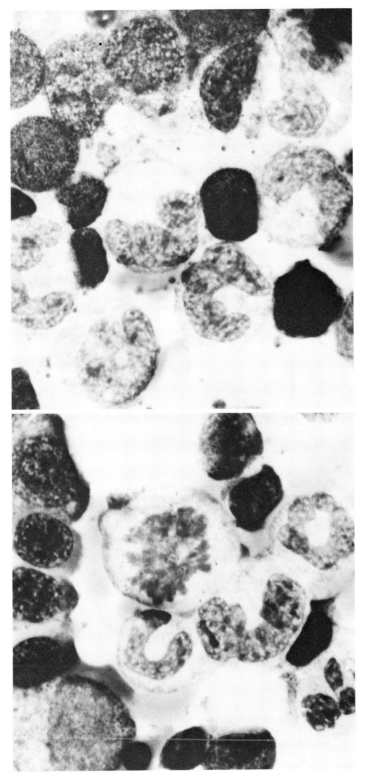

Figure 2–103   *Giant, bizarre-appearing metamyelocytes in pernicious anemia.*

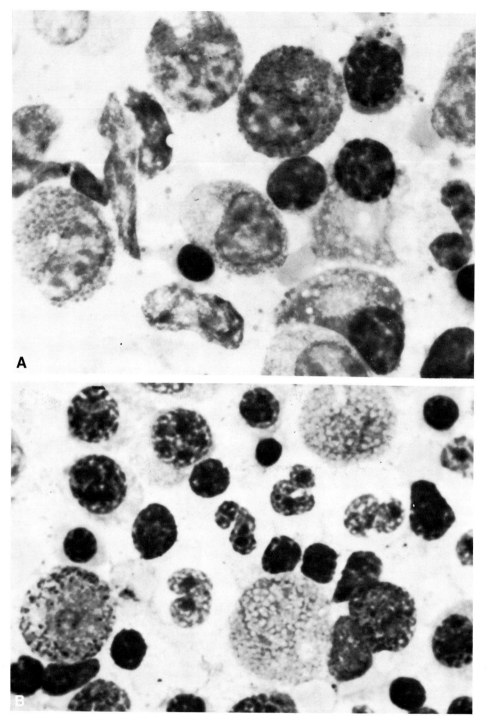

Figure 2–104   (A) *Eosinophilia and plasmacytosis in pernicious anemia.* (B) *Eosinophilia and early megaloblastic changes in erythroblasts in mild pernicious anemia.*

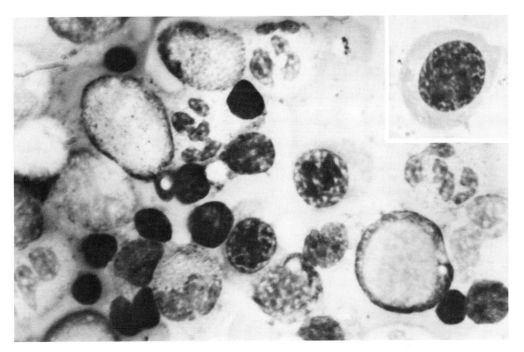

Figure 2–105   *Early megaloblastic changes in erythroblasts, pernicious anemia. Increased numbers of eosinophils also occur.*

loblastic anemia is a loss of the normal chromatin circularity and its replacement by a more disorganized pattern of nuclear chromatin (Fig. 2–106).

As megaloblastosis becomes more severe, these changes become more pronounced (Fig. 2–107). Erythroblastic proliferation becomes more intense, and in severe cases large numbers of proerythroblasts and early intermediate megaloblasts are found (Fig. 2–108 through 2–110). In erythroblasts, megaloblastic changes are noted first in the early intermediate stages of maturation when evidence of hemoglobinization is first detectable. Multinuclear erythroblasts may be observed, although the degree of gigantism and number of bizarre-appearing erythroblasts are substantially less compared to those found in erythroleukemia.

Multipolar and bizarre-appearing mitotic figures are found (Fig. 2–111). Evidence for abnormal karyorrhexis and accelerated pyknosis is often observed, and these processes contribute to the pathogenesis of multiple Howell-Jolly bodies.

Degenerating megaloblasts are frequently seen. In these cells, nuclear chromatin and cytoplasmic features are obliterated, imparting a smudged appearance to the cell (Fig. 2–112). In other degenerating megaloblasts, nuclear chromatin appears vacuous and tenuous, causing the nucleus to appear unusually fenestrated (Fig. 2–113, upper right).

Hemoglobin lakes in which areas of apparent hemoglobinization seem to be sequestered from the polychromatophilic cytoplasm constitute evidence of defective hemoglobinization (Fig. 2–113 and inset, lower left). Macrophages showing erythrocytophagy of mature erythroblasts and/or degenerating megaloblasts are cytologic indicators of ineffective erythropoiesis (Fig. 2–114). It is thought that intermediate (polychromatophilic) megaloblasts are unusually susceptible to intramedullary cell death.

Precursors of or actual Cabot's rings may be found in megaloblasts, particularly late intermediate megaloblasts that have unusually intense basophilic stippling. Coarse basophilic stippling in megaloblasts is often found in erythroblasts that have nuclear pyknosis or nuclear degeneration. In these cells, basophilic stippling is thought to indicate faulty incorporation of iron into hemoglobin.

(Text continued on page 106)

Figure 2–106   *Megaloblasts, pernicious anemia, showing early megaloblastic changes.*

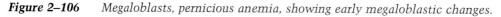

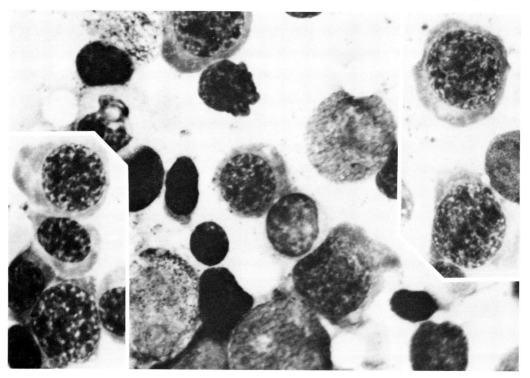

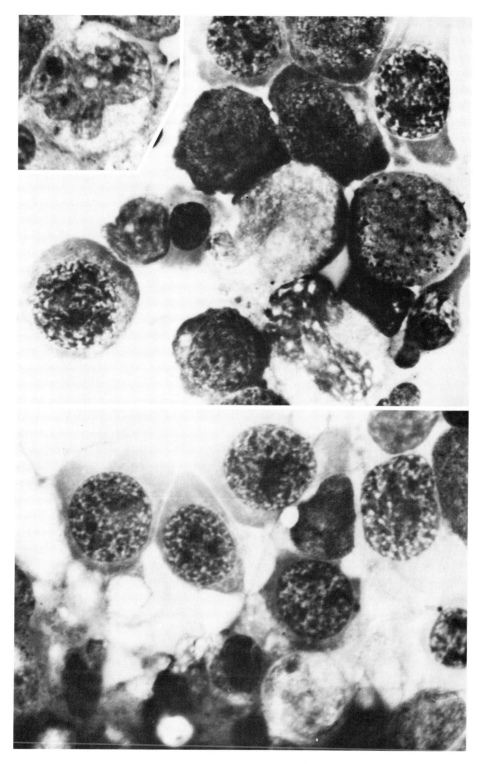

Figure 2–107   *Megaloblasts, pernicious anemia. Inset shows aberrant metamyelocyte.*

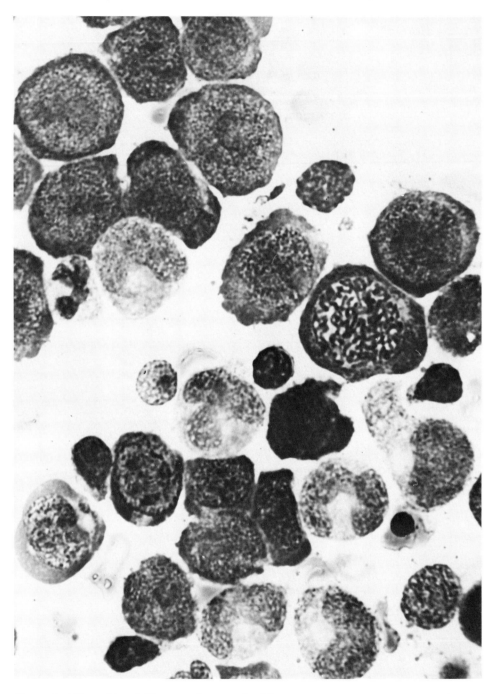

Figure 2–108 *Megaloblasts and proerythroblasts, severe pernicious anemia. (Kass L: Pernicious Anemia. Philadelphia, WB Saunders, 1979)*

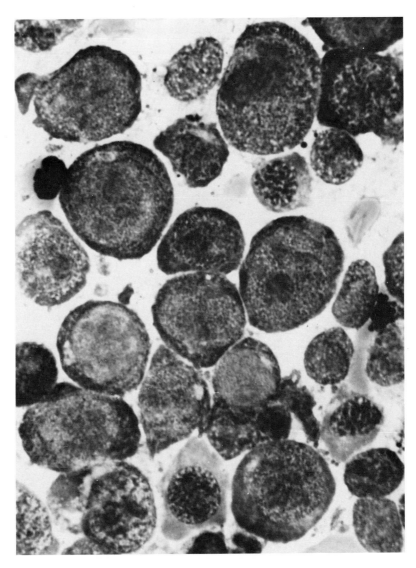

Figure 2–109   *Megaloblasts and proerythroblasts, pernicious anemia. (Kass L: Pernicious Anemia. Philadelphia, WB Saunders, 1976)*

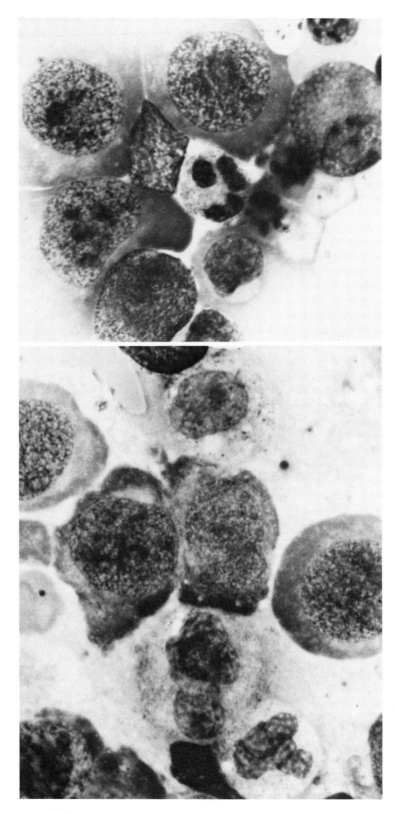

Figure 2–110   *Megaloblasts, severe pernicious anemia.*

104

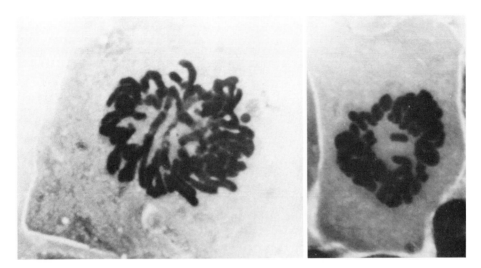

Figure 2–111 *Aberrant mitotic figures in pernicious anemia megaloblasts, showing elongated chromosomes and abnormal karyorrhexis.*

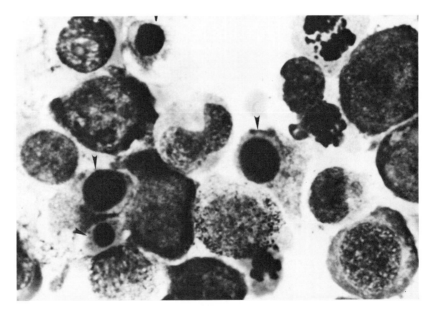

Figure 2–112 *Degenerating megaloblasts, pernicious anemia, showing dense nuclear chromatin and ragged-appearing cytoplasm.*

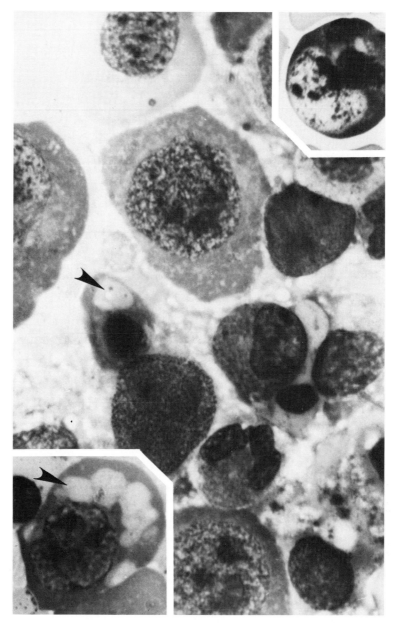

Figure 2–113 *Hemoglobin lakes* (arrows) *in megaloblast* (lower left inset). *Inset at upper right shows megaloblast with vacuous-appearing nuclear chromatin.*

In severe megaloblastic anemias, nuclear chromatin patterns are unusually attenuated and chromatin aggregates are virtually absent. Megaloblasts with these characteristics are large and their nuclei have a reticular appearance (see Fig. 2–110 and Plate 1*D*).

Megaloblastic erythropoiesis occurs in part as the result of abnormalities in the biosynthesis of DNA. Most of the effects of vitamin B_{12} on DNA synthesis are believed to be mediated by folate.

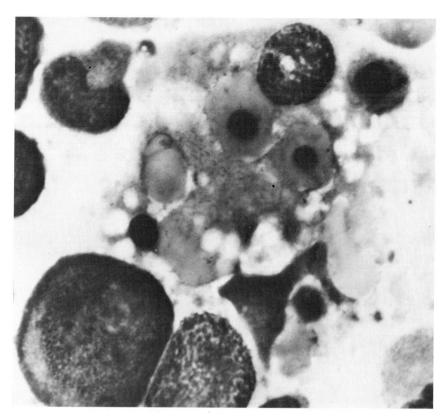

Figure 2–114   *Erythrocytophagy by macrophage in pernicious anemia.*

Pathogenesis of abnormalities of DNA synthesis resulting from a lack of folate intermediates in untreated deficiency of vitamin B_{12} has been conceptualized as the "methyltetrahydrofolate trap" hypothesis. According to current theory, decreased activity of 5-methyltetrahydrofolate homocysteine cobalamin methyltransferase in untreated pernicious anemia leads to decreased tetrahydrofolate available for conversion to various folate derivatives. Of these, 5, 10-methylenetetrahydrofolate occupies a pivotal role, since it is the cofactor for thymidylate synthetase, an enzyme that catalyzes conversion of deoxyuridine monophosphate to deoxythymidine in the biosynthesis of DNA. In untreated folate deficiency, lack of tetrahydrofolate and folate intermediates that function as cofactors for enzymes involved in DNA synthesis contribute to the pathogenesis of megaloblastic erythropoiesis. Additionally, abnormalities in the type and composition of histones as well as abnormalities of histone acetylation and methylation may contribute to the pathogenesis of megaloblastic erythropoiesis.

Granulocytic aberrations are noted first in metamyelocytes and are more prominent in metamyelocytes throughout the increasing severity of the anemia. A variety of shapes and configurations of these cells are seen. Metamyelocytes are gigantic and have abundant

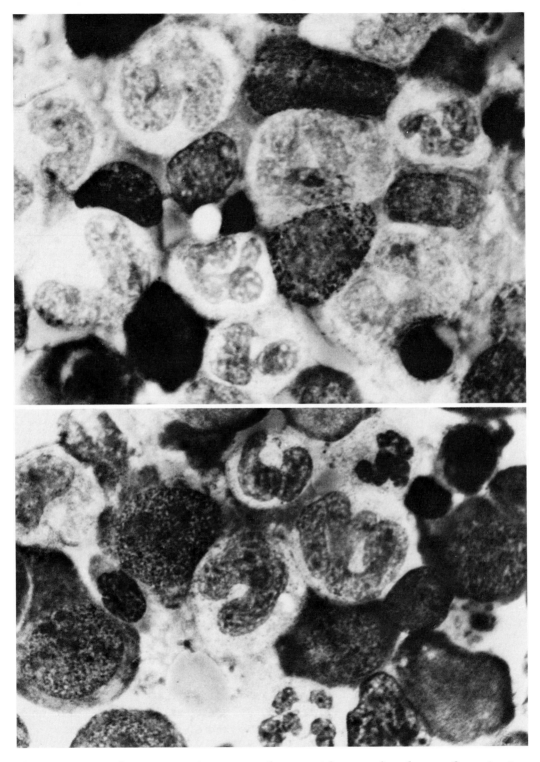

Figure 2–115 *Aberrant-appearing metamyelocytes with unusual nuclear configuration in untreated pernicious anemia.*

cytoplasm and in some instances increased granularity. Nuclei show aberrations of shape, including bulbous ends, "E" shape or sigma shape in which there is a central protrusion between the two ends of the nucleus, a square-shaped nucleus with focal constrictions at the right-angle bends of the nucleus, focal constrictions of the nucleus, and unusual serpentine twistings and convolutions of the nucleus. In band and segmented cells, twistings and convolutions of this type are observed frequently. Polymorphonuclear leukocytes are usually hypersegmented with multiple connections between adjacent nuclear lobulations (Fig. 2–115).

Granulocytic abnormalities are thought to be recognizable under the light microscope before the appearance of erythroblastic abnormalities. They are also the last of the marrow abnormalities to disappear after specific treatment. Increased numbers of eosinophil myelocytes and mature eosinophils are also seen in megaloblastic anemias due to deficiency of vitamin B_{12} or folate.

Increased numbers of plasma cells are also found. In some instances, these cells contain numerous cytoplasmic vacuoles in which antibodies to intrinsic factor–B_{12} complex and parietal cell antigens are localized (Fig. 2–116A). In other instances, plasma cells appear normal (Fig. 2–116B). Plasma cells and lymphocytes are believed to be spared megaloblastic alterations because they proliferate slowly. Abnormalities of megakaryocytes include large cells with multiple small, detached nuclear lobulations, unusually attenuated nuclear chromatin, and pale hypogranular cytoplasm.

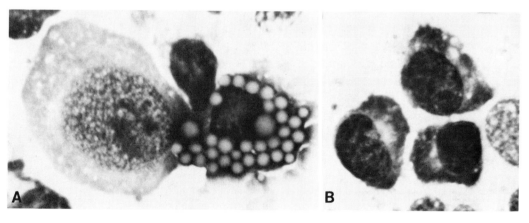

Figure 2–116   *Vacuolated plasma cell (A) and normal-appearing plasma (B) in untreated pernicious anemia.*

Cytochemistry of Nutritional Megaloblastic Anemias

In megaloblastic anemias due to deficiency of vitamin B_{12} or folate, a number of cytochemical abnormalities provide evidence of metabolic aberrations within the cells.

Ammoniacal silver reagent indicates abundant lysine-rich histone in the nuclei of megaloblasts (Fig. 2–117). *Prussian blue* reagent demonstrates siderotic granules in megaloblasts, indicating abnormalities of iron storage and mobilization (Fig. 2–118). *PAS reagent* detects punctate deposits of glycogen in the cytoplasm of proerythroblasts and early intermediate megaloblasts and diffuse cytoplasmic staining in late intermediate megaloblasts (Fig. 2–119). The activity of *phosphorylase* is increased in megaloblasts (Fig. 2–120).

Figure 2–117 *Megaloblast stained with ammoniacal silver. The nucleus stains yellow, indicating predominance of lysine-rich histone.*

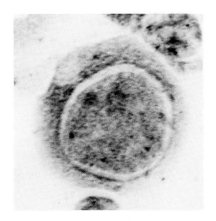

Figure 2–118 *Siderotic granules in megaloblast. (Prussian blue stain)*

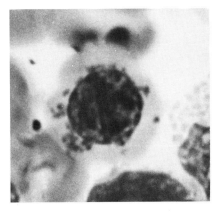

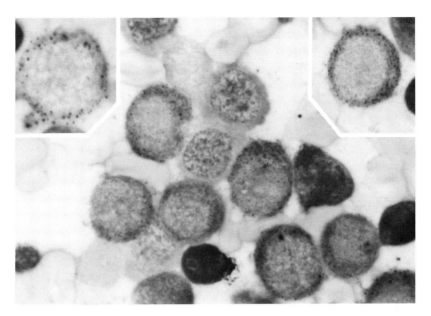

Figure 2–119   *PAS-positive material in pernicious anemia megaloblast. PAS material is punctate in proerythroblasts and early intermediate megaloblasts (insets) and more diffuse in later megaloblasts.*

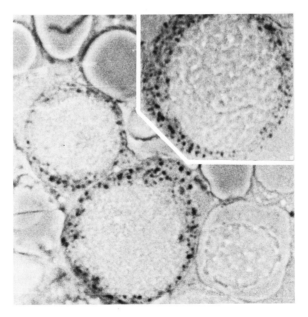

Figure 2–120   *Increased phosphorylase activity in pernicious anemia megaloblasts.*

Nonspecific esterase activity utilizing alpha naphthyl acetate as the substrate is intense in megaloblasts from patients with untreated pernicious anemia. On isoenzymatic analysis, this nonspecific esterase is not distinctive. *Pyronine* stain demonstrates intense cytoplasmic pyroninophilia, indicating abundant amounts of ribosomal RNA (Fig. 2–121). Using *alizarin red S*, cytoplasm of megaloblasts from patients with untreated pernicious anemia stains pink (Fig. 2–122). The pink color is believed to be due in part to accumulation of methylmalonyl CoA in these cells. Methylmalonyl CoA accumulates as a result of decreased activity of coenzyme B_{12}-dependent methylmalonyl CoA mutase, an enzyme that catalyzes conversion of methylmalonyl CoA to succinyl CoA.

Several cytochemical abnormalities have been identified in a metabolic reaction that is catalyzed by 5-methyltetrahydrofolate

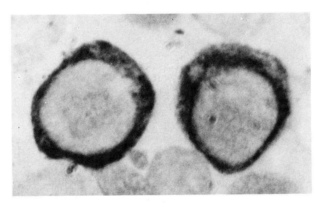

Figure 2–121   *Pyronine stain, demonstrating intense staining of cytoplasm of pernicious anemia megaloblasts. This pyroninophilia indicates the presence of abundant RNA.*

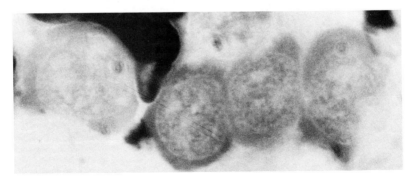

Figure 2–122   *Pink staining of cytoplasm of pernicious anemia megaloblasts by alizarin red S.*

homocysteine cobalamin methyltransferase. In this reaction, the methylcobalamin-dependent methyltransferase catalyzes the enzymatic transfer of the methyl group of 5-methyltetrahydrofolate to homocysteine to form methionine and tetrahydrofolate.

In one reaction, *homocysteine* was identified with the use of nickel chloride. Nickel forms an insoluble yellow brown precipitate with homocysteine, and the precipitate is composed of both nickel and homocysteine in a ratio of 2:1. In untreated pernicious anemia, increased amounts of homocysteine are believed to occur as a result of decreased activity of methylcobalamin methyltransferase and subsequent reduced conversion of homocysteine to methionine. With nickel salts, yellow brown staining of erythroblast cytoplasm occurs and is believed to indicate accumulations of homocysteine within the cells.

In another cytochemical test, *methionine* was identified with the use of a bacterial-overlay technique using the bacterium *Leuconostoc mesenteroides*, a microorganism that has an absolute growth requirement for methionine. In pernicious anemia, decreased activity of methylcobalamin methyltransferase leads to decreased generation of methionine. Decreased amounts of this substance are reflected in decreased growth of the methionine-requiring microorganism in contact with pernicious anemia megaloblasts (Fig. 2–123).

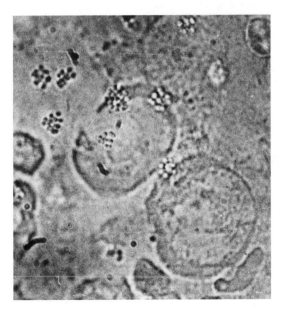

Figure 2–123   *Reaction for methionine using* Leuconostoc mesenteroides. *Scant bacterial growth indicating a decreased amount of methionine is found near pernicious anemia megaloblasts.*

In pernicious anemia, decreased amounts of *tetrahydrofolate* are formed because of decreased activity of methylcobalamin methyltransferase. Tetrahydrofolate can be detected in the cytoplasm of cells with the use of molybdenum dichloride dioxide, a substance that forms an insoluble black precipitate with tetrahydrofolate (Fig. 2–124*A*). A compound formed by interaction of these two substances is composed of tetrahydrofolate and molybdenum in the ratio of 1:3. Using this reaction, tetrahydrofolate is markedly reduced and in some instances absent from the cytoplasm of polymorphonuclear leukocytes from patients with untreated pernicious anemia (Fig. 2–124*B*).

Figure 2–124   *Molybdenum dichloride dioxide test for tetrahydrofolate. Tetrahydrofolate appears as black punctate areas in cytoplasm of normal cells (A) and is missing from cytoplasm of polymorphonuclear leukocytes of patients with untreated pernicious anemia (B).*

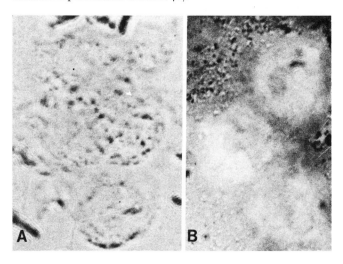

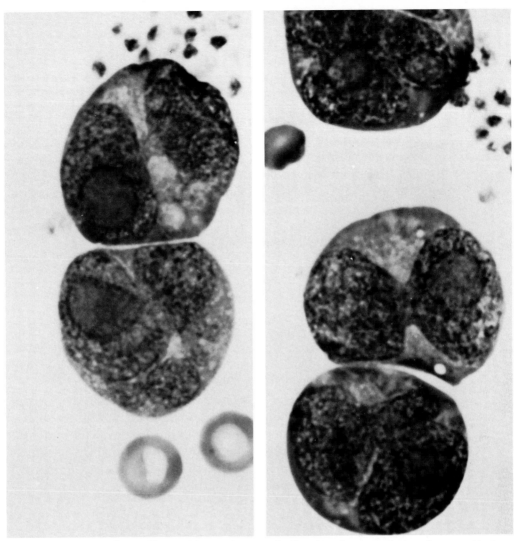

Leukemic blasts with prominent nucleoli and nuclear convolutions from a patient with adult T-cell leukemia.

3   *Lymphocytosis*

Lymphocytes constitute less than 25% of the differential cell count in normal bone marrows. Increased numbers of normal lymphocytes in the marrow are found in disorders of presumed immune etiology, like rheumatoid arthritis, and in other chronic disorders like chronic ulcerative colitis and cirrhosis of the liver. Presumably, lymphocytosis of the marrow in these conditions reflects an activated immune response to the underlying condition. Increased numbers of neoplastic lymphocytes are found in marrows of patients with acute lymphoblastic leukemia, chronic lymphocytic leukemia, lymphocytic lymphoma, and Waldenström's macroglobulinemia.

Types of Lymphocytes

Normal Lymphocytes. Normal intermediate-sized lymphocytes have nuclear chromatin with characteristic striped-shaped aggregates that extend in a linear fashion throughout the nucleus (Fig. 3–1). Between these aggregates there are areas of euchromatin that vary in size and stain darkly. Indistinct masses of chromatin connect adjacent aggregates. The cytoplasm is basophilic and devoid of granules. Rarely, an occasional azurophilic granule can be found in the cytoplasm. The nuclear chromatin in small lymphocytes appears denser than in intermediate-sized lymphocytes.

Figure 3–1   *Normal lymphocytes.*

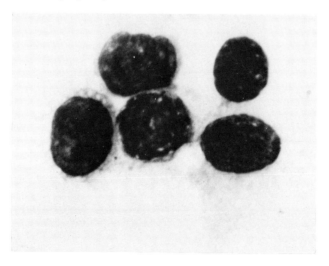

Atypical Lymphocytes. Lymphocytes possessing abundant pale cytoplasm with basophilic striations radiating toward the nucleus and a nucleus with prominent aggregates of chromatin are found in the peripheral blood of patients with infectious mononucleosis and in the bone marrows of patients with chronic lymphocytic leukemia and subleukemic lymphocytic lymphoma (Fig. 3–2).

Immunoblasts. These cells are believed to be transformed lymphocytes. An immunoblast has a large, pale, vesicular nucleus containing a prominent irregularly shaped nucleolus connected to adjacent strands of chromatin and to the nuclear membrane by thin webs of chromatin (Fig. 3–3). Cytoplasm is intensely basophilic and stains intensely positive for RNA using the pyronine stain. Immunoblasts are increased in marrows from patients with infectious mononucleosis and angioimmunoblastic lymphadenopathy.

Figure 3–2　　*Atypical lymphocyte.*

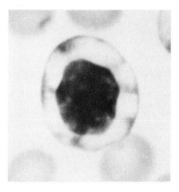

Figure 3–3　　*Immunoblasts.*

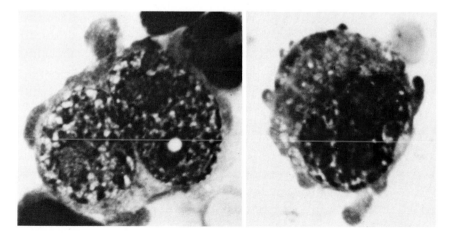

T and B Cells. Lymphocytes in the marrow have been classified as T cells, or thymus-derived lymphocytes, and B cells, or bursa-derived lymphocytes, on the basis of immunologic and immunochemical reactions.

Morphologically, B-lymphocytes from normal peripheral venous blood or from bone marrow are round to oval and, in most instances, larger than T-lymphocytes. In B cells, nuclei contain chromatin that appears diffuse, and aggregates are poorly defined and small. Nucleoli are indistinct. Cytoplasm of B cells is deeply basophilic and does not contain any granular structures visible with standard panoptic stains. Sometimes, B cells demonstrate radial striations of the cytoplasm and a plasmacytoid appearance of the nucleus with eccentric placement of the nucleus in the cell. A cytocentrifuge preparation of normal human B cells isolated by F(ab)$_2$ surface-marker labeling in a flow cytometer is shown in Figure 3–4A, *top*.

Cytochemically, normal B cells contain activities of nonspecific esterase and acid phosphatase. Using conventional cytochemical stains for these enzymes, reaction products are distributed randomly throughout the cytoplasm. Immunologically, B cells form rosettes with sheep erythrocytes that have been coated with complement. B cells possess surface immunoglobulin markers for IgG and complement and also receptors for the Fc fragment of IgG immunoglobulin. B cells are believed to be involved in humoral immunity and in the biosynthesis of immunoglobulins.

In contrast to normal B cells, normal T cells can be divided into several distinct populations, based on immunologic differences. T cells are smaller than B cells. In T cells, nuclei are round to oval and stain deeply with routine panoptic stains. Compared to the diffuse-appearing nuclear chromatin of normal B cells, nuclei of T cells demonstrate well-defined blocklike aggregates of nuclear chromatin. In T helper cells the cytoplasm is deeply basophilic and devoid of granules (Fig. 3–4A, *center*). Using traditional stains, like Wright's or Giemsa's, T helper cells cannot be distinguished from T suppressor cells. Cytochemically, T cells may show focal activities of acid phosphatase and nonspecific esterase. Immunologically, T cells form rosettes with untreated sheep erythrocytes. T cells respond to mitogens such as phytohemagglutinin and are believed to participate in cell-mediated immunity.

In addition to T and B cells, normal persons also have natural killer cells in the peripheral blood. Corresponding to large granular lymphocytes, these natural killer cells can be identified with specific monoclonal antibodies (leu 7 and leu 11) and constitute up to 10% to 15% of the total number of lymphocytes in the peripheral blood.

In the large granular lymphocyte, the nucleus contains diffuse-appearing nuclear chromatin strands, as well as sharply defined aggregates of chromatin. The cytoplasm is abundant and contains 8 to 20 red to pink granular structures of varying sizes (Fig. 3–4*A, bottom*). These granules contain acid phosphatase and most likely represent lysosomes. Currently, it is believed that natural killer cells constitute the body's first-line defense against malignancies, and the physiology and pathology of natural killer cells is a topic of active investigation in many laboratories.

Analysis of T- and B-cell properties of marrow lymphocytes in lymphocytic lymphomas has indicated that most lymphocytic lymphomas are of the B-cell, or follicular center, type and that only rarely are lymphocytic lymphomas of the T-cell type. Corresponding to their normal counterparts, lymphocytic lymphomas can be T-helper or T-suppressor types. In time, immunologic characterization of lymphocytic lymphomas may have direct diagnostic and therapeutic implications, based on greater understanding of the origin and differentiation of neoplastic lymphocytes.

Lymphoid Follicles. Lymphoid follicles are found in normal marrows (Fig. 3–4*B* through *D*). In most instances, a follicle is composed of a germinal center containing mostly B-lymphocytes, macrophages, and immunoblasts or transformed lymphocytes and a corona containing primarily T-lymphocytes. These lymphoid follicles are usually well demarcated, with cords of lymphocytes infiltrating adjacent marrow to only limited degree. Lymphoid aggregates are composed of well-differentiated lymphocytes. In typical lymphoid aggregates, germinal centers are not seen. In normal bone marrows, lymphoid aggregates are seen more frequently than typical lymphoid follicles; in lymphocytic lymphomas, lymphoid aggregates appear nodular and are often larger and more numerous than in normal marrows. The margins of a lymphoid follicle or lymphoid aggregate are usually well demarcated, with cords of lymphocytes infiltrating adjacent marrow to only a limited degree.

The presence of a lymphoid follicle or lymphoid aggregate on a routine aspirate can lead to the erroneous diagnosis of chronic lymphocytic leukemia if large numbers of lymphocytes and few other marrow elements are present. With the use of marrow biopsies and inspection of several films of marrow aspirates, it may be possible to conclude that lymphocytosis on one specimen was most likely due

(Text continued on page 122)

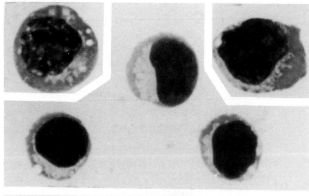

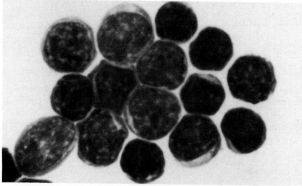

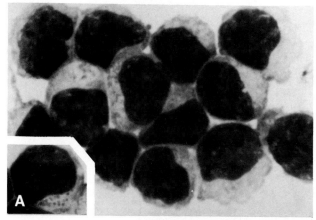

Figure 3–4

(A) *Cytocentrifuge preparations of lymphocyte subpopulations from normal heparinized peripheral venous blood. Lymphocytes were sorted on a commerical cell sorter and identified with appropriate monoclonal antibodies. (Top) Normal B-lymphocytes, showing nuclei with indistinct nuclear chromatin and basophilic cytoplasm devoid of granules [F(ab)₂ surface maker used for B-cell identification]. (Center) Normal T helper cells, demonstrating small lymphocytes with sharply defined aggregates of nuclear chromatin and deeply basophilic cytoplasm devoid of inclusions (OKT4 antibody for identification of T helper cells). (Bottom) Normal natural killer (NK) cells identified with leu 7 antibody, depicting large lymphocytes with both indistinct nuclear chromatin and well-defined aggregates of chromatin. Cytoplasm is abundant and poorly stained and contains 8 to 20 coarse-appearing granular structures that appear red to purple with conventional panoptic stains. (B) Normal marrow biopsy section stained with H and E, depicting a lymphoid follicle.*

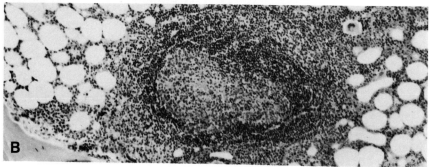

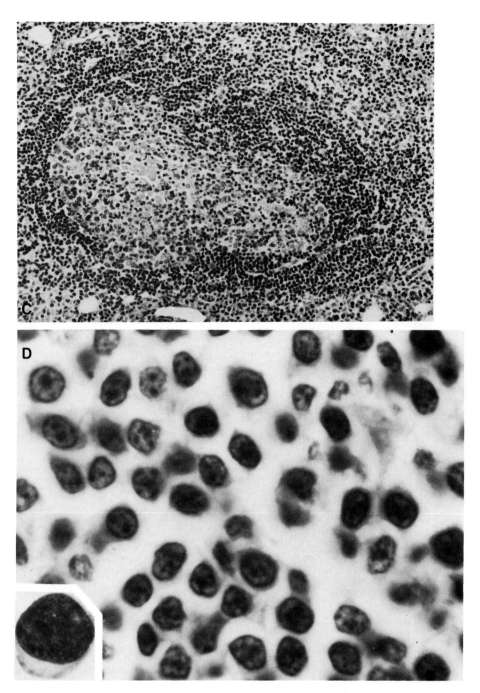

(C) *Higher-power view of biopsy section, showing uniform-appearing lymphocytes and germinal center.* (D) *Higher-power view of biopsy section, showing uniform-appearing lymphocytes with prominent nuclear chromatin aggregates and round to oval nuclei. Inset shows Wright's-stained lymphocyte from normal marrow aspirate, illustrating typical lymphoid nuclear chromatin pattern.*

to the presence of a lymphoid follicle or aggregate, since the lymphocytosis was not universal.

With immunoperoxidase techniques using monoclonal antibodies, it may now be possible to distinguish between increased numbers of normal lymphocytes and increased numbers of neoplastic lymphocytes in a bone marrow specimen. Using these techniques, normal lymphocytes show a mixture of cell types, whereas neoplastic lymphocytes demonstrate a monoclonal pattern. Studies of this type may be particularly useful in determining whether or not modest lymphocytosis in a bone marrow specimen represents involvement by lymphocytic lymphoma.

Infectious Mononucleosis

Infectious mononucleosis is thought to be a disease of T-lymphocytes. Atypical lymphocytes in the blood may superficially resemble lymphoblasts, and bone marrow aspirations may be performed in atypical cases. Marrows may contain a modest lymphocytosis, usually less than 25%, and lymphocytes appear normal or demonstrate prominent nucleoli and basophilia (immunoblasts). In some cases of infectious mononucleosis, marrows contain granulomas composed of plasma cells, fibroblasts, reticulum cells, histiocytes, and eosinophils (Fig. 3–5*A* and *B*).

Nuclear Abnormalities

Well-Differentiated Neoplastic Lymphocyte. The well-differentiated lymphocyte is seen in cases of well-differentiated chronic lymphocytic leukemia and subleukemic well-differentiated lymphocytic lymphoma in which lymphocytes have invaded the marrow but leukemia has not yet developed. Lymphocytes appear normal (Fig. 3–6).

Attenuation of Nuclear Chromatin. As lymphocytes develop neoplastic characteristics, nuclear chromatin strands appear more attenuated and more diffuse, with fewer aggregates of chromatin (Fig. 3–7).

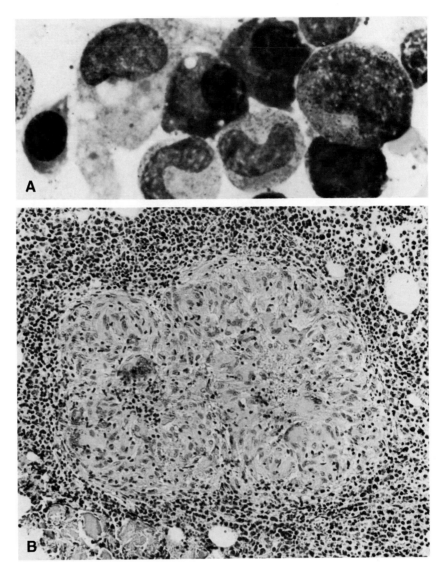

Figure 3–5 (A) *Histiocyte and plasma cells in a granuloma from a patient with infectious mononucleosis.* (B) *H and E stained section of granuloma. Epithelioid cells and multinuclear giant cells can be seen. Granulomas of this type can be found in patients with histoplasmosis and in patients with sarcoidosis.*

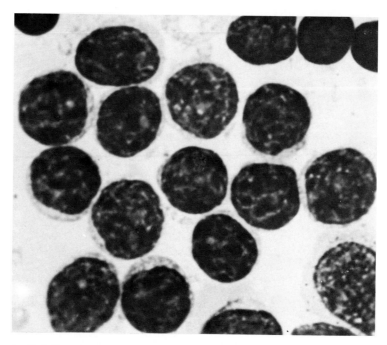

Figure 3–6   *Well-differentiated neoplastic lymphocytes.*

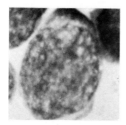

Figure 3–7   *Neoplastic lymphocyte with finely attenuated nuclear chromatin strands.*

Prominent Nucleolus. Although normal lymphocytes may possess a small nucleolus, neoplastic lymphocytes often demonstrate a prominent nucleolus with perinucleolar condensation of chromatin (Fig. 3–8).

Nuclear Cleft. A valuable sign of neoplasia in the lymphocyte is the presence of a deep cleft in the nucleus, extending at least one third through the nucleus itself (Fig. 3–9).

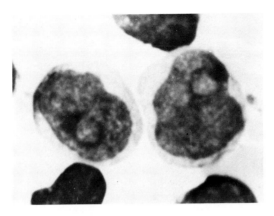

Figure 3–8   *Large neoplastic lymphocytes with large nucleoli and prominent perinucleolar condensations of chromatin. Cells similar in appearance to these have also been called "prolymphocytes."*

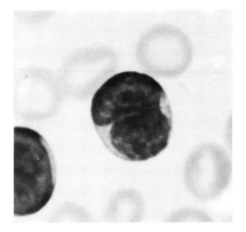

Figure 3–9   *A neoplastic lymphocyte with a prominent nuclear cleft.*

Binuclearity. Presumably, as the nuclear cleft deepens, it severs connections between the halves of the nucleus, leading to a binuclear cell (Fig. 3–10).

Polar Body. Polar bodies are the remains of asynchronous nuclear divisions and are found in neoplastic lymphocytes that demonstrate abnormalities of cellular replication and division (Fig. 3–11).

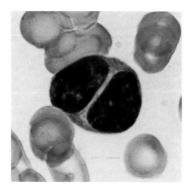

Figure 3–10   *Binuclear neoplastic lymphocyte.*

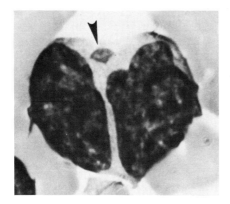

Figure 3–11   *Neoplastic lymphocyte with polar body* (arrow).

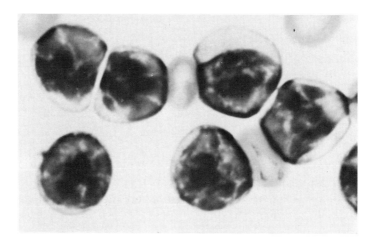

Figure 3–12   *Neoplastic lymphocytes with large, dense-appearing aggregates of chromatin.*

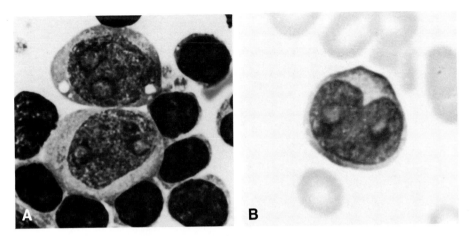

Figure 3–13   (A) *Prolymphocytes from a patient with prolymphocytic leukemia.*
(B) *Lymphosarcoma cell with prominent nucleoli and perinucleolar*
condensations of chromatin.

Hyperaggregated Chromatin. Some neoplastic lymphocytes show unusually intense and large aggregates of nuclear chromatin, separated from one another by vacuous areas that contain little or no chromatin (Fig. 3–12).

Prolymphocyte. Occurring in the blood and bone marrow of patients with prolymphocytic leukemia, prolymphocytes are large mononuclear cells with a round to oval nucleus, a large prominent nucleolus with perinucleolar condensations of chromatin, linear and stripelike aggregates of nuclear chromatin, and abundant cytoplasm containing few if any vacuoles (Fig. 3–13*A* and Plate 3*A*). Usually, granules are not identified in the cytoplasm.

Lymphosarcoma Cell. The lymphosarcoma cell is a neoplastic lymphocyte that has a large nucleus, with prominent indentation and in some instances folding resembling that seen in a cell of monocytic origin (Fig. 3–13*B*). The nuclear chromatin has a spongy appearance. One or more prominent nucleoli with perinucleolar condensation of chromatin are observed. The cytoplasm is deeply basophilic with numerous small vacuoles. Oat cell carcinoma cells (Fig. 3–14) and prostatic carcinoma cells (Fig. 3–15) metastatic to the marrow can resemble lymphosarcoma cells. However, carcinoma cells show more pleomorphism and increased nuclear stainability compared to lymphosarcoma cells. Also, carcinoma cells often have indistinct cellular borders, causing them to look like a syncytium, and they

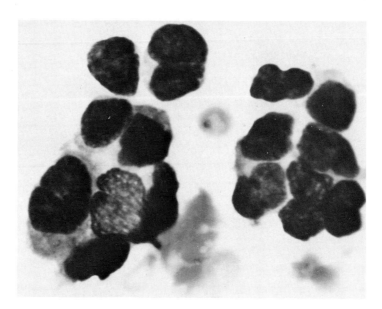

Figure 3–14   *Oat cell carcinoma cells in marrow.*

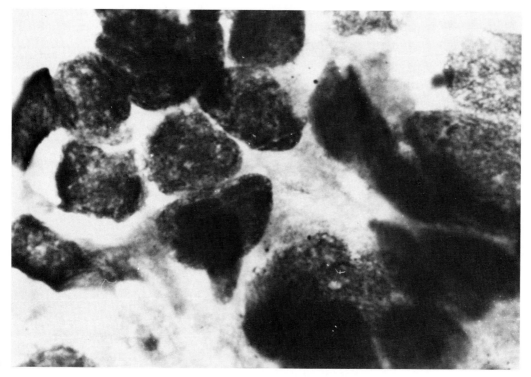

Figure 3–15   *Prostatic carcinoma cells in marrow.*

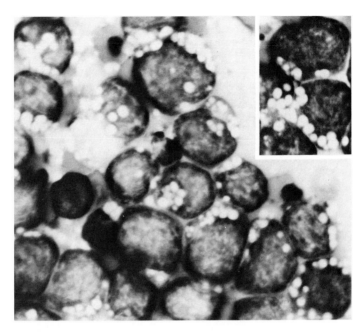

Figure 3–16   *Neoplastic lymphoid cells with multiple cytoplasmic vacuoles in Burkitt's lymphoma.*

occur in discrete clumps that are readily discernible under low magnification.

Burkitt's Lymphoma Cells. Burkitt's lymphoma cells are poorly differentiated lymphocytes that have characteristic lymphoid-type striping of nuclear chromatin, a small inconspicuous nucleolus, and basophilic cytoplasm containing numerous vacuoles. Because of their high content of RNA, Burkitt cells are intensely pyroninophilic (Fig. 3–16).

Small, Multiclefted Lymphocytes. Cytoplasm is scant and in some instances barely visible. The nucleus contains numerous clefts that penetrate the nucleus to varying depths (Fig. 3–17).

Large, Multiclefted Lymphocytes. Nuclei have been described as cerebriform because of numerous convolutions and clefts. The cells resemble the abnormal mononuclear cells found in the peripheral blood of patients with Sézary syndrome (Fig. 3–18).

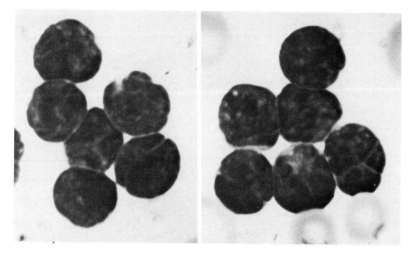

Figure 3–17   *Small, poorly differentiated lymphocytes with multiple nuclear clefts and scant cytoplasm.*

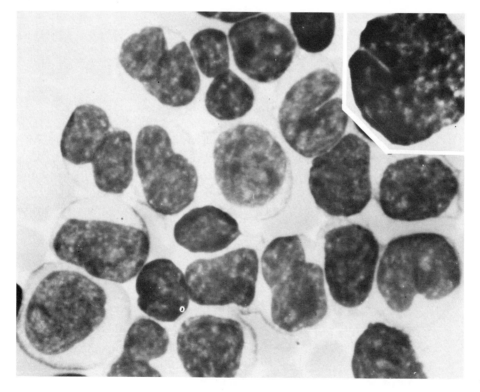

Figure 3–18   *Large neoplastic lymphoid cells with prominent nucleoli and large, dense, multiple aggregates of nuclear chromatin and nuclear clefts.*

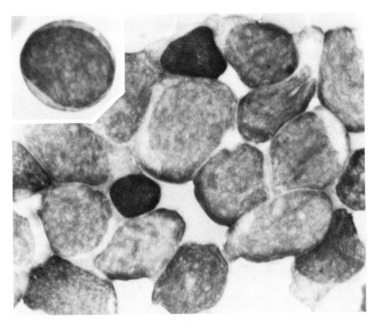

Figure 3–19   *Leukemic lymphoblasts, L2 type of acute lymphoblastic leukemia.*

Lymphoblasts. Lymphoblasts are large lymphoid cells that have characteristic lymphoid-type stripe aggregates of nuclear chromatin and prominent nucleoli (Fig. 3–19). Typical chromatin patterns of lymphoblasts are most evident in large, well-stained and well-spread lymphoblasts in contrast to small lymphoblasts in which these features may not be apparent. Cytoplasm is usually deeply basophilic and devoid of granularity. Rarely, several small azurophilic inclusions are found. Cytochemically, these inclusions do not demonstrate activities of peroxidase or specific esterase. Auer rods are never found in leukemic lymphoblasts. Lymphoblasts are found in acute lymphoblastic leukemia and rarely in lymphocytic lymphoma and chronic lymphocytic leukemia.

Histiocytic Lymphoma Cells In some patients with large cell lymphocytic lymphoma (histiocytic lymphoma), neoplastic cells occur in the marrow (Fig. 3–20). Once thought to be derived from the reticuloendothelium, these cells have been found to possess immunoglobulin markers and are currently regarded as large neoplastic cells of lymphoid origin. Histiocytic lymphoma cells have a large round to oval nucleus that sometimes shows convolutions. Nuclear chromatin is coarse, and chromatin strands appear widely separated. Char-

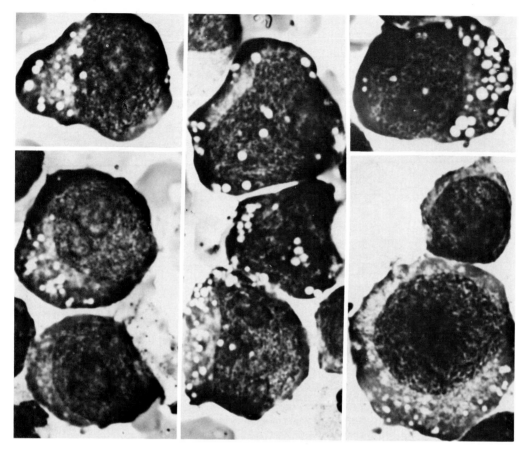

Figure 3–20   *Neoplastic cells, lymphocytic lymphoma, large cell type (diffuse histiocytic lymphoma).*

acteristically, nucleoli are unusually large and may be hexagonal in shape. Perinucleolar condensations of chromatin can be found. Cytoplasm is abundant and deeply basophilic due to increased content of ribosomal RNA. Multiple vacuoles are usually found in the cytoplasm.

Cytoplasmic Abnormalities

Lymphoblasts With Azurophilic Inclusions. Rarely, leukemic lymphoblasts have 8 to 10 large, coarse-appearing azurophilic cytoplasmic inclusions (Fig. 3–21A). These inclusions do not contain activity of either myeloperoxidase or specific esterase.

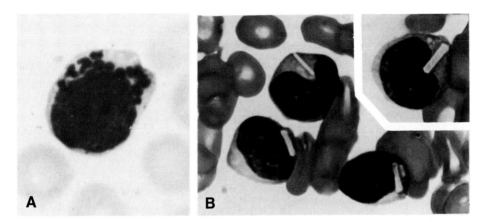

Figure 3–21 (A) *Leukemic lymphoblast with large azurophilic inclusions.* (B) *Leukemic lymphocytes, chronic lymphocytic leukemia, containing pale-staining rectangular-shaped crystal. Immunologically, the crystals contained IgA immunoglobulin.*

Lymphocytes With Crystalloid Inclusions. In a rare variant of chronic lymphocytic leukemia, leukemic lymphocytes contain one or more pale-staining rectangular-shaped crystals (Fig. 3–21B). Usually, the crystals contain immunoglobulin demonstrable with immunoperoxidase techniques.

Histiocytoid Lymphocyte. In some patients with poorly differentiated lymphocytic lymphoma in a leukemic phase, lymphocytes show dense nuclear chromatin and abundant cytoplasm containing pseudopodia, similar to that seen in a macrophage (Fig. 3–22). Cytoplasm of these cells often contains small nonspecific azurophilic inclusions.

Figure 3–22 *Histiocytoid lymphocytes with voluminous cytoplasm.*

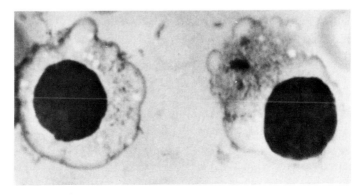

Chronic Lymphocytic Leukemia

——————
——————
——————   Once regarded as a single disease entity, chronic lymphocytic leukemia is now believed to be the leukemic phase of lymphocytic lymphoma and to have a wide spectrum of morphologic and immunologic variants. These variants can also be found in subleukemic
lymphocytic lymphomas. Marrows from patients with these disorders show invasion by neoplastic lymphocytes, although few or no
neoplastic lymphocytes appear in the blood.

Corresponding to normal B cells, chronic lymphocytic leukemia
can be of the B-cell type immunologically. In fact, most of the examples of chronic lymphocytic leukemia are B-cell variants. In a similar way, T-cell variants of chronic lymphocytic leukemia have been
described. Immunologically, it has been possible to identify both T-
suppressor-cell and T-helper-cell variants. Recently, a natural killer-
cell variant of chronic lymphocytic leukemia has been described and
identified with the use of monoclonal antibodies specific for natural
killer cells, such as the leu 7 antibody. Like the normal large granular lymphocyte, the leukemic natural killer lymphocyte also has
voluminous cytoplasm containing substantial numbers of azurophilic granules that contain acid phosphatase.

Morphologic variants of lymphocytes seem to bear relationship
to the clinical course. Serious complications such as autoimmune
hemolytic anemia, autoimmune thrombocytopenia, and extensive
tumefaction occur more frequently in patients who have the highest
proportion of lymphocytes showing abnormal and perhaps neoplastic
characteristics than in patients whose lymphocytes appear well differentiated. From both prognostic and therapeutic standpoints, it is
advantageous to characterize the state of differentiation of the lymphocytes as precisely as possible at the time of diagnosis and
throughout the clinical course.

Chronic Lymphocytic Leukemia, Well-Differentiated Type

Lymphocytes appear relatively normal. Some have prominent
nucleoli. Normal marrow cells are greatly reduced in number. On H
and E section, the nuclei of lymphocytes are uniform in size and
shape and have prominent aggregates of chromatin, some of which
adhere to the nuclear membrane (Fig. 3–23). In chronic lymphocytic
leukemia, bone marrow involvement by leukemic lymphocytes is
usually diffuse, but can be nodular in some cases.

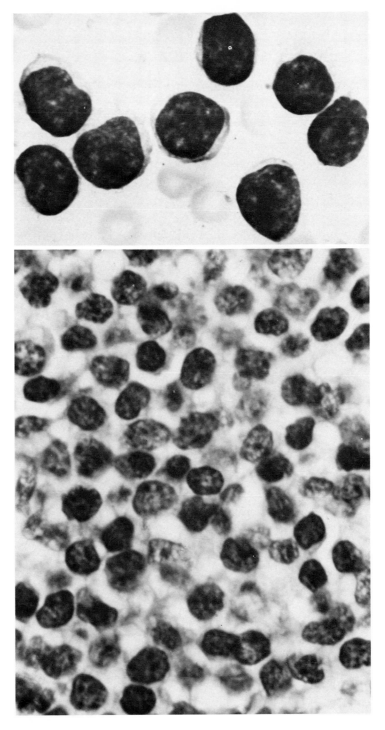

Figure 3–23   *Chronic lymphocytic leukemia. (A) Wright's-stained cells from marrow aspirate. The cells appear well differentiated. (B) H and E section of a marrow biopsy, showing cells with round to oval nuclei and a few cells with nuclear indentations or clefts.*

Chronic Lymphocytic Leukemia, Moderately Poorly Differentiated Type

Lymphocytes show deep nuclear clefts and indentations. Usually, only one cleft or indentation is seen in an individual nucleus. The nuclear chromatin pattern looks spongy. Some of the cells are so-called lymphosarcoma cells. These cells have prominent nucleoli having perinucleolar condensations of chromatin and deeply basophilic cytoplasm containing numerous small vacuoles. Normal marrow cells are greatly reduced. On H and E section, lymphocyte nuclei have clefts of varying sizes and depths. Nuclei are irregular in shape and size (Fig. 3–24). Cytochemically, these neoplastic lymphocytes possess intense unipolar activities of nonspecific esterase and acid phosphatase.

Chronic Lymphocytic Leukemia, Poorly Differentiated Type

Lymphocytes vary considerably in size and shape. On Wright-stained aspirate, cells are small with multiple micellar clefts of varying depths. Cytoplasm is scant and agranular. Numerous disrupted or smudge cells are found. Normal marrow cells are greatly reduced. On H and E section, lymphocyte nuclei vary considerably in size and shape and have irregular nuclear outlines. Chromatin is dispersed throughout the nucleus, and several prominent nucleoli are found. Nuclear clefts are numerous and extend to varying depths into the nucleus (Fig. 3-25). Lymphocytes of this type have been described in patients with the T-cell variant of chronic lymphocytic leukemia.

Lymphocytes of varying degrees of differentiation may be seen in all of the varieties of chronic lymphocytic leukemia and/or lymphocytic lymphoma in the subleukemic stage. In the three morphologic varieties of chronic lymphocytic leukemia described, one or more types of lymphocytes showing characteristic nuclear and cytoplasmic features predominate in each instance, although in some cases an entire spectrum of poorly differentiated lymphocytes can be observed.

(Text continued on page 140)

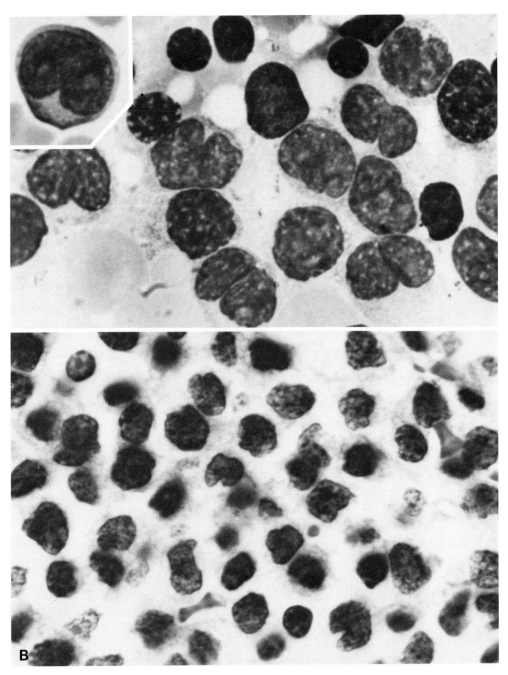

Figure 3–24 *Moderately poorly differentiated lymphocytic lymphoma involving marrow. (A) Large poorly differentiated lymphocytes with prominent nuclear clefts and large nucleoli (inset). (B) H and E section of marrow biopsy, showing large lymphoid cells with nuclear clefts and convolutions. Cells similar to these may be seen in T-cell convoluted type lymphocytic lymphoma and in prolymphocytic leukemia.*

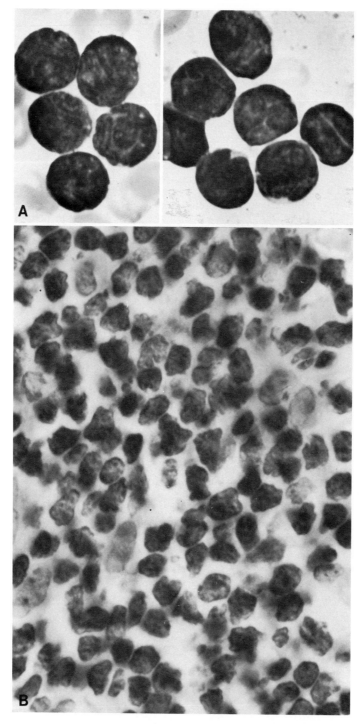

Figure 3–25   *Poorly differentiated lymphocytic lymphoma involving marrow. (A) Small poorly differentiated lymphocytes with multiple nuclear clefts and scant cytoplasm. (B) H and E section of marrow, showing lymphoid cells with multiple nuclear clefts.*

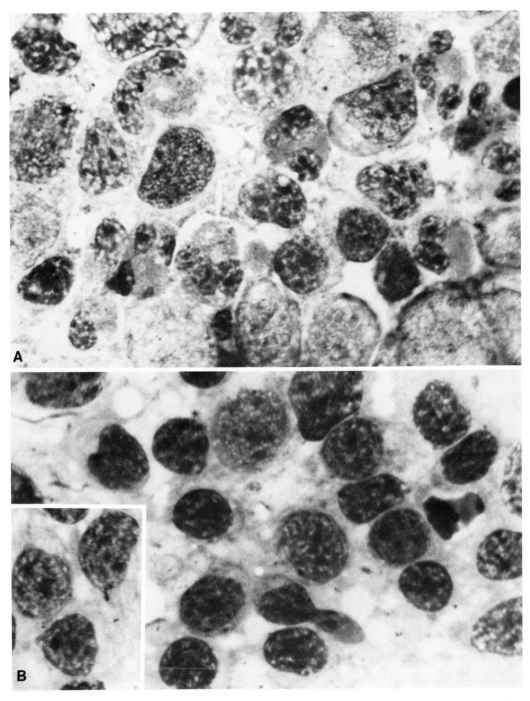

Figure 3–26   *Eosinophilia and lymphocytosis of marrow (A) in patients who have poorly differentiated lymphocytic lymphoma involving bone marrow (B and inset).*

In some patients with lymphocytic lymphoma, particularly poorly differentiated varieties, neoplastic lymphocytes coexist in the marrow with increased numbers of other types of cells. Increased numbers of mature eosinophils are found in conjunction with increased numbers of neoplastic lymphocytes in poorly differentiated lymphocytic lymphoma (Fig. 3–26). The pathogenetic significance of this eosinophilia has not yet been defined.

Increased numbers of intermediate normoblasts occur in marrows having increased numbers of neoplastic lymphocytes in patients who have chronic lymphocytic leukemia and concomitant autoimmune hemolytic anemia (Fig. 3–27).

Increased numbers of mature-appearing plasma cells are associated with increased numbers of neoplastic lymphocytes in patients who have Waldenström's macroglobulinemia. Coexistence of plasma cells and neoplastic lymphocytes also occurs in patients who have chronic lymphocytic leukemia and concomitant hyperglobulinemia, either monoclonal or polyclonal (Fig. 3–28).

Prolymphocytic Leukemia

This unusual variant within the spectrum of chronic lymphocytic leukemia is characterized hematologically by the occurrence in the blood and bone marrow of prolymphocytes and clinically by marked splenomegaly and lymphadenopathy. As depicted in Figure 3–29*A* and Plate 3*A*, prolymphocytes are large mononuclear cells with oval to round nuclei, coarse-appearing chromatin strands with linear and stripelike aggregates, and one or two large nucleoli with perinucleolar condensations of chromatin. The cytoplasm of prolymphocytes is abundant and basophilic when stained with a conventional panoptic stain. Usually, granules are not identified in the cytoplasm. From patient to patient, the number of prolymphocytes in the blood varies, and prolymphocytes may constitute a small or major portion of the differential cell count. Smaller prolymphocytes can be identified and usually have a prominent nucleolus and multiple linear-appearing aggregates of nuclear chromatin.

Figure 3–27
(opposite)

Lymphocytosis of marrow along with proliferation of erythroblasts in patients who have lymphocytic lymphoma and concomitant autoimmune hemolytic anemia.

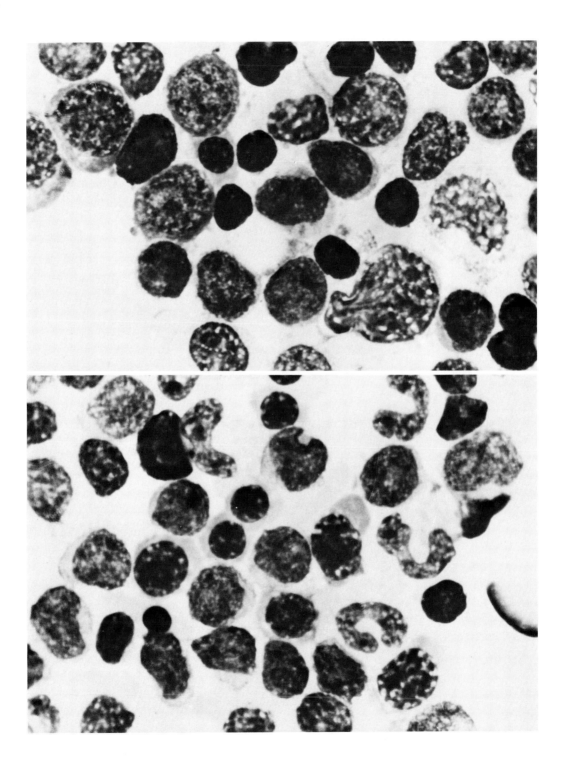

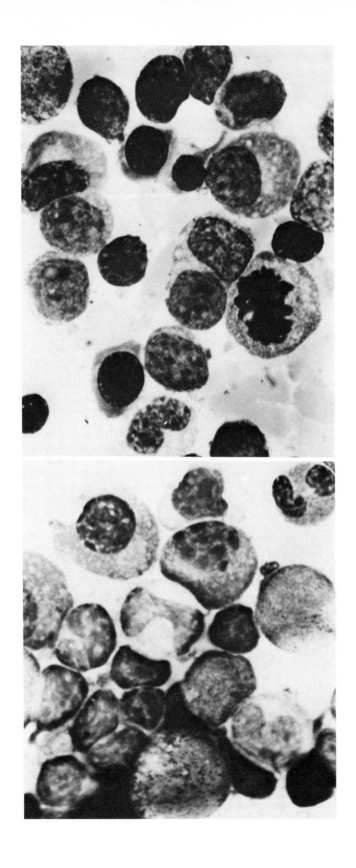

In bone marrows from patients with prolymphocytic leukemia, most of the cells are prolymphocytes. Megakaryocytes, granulocytic cells, and erythroblasts are markedly reduced in number. On H and E–stained sections of bone marrow biopsies, marrows are hypercellular and are largely replaced by mononuclear cells having round to oval nuclei and prominent aggregates of nuclear chromatin. Most of the prolymphocytes have large, oval-shaped nucleoli. Cytochemically, prolymphocytes have variable amounts of glycogen identified with the PAS reagent and weak activities of acid phosphatase and nonspecific esterase. In at least one instance, the author has observed the evolution of prolymphocytic leukemia into immunoblastic sarcoma (Fig. 3–29*B*).

Figure 3–29*C* depicts differences between prolymphocytes, leukemic lymphoblasts, "lymphosarcoma cells," and histiocytic lymphoma cells. Compared to lymphosarcoma cells, prolymphocytes have a larger nucleolus, more prominent perinucleolar aggregations of chromatin, more delicate-appearing nuclear chromatin strands, and more abundant cytoplasm. Compared to neoplastic cells in histiocytic lymphoma, prolymphocytes have smaller nucleoli, more pronounced perinucleolar aggregations of chromatin, and less cytoplasm. In histiocytic lymphoma cells, nucleoli are often gigantic and appear irregular and lobulated. The cytoplasm of histiocytic lymphoma cells stains deeply basophilic and contains multiple vacuoles of varying sizes and shapes, in contrast to the cytoplasm of prolymphocytes, which stains less deeply basophilic and contains few if any vacuoles. Compared to leukemic lymphoblasts, prolymphocytes have larger nucleoli, fewer aggregates of nuclear chromatin, and more abundant cytoplasm.

(Text continued on page 147)

Figure 3–28
(opposite)   *Plasmacytosis of marrow along with lymphocytosis in patients who have lymphocytic lymphoma and concomitant dysproteinemia.*

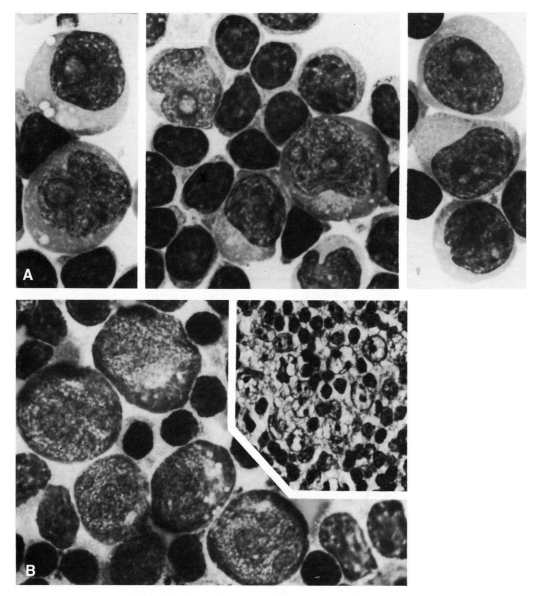

Figure 3–29   (A) *Prolymphocytes in prolymphocytic leukemia. Large and small prolymphocytes are seen. Nucleoli are prominent, and there are perinuclear condensations of chromatin. Cytoplasm is abundant. (B) Immunoblasts in imprint of lymph node of patient with prolymphocytic leukemia who evolved into immunoblastic sarcoma. Inset shows low-power view of H and E stained section of lymph node biopsy, illustrating malignant immunoblasts.*

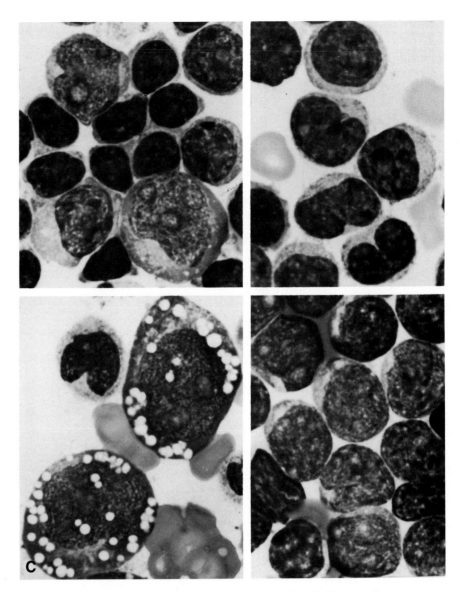

(C) *Prolymphocytes in prolymphocytic leukemia* (top left). *Lymphosarcoma cells in leukemic phase of poorly differentiated lymphocytic lymphoma* (top right). *Histiocytic lymphoma cells in bone marrow* (bottom left). *Leukemic lymphoblasts, acute lymphoblastic leukemia (L1)* (bottom right).

Figure 3–30
Burkitt's lymphoma. (A)
Wright's-stained aspirate of
marrow, showing a large
histiocyte surrounded by
neoplastic lymphoid cells.
(Inset shows a higher-power
view of Burkitt L3) cells
containing many cyto-
plasmic vacuoles. (B) H and
E section of marrow biopsy,
showing a central histiocyte
containing cellular debris
and surrounded by neoplastic lymphoid cells. Histiocytes like these impart a
starry sky appearance to
the marrow of patients with
Burkitt's lymphoma who
have involvement of the
marrow.

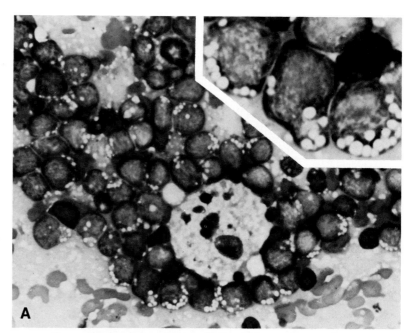

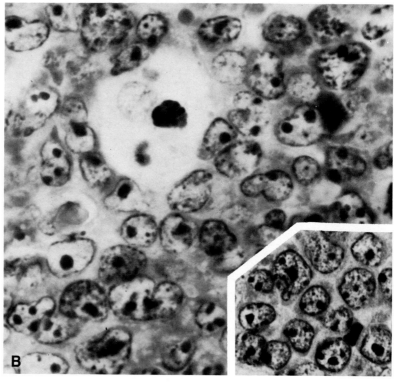

Burkitt's Lymphoma

In cases in which Burkitt's lymphoma has invaded the marrow, characteristic types of lymphocytes and macrophages are found in the marrow (Fig. 3–30A and B). On Wright's-stained aspirates, lymphocytes are large and have typical nuclear chromatin striping found in lymphoid cells (Fig. 3–30A). Nucleoli are usually small and inconspicuous. Cytoplasm is deeply basophilic and contains numerous small vacuoles. Large macrophages containing nuclear and cytoplasmic debris are scattered throughout the neoplastic lymphoid cells, imparting the characteristic "starry sky" appearance to the marrow preparation (Fig. 3–30).

On H and E section, Burkitt's lymphoma cells show large round nuclei with prominent aggregates of chromatin and small nucleoli (Fig. 3–30B). Cytoplasm is scant. Most of the cells appear similar, and marked irregularities in nuclear size and shape are infrequent. Typical dendritic macrophages containing nuclear and cytoplasmic debris are found. Cytochemically, Burkitt's lymphoma cells are PAS negative and contain abundant RNA that is detectable with the pyronine reagent. According to the FAB (French-American-British) classification, acute leukemia with Burkitt cells has been named L3.

Acute Lymphoblastic Leukemia

According to the FAB classification of the acute leukemias, there are three morphologic subtypes of acute lymphoblastic leukemia. In the first, or L1 type, lymphoblasts are small and uniform in size and show linear aggregates of nuclear chromatin and few, small nucleoli. The cytoplasm is scant and devoid of granules (Fig. 3–31A). In the L2 variant, cellular pleomorphism is more obvious, and there are both large and small leukemic lymphoblasts. Nuclear chromatin shows prominent aggregates, and nucleoli may be large and have perinucleolar condensations of chromatin. The cytoplasm is basophilic with panoptic stains and does not contain granules (Fig. 3–31B). In the L3 or Burkitt's leukemia variant of acute lymphoblastic leukemia, the leukemic lymphoblasts show prominent aggregates of nuclear chromatin, one or more nucleoli, and deeply basophilic cytoplasm containing numerous vacuoles of varying sizes and shapes (see Fig. 3–29A and B). Immunologically, acute lympho-

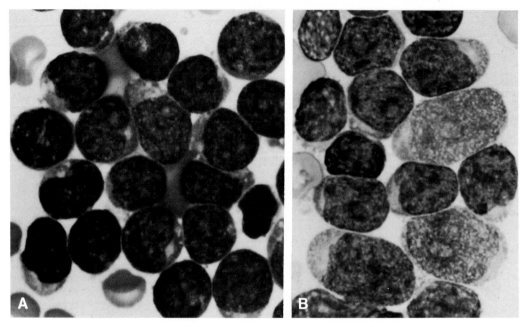

Figure 3–31   (A) *Lymphoblasts, acute lymphoblastic leukemia, L1 variant. Lymphoblasts are uniform in size, are small, and have darkly stained chunklike aggregates of nuclear chromatin. Nucleoli are small and inconspicuous. Cytoplasm is deeply basophilic and devoid of inclusions. (B) Lymphoblasts, acute lymphoblastic leukemia, L2 variant. Lymphoblasts show variation in size and shape, ranging from small lymphoblasts to large lymphoblasts with prominent chromatin pattern. Nucleoli are conspicuous, and there are perinucleolar condensations of chromatin. Chromatin strands appear coarse and resemble stripes.*

blastic leukemia can be characterized as to B-cell, T-cell, or null-cell type. On H and E–stained sections, leukemic lymphoblasts cannot be distinguished with certainty from leukemic myeloblasts. Usually, leukemic lymphoblasts are large mononuclear cells with irregular outlines and prominent aggregates of chromatin. Nucleoli are inconspicuous and the cytoplasm is scant (Fig. 3–32).

Cytochemically, leukemic lymphoblasts often have prominent PAS-positive material representing glycogen in the cytoplasm (Fig. 3–33*A* and *B* and Plate 4*B*). Diffuse staining is seen rarely. Activities of specific esterase and peroxidase cannot be demonstrated in leukemic lymphoblasts, since these enzymes are properties of granulocytic cells. Immunologically, various subtypes of leukemic lymphoblasts can be distinguished. Currently, these include T-cell, B-cell, and null-cell types. Based on these characterizations, it has become apparent that certain immunologic subtypes of leukemic lymphoblasts are associated with distinctive clinical manifestations and response to specific treatment. This is particularly true in the

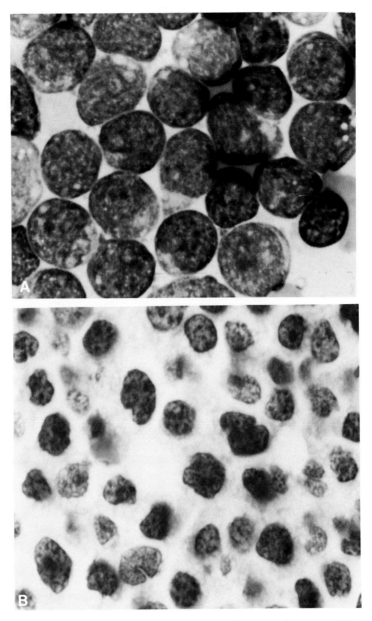

Figure 3–32 *Lymphoblasts, acute lymphoblastic leukemia, L2 variant, Wright's stain. (A) Lymphoblasts, acute lymphoblastic leukemia. (B) H and E section, demonstrating mononuclear cells with irregular nuclear outlines and prominent aggregates of chromatin.*

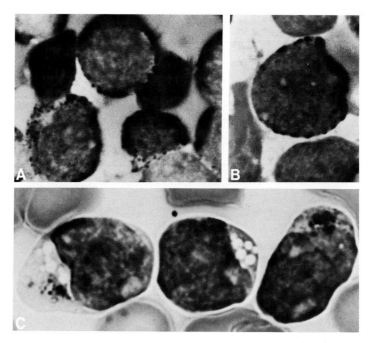

Figure 3–33   *Lymphoblasts, acute lymphoblastic leukemia. (A and B) Prominent PAS-positive material in cytoplasm of leukemic lymphoblasts. (C) Unipolar acid phosphatase activity in T-cell convoluted leukemic lymphoblasts.*

case of T-cell convoluted type of acute lymphoblastic leukemia, a disorder seen in younger persons and often associated with mediastinal lymphadenopathy and an aggressive clinical course. Combining cytochemical and immunologic techniques, unique patterns and distributions of activities of several enzymes can be correlated with immunologic subtypes. For example, T-cell convoluted type of leukemic lymphoblasts contain unipolar localizations of acid phosphatase and nonspecific esterase activities (Fig. 3–33C and Plate 4D).

Enzymologic markers have also been used to distinguish leukemic lymphoblasts from other types of leukemic blasts. Recently, the enzyme terminal deoxyribonucleotidyl transferase has been identified in leukemic lymphoblasts and in thymic lymphocytes. It has been suggested that this enzyme may be a unique marker for cells of lymphoid origin. Assay of suspensions of leukemic blasts for terminal transferase activity may aid in classifying them as lymphoblastic or nonlymphoblastic, particularly when morphologic and cytochemical studies are equivocal, as in some patients with the blast phase of chronic granulocytic leukemia.

Hairy Cell Leukemia

Hairy cell leukemia is a controversial disorder characterized by pancytopenia, splenomegaly, and the occurrence in the bone marrow and visceral organs of characteristic cells. Classified variously as lymphoreticular, monocytoid, and lymphocytoid, hairy cells have a finely reticular nucleus that is round to oval with small round nucleoli. Cytoplasm stains faint lilac to light gray and demonstrates numerous hairlike projections of various shapes and sizes seeming to originate from the cytoplasmic membrane.

Routine aspirates of bone marrow often result in a "dry tap," necessitating a biopsy of marrow. On marrow biopsies, touch preparations show only a few characteristic-appearing hairy cells. Other hairy cells appear in clumps and demonstrate linear aggregates of chromatin and abundant clear-appearing cytoplasm that lacks the characteristic hairy projections (Fig. 3–34). Erythropoiesis is often megaloblastoid, perhaps explaining in part the macrocytic anemia that sometimes occurs in patients with hairy cell leukemia. Other marrow cells are greatly reduced in number.

Figure 3–34   *Hairy cells in marrow from patient with hairy cell leukemia. Nuclear chromatin is reticular with few aggregates, and cytoplasm is abundant with excrescences.*

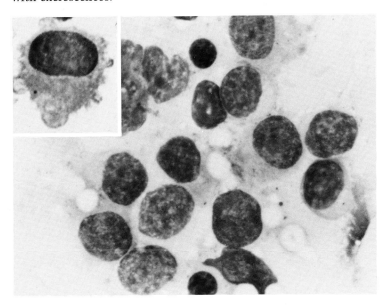

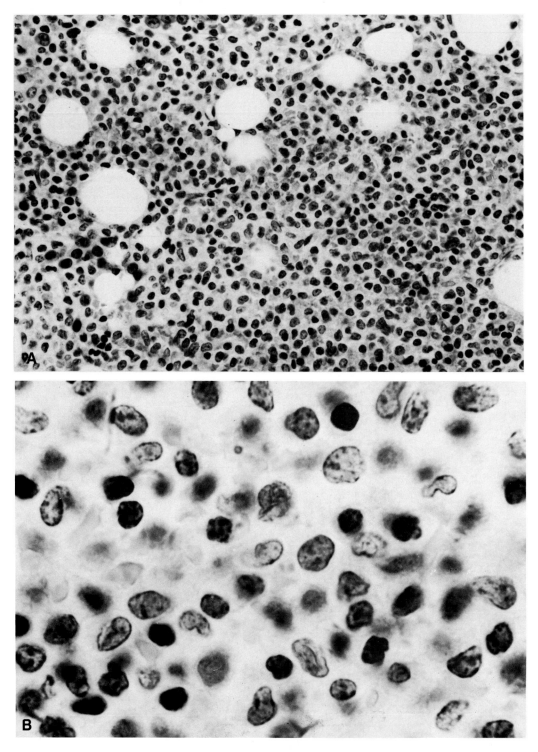

Figure 3–35   *Hairy cell leukemia (A) A low-power view of the marrow, showing nuclei that are widely separated. (B) A higher-power view, demonstrating round to oval nuclei of hairy cells and indistinct cytoplasmic borders.*

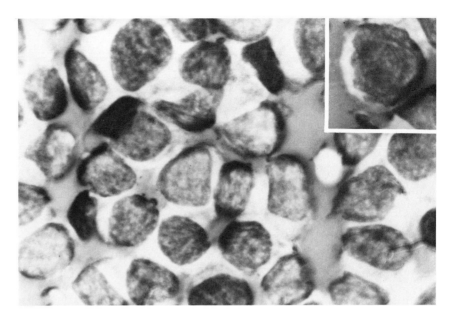

Figure 3–36   *Hairy cells in the spleen of a patient with hairy cell leukemia. Cells lack the characteristic hairy projections.*

H and E sections of marrows from patients with hairy cell leukemia are hypercellular and demonstrate replacement by cells with round to oval nuclei, irregular nuclear membranes, and variability in size and shape of the nuclei (Fig. 3–35). Nucleoli are small and inconspicuous. Cytoplasm is lightly eosinophilic, and cytoplasmic borders are indistinct. Cytoplasm is also relatively abundant, causing the nuclei to appear widely separated. Normal marrow elements are greatly reduced in number. Hairy cells in spleens from patients with hairy cell leukemia have typical nuclear features of hairy cells but lack the characteristic cytoplasmic projections (Fig. 3–36).

Cytochemically, the activity of acid phosphatase is increased in hairy cells. Characteristically, the activity of this acid phosphatase is not inhibited by the addition of L-tartrate to the incubation medium. In fact, the activity of tartrate-resistant acid phosphatase may actually be stronger than acid phosphatase not containing tartrate in the medium (Fig. 3–37, *top right inset,* and Plate 4C).

Activity of nonspecific esterase using either alpha naphthyl acetate or alpha naphthyl butyrate is increased in hairy cells, and enzymatic activity is sensitive to inhibition by sodium fluoride (Fig. 3–37, *bottom right inset*).

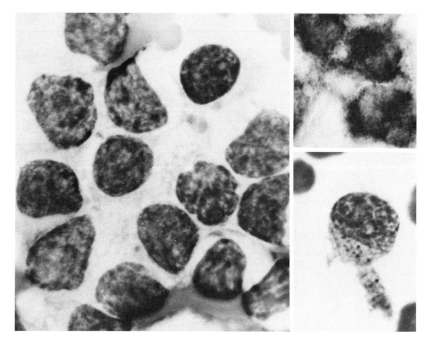

Figure 3–37   *Hairy cells in the marrow of a patient with hairy cell leukemia. Top right inset shows strong tartrate-resistant acid phosphatase activity. Bottom right inset shows increased activity of nonspecific esterase using alpha naphthyl acetate as the substrate and fast garnet GBC as the dye indicator.*

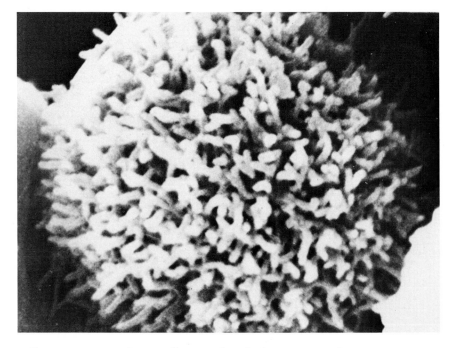

Figure 3–38   *Villous processes in hairy cell, viewed with the scanning electron microscope.*

154

At present, the origin of hairy cells is controversial. Certain properties such as the presence of microvilli (Fig. 3–38) and surface immunoglobulins favor a lymphocytic origin. Most of the evidence to date suggests that hairy cells are of B cell origin. Yet, other properties such as phagocytosis suggest relationships to monocytic cells. Cytochemically, the presence of fluoride-sensitive nonspecific esterase activity is characteristic of cells of monocytic origin. The presence of this type of enzymatic activity in hairy cells suggests that these cells share properties of cells of monocytic origin.

Hodgkin's Disease Involving Bone Marrow

Detection of the presence of Hodgkin's disease in the bone marrow is an important aspect in the staging of this disorder. Generally, foci of Hodgkin's disease can be found more easily on marrow biopsy than marrow aspirate. However, in some instances, involvement of marrow by Hodgkin's disease can be observed in routine marrow aspiration. In these cases, typical Sternberg-Reed cells are found (Fig. 3–39). On Wright's-stained films of marrow, Sternberg-Reed cells are giant multinuclear cells with large blue-staining nucleoli and a vacuous-appearing nucleus with a coarse, irregular-appearing, disorganized nuclear chromatin pattern. Cytoplasm is faintly basophilic and appears opaque. Sternberg-Reed cells are often fragile and can be disrupted during the process of making a film of marrow.

Cytochemically, Sternberg-Reed cells show a characteristic yellow staining of the cytoplasm when the ammoniacal silver reagent is used, indicating an abundance of lysine-rich histone in the cytoplasm (Fig. 3–40*B*). Sternberg-Reed cells also demonstrate intense pyroninophilia using methyl green-pyronin, and they show intense cytoplasmic basophilia when Giemsa stain is used.

Other cells that constitute part of the microenvironment of Hodgkin's disease are also found on routine marrow aspiration. These include plasma cells, eosinophils, fibroblasts, and large primitive-appearing cells with nucleolar features and nuclear chromatin patterns similar to those seen in typical Sternberg-Reed cells (Fig. 3–41 and 3–42). These cells are probably malignant histiocytes (see Fig. 3–42).

On H and E section, foci of Hodgkin's disease are detectable at low magnification. They appear as areas of fibrosis and hypocellularity in some instances and in other instances as areas of hypercellularity in which normal elements are depleted and replaced with cells

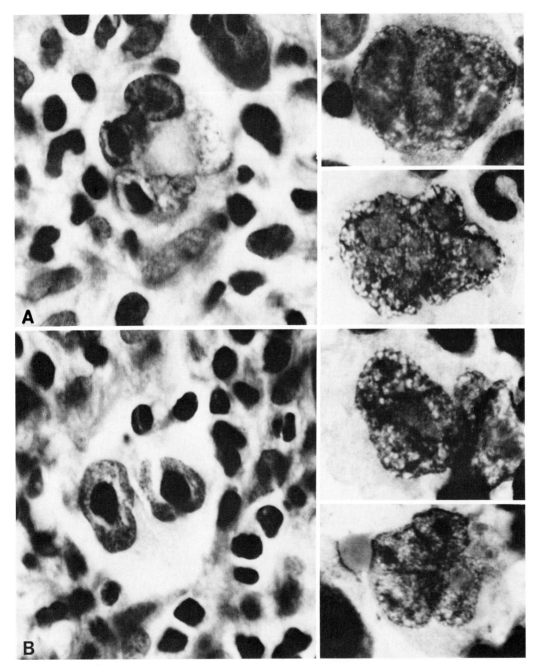

Figure 3–39   (A *and* B) *Sternberg-Reed cells in the marrow of patients with Hodgkin's disease, H and E stain of biopsy section. Insets, right, top to bottom, show Wright's-stained Sternberg-Reed cells on marrow aspirate from patients with Hodgkin's disease.*

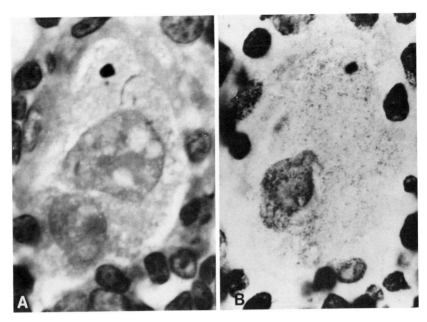

Figure 3–40   *Sternberg-Reed cell (A) stained with H and E; same cell in adjacent section (B) stained with ammoniacal silver to demonstrate lysine-rich histone, as reflected by the yellow staining of the cytoplasm. Punctate brown particles represent arginine-rich histone.*

noted above (Fig. 3–43). On higher magnification, typical Sternberg-Reed cells may be found but are infrequent. Strands of collagen, plasma cells, fibroblasts, large malignant histiocytes, and eosinophils are found (Figs. 3–44 and 3–45).

Histiocytic Lymphoma Involving Bone Marrow

Once believed to be a disorder of malignant histiocytes, histiocytic lymphoma is now regarded as a disorder of neoplastic B lymphocytes that have distinctive nuclear and cytoplasmic features. As in Hodgkin's disease, marrow involvement by histiocytic lymphoma is detected best with marrow biopsy. Histiocytic lymphoma cells are large and have prominent nuclei (Fig. 3–46). Nuclear chromatin has a coarse appearance, and nucleoli are unusually large with perinucleolar condensations of chromatin. Nucleoli are single or multiple. Cytoplasm is deeply basophilic and devoid of granularity. Characteristically, multiple small and large cytoplasmic vacuoles may be found. Cytoplasm is abundant and sometimes demonstrates a cyto-

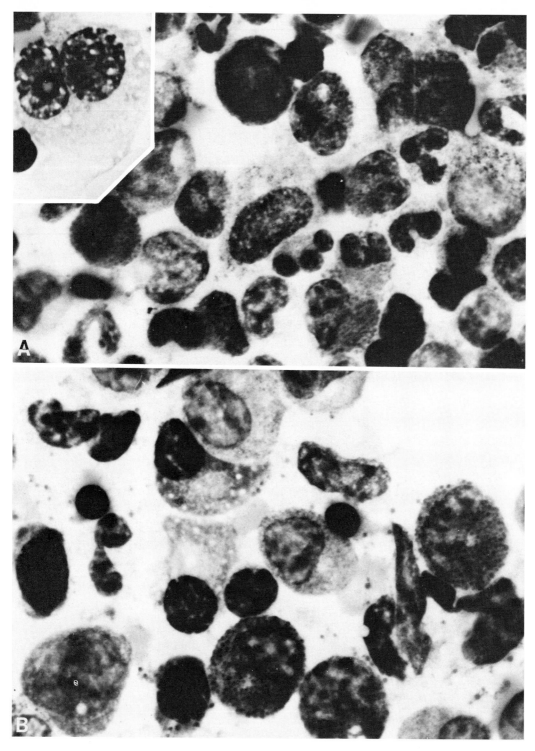

Figure 3–41 *Hodgkin's disease, showing increased numbers of eosinophils and malignant histiocytes* (A *and* inset) *and increased numbers of plasma cells and eosinophils* (B).

158

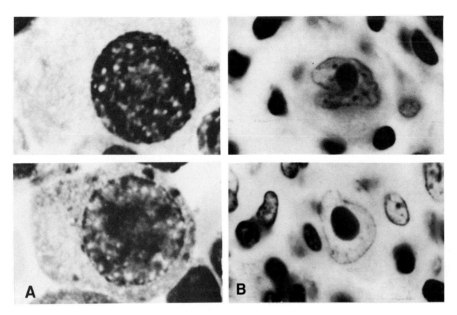

Figure 3–42   *Malignant histiocytes in Hodgkin's disease. On Wright's stain (A), these cells have large nuclei with prominent nucleoli. Similar cells are seen on H and E section of marrow biopsies (B).*

plasmic "tail." Using alpha naphthyl acetate as a substrate, these cells often possess intense nonspecific esterase activity localized in a perinuclear area (Fig. 3–46, *insets*).

On H and E section, normal marrow elements are reduced in number. Histiocytic lymphoma cells contain pale vesicular nuclei having numerous aggregates of chromatin and prominent nucleoli that stain deeply acidophilic (Fig. 3–47). Cytoplasm is abundant and stains deeply eosinophilic. Nuclei vary considerably in size and shape. As in marrow aspirates, multinuclear giant malignant cells may be found.

Angioimmunoblastic Lymphadenopathy

Also called immunoblastic lymphadenopathy, this disorder is characterized by lymphadenopathy, immune hemolytic anemia, splenomegaly, and fever. The clinical course may be brief in some instances and protracted in others. Marrow aspirates and biopsies

(Text continued on page 167)

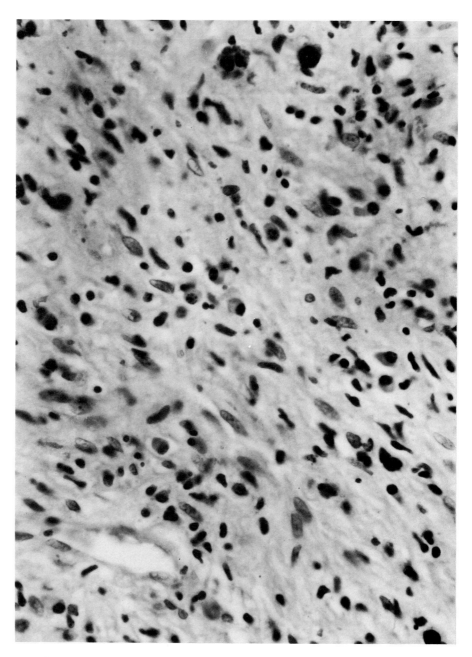

Figure 3–43   *H and E section of marrow biopsy from a patient with Hodgkin's disease who had marrow involvement. Areas of involvement appear densely cellular and fibrotic, with many fibroblasts and plasma cells.*

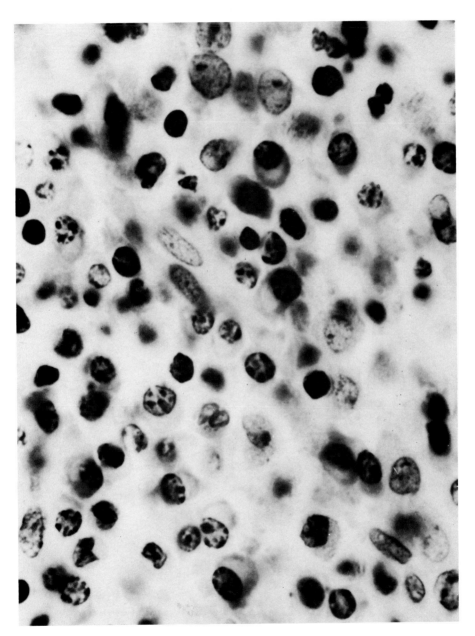

Figure 3–44   *Hodgkin's disease with bone marrow involvement, demonstrating increased numbers of plasma cells and fibroblasts.*

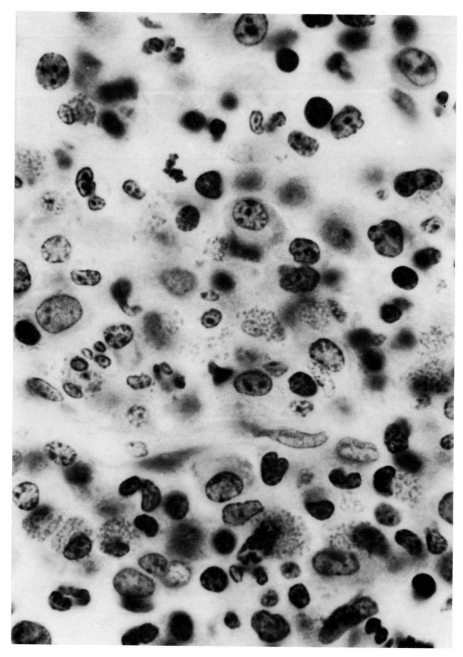

Figure 3–45   *Hodgkin's disease with bone marrow involvement, showing increased numbers of eosinophils, plasma cells, and fibroblasts.*

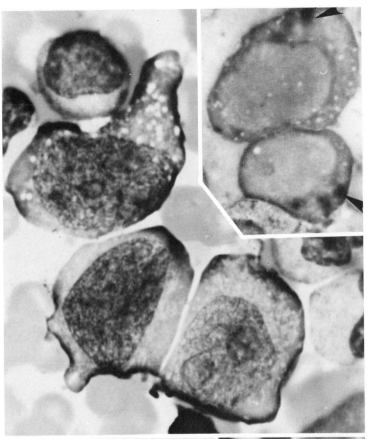

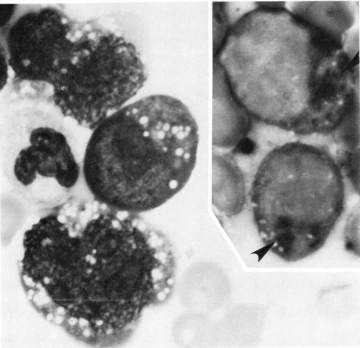

Figure 3–46

Malignant cells in marrow aspirates of patients with leukemic phase of histiocytic lymphoma. Insets show distinctive unipolar nonspecific esterase activity (arrows) typical of these cells, using alpha naphthyl acetate and pararosaniline.

Neoplastic lymphoid cells in histiocytic lymphoma can be confused with other types of malignant cells, such as those found in poorly differentiated multiple myeloma, anaplastic carcinoma, amelanotic melanoma, or chloroma (granulocytic sarcoma). Ultrastructural and cytochemical techniques may help to distinguish between these disorders.

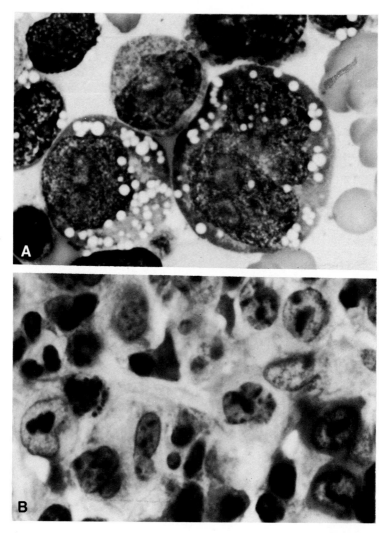

Figure 3–47   *Large bizarre-appearing histiocytic lymphoma cells on Wright's-stained aspirate of bone marrow. Cells show irregular nuclear configurations, prominent nucleoli with perinucleolar condensations of chromatin, and multiple cytoplasmic vacuoles (A). On H and E section (B), these cells show large, vacuous-appearing nuclei with large, prominent nucleoli and darkly staining aggregates of nuclear chromatin. Cytoplasm is abundant, and cytoplasmic margins are indistinct.*

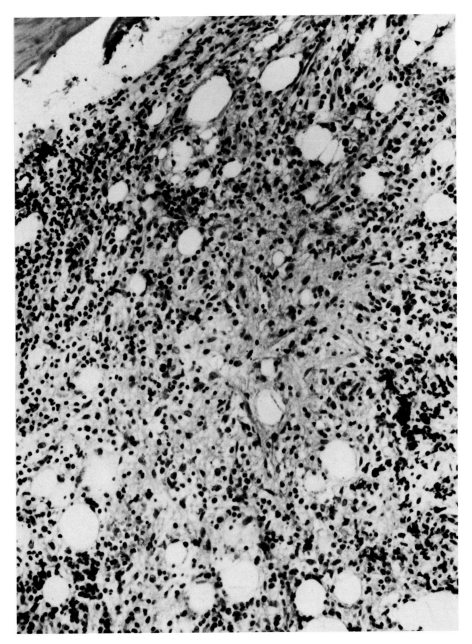

Figure 3–48   *Angioimmunoblastic lymphadenopathy. Low-power view of H and E section of marrow biopsy, illustrating fibrosis in area of involvement.*

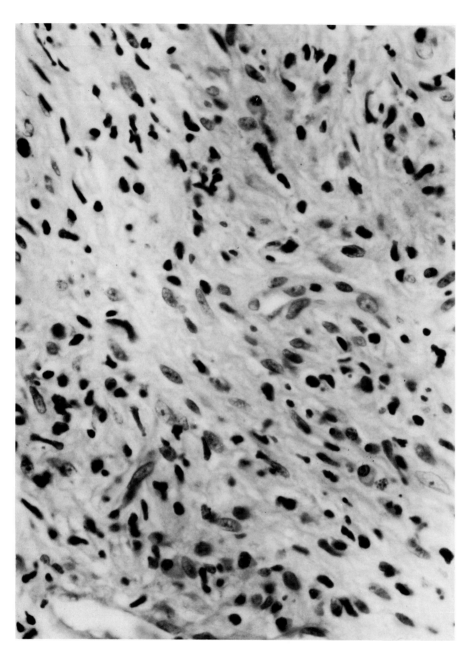

Figure 3–49   *Angioimmunoblastic lymphadenopathy, showing increased numbers of plasma cells and fibroblasts on H and E section of biopsy.*

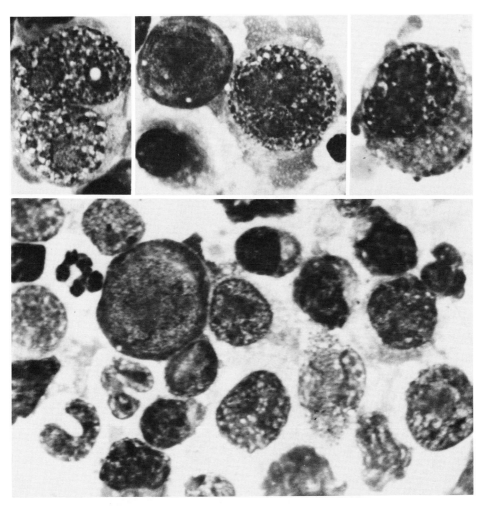

Figure 3–50   *Angioimmunoblastic lymphadenopathy, showing increased numbers of large immunoblasts, plasma cells, reticulum cells, and eosinophils. Insets show large immunoblasts.*

from patients with this disorder often show abnormalities similar to those found in lymph nodes. Paratrabecular fibrosis is observed frequently on H and E section (Figs. 3–48 and 3–49).

On aspiration, increased numbers of immunoblasts are found. These are plasmacytoid cells of varying size and shape, with prominent nucleoli and deeply basophilic cytoplasm (Fig. 3–50). In some instances, numerous cytoplasmic excrescences are found. Other immunoblasts have primitive-appearing nuclei with nucleoli and deeply basophilic cytoplasm containing vacuoles (Figs. 3–50 through 3–52).

(Text continued on page 170)

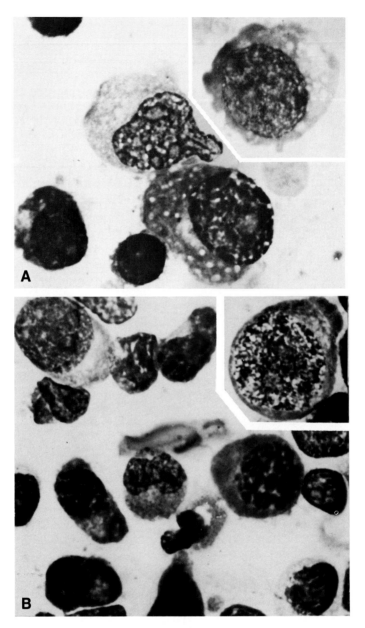

Figure 3–51   *Angioimmunoblastic lymphadenopathy with bone marrow involvement, illustrating large plasmacytoid-appearing cells (immunoblasts) (A, B, and insets) and increased numbers of plasma cells and eosinophils (B).*

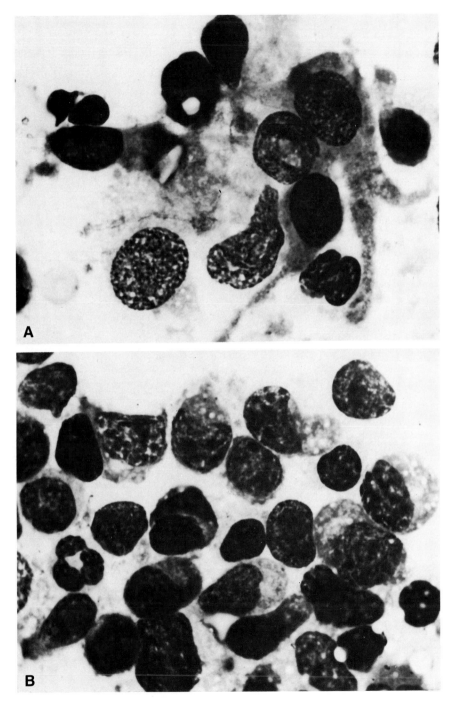

Figure 3–52   *Angioimmunoblastic lymphadenopathy with bone marrow involvement, illustrating a large macrophage containing cytoplasmic debris (A) and increased numbers of lymphocytes, plasma cells, and immunoblasts (B).*

Increased numbers of plasma cells, eosinophils, reticulum cells, and macrophages are also found (Figs. 3–52 and 3–53). On H and E sections of marrow biopsies, numerous eosinophils, plasma cells, and fibroblasts are seen (Fig. 3–54). Characteristically, arborizing small blood vessels and immunoblasts are observed (Fig. 3–55*A*). Immunoblasts demonstrate large nuclei with prominent aggregates of nuclear chromatin, large nucleoli, and deeply stained cytoplasm (Fig. 3–55*B*).

(Text continued on page 174)

Figure 3–53   *Angioimmunoblastic lymphadenopathy, showing increased numbers of plasma cells and reticulum cells.*

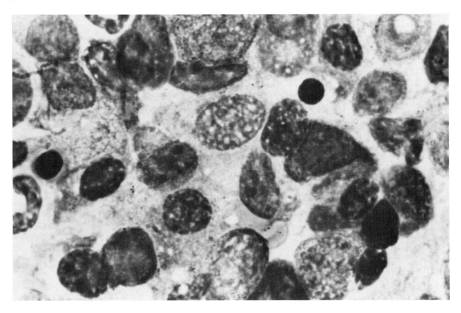

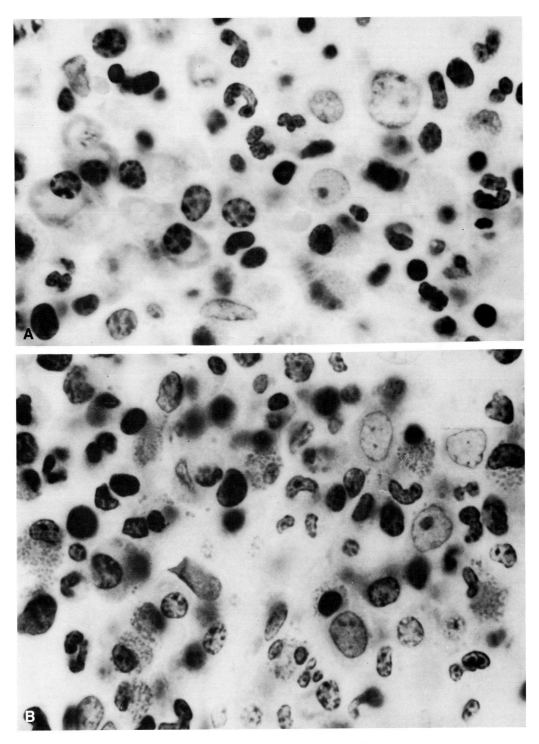

Figure 3–54   *Angioimmunoblastic lymphadenopathy with bone marrow involvement, showing increased numbers of mature-appearing plasma cells (A) and increased numbers of eosinophils along with plasma cells (B).*

171

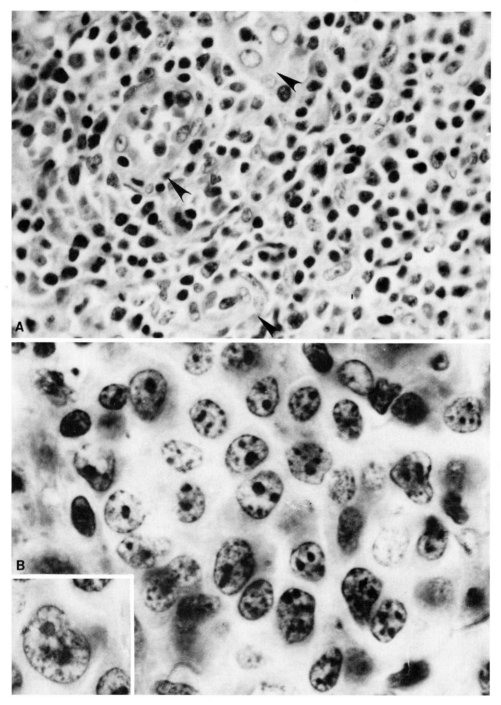

Figure 3–55   *Angioimmunoblastic lymphadenopathy. (A) Low-power view of marrow, showing small capillaries (arrows) and immunoblasts. (B) Large immunoblasts with prominent nucleoli and large aggregates of nuclear chromatin, some of which are adherent to the nuclear membrane. Inset shows large immunoblast with several nucleoli.*

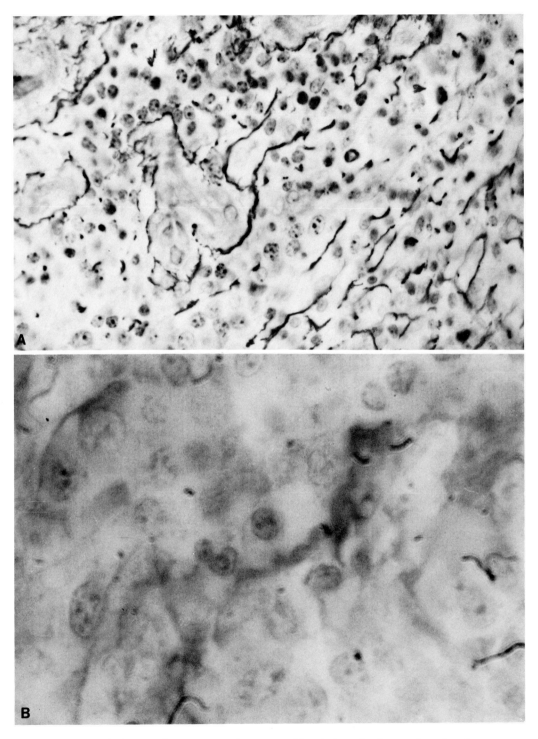

Figure 3–56 (A) *Reticulin stain, angioimmunoblastic lymphadenopathy, showing increased numbers of delicate reticulin fibers. (B) PAS stain of marrow, showing faint staining of diastase-resistant PAS-positive material (gray).*

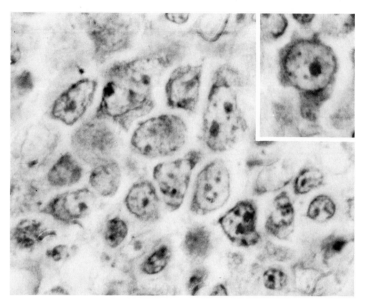

Figure 3–57   *Intense pyroninophilia of immunoblasts in the marrow of a patient with angioimmunoblastic lymphadenopathy, methyl green-pyronine stain.*

Cytochemically, increased reticulin fibers are seen using reticulin stains (Fig. 3–56*A*). Faint diastase-resistant PAS-positive material is also detectable in the fibrotic lesions (Fig. 3–56*B*). Immunoblasts stain deeply for RNA, using the methyl green-pyronine reagent, and detection of pyroninophilia is a useful identifying feature for these immunoblasts (Fig. 3–57).

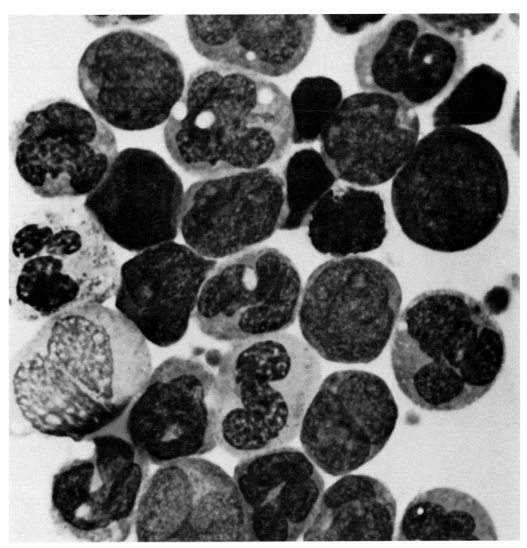

Leukemic monocytes in acute myelomonocytic leukemia, M4 type.

4   *Monocytosis*

In normal bone marrow, monocytes comprise less than 1% of the cells in a differential count. Monocytosis of the marrow occurs in acute infections and in the recovery phase of drug-induced hypoplasia of the bone marrow. Most often, monocytosis of the marrow occurs as the result of monocytic leukemia.

Normal Monocyte. Normally, monocytes are believed to arise from promyelocytes in the bone marrow. Precursors of monocytes are difficult to identify as such in the marrow. Promyelocytes that have indentations and convolutions of their nuclei may represent cells that have differentiated along monocytic lines (Fig. 4–1). In the marrow, normal monocytes show typical convolutions and lobulations of the nucleus and pale gray-staining cytoplasm containing numerous pink dustlike granules (Figs. 4–2 and 4–3).

Figure 4–1   *Promyelocytes in normal marrow, showing monocytoid-type convolutions and lobulations of the nucleus. These cells may be precursors of monocytes.*

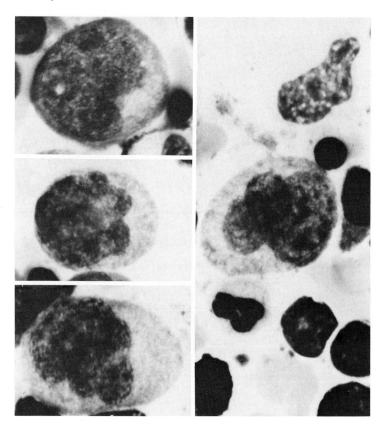

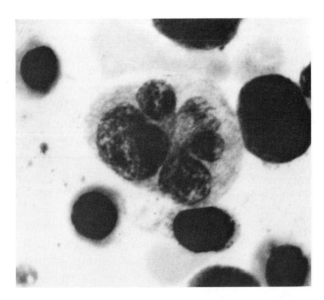

Figure 4–2   *Monocyte, normal marrow, showing multiple nuclear lobulations.*

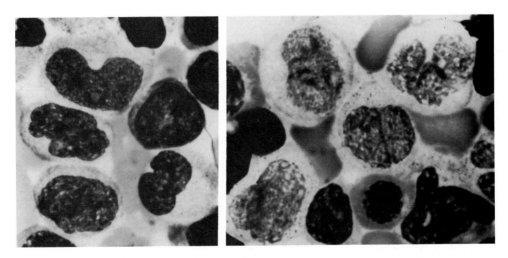

Figure 4–3   *Monocytes, normal marrow.*

Spectrum of Abnormal Monocytes. Monocytosis of the blood is defined as greater than 600 monocytes per cubic millimeter. It can occur in a wide variety of non-neoplastic disorders like tuberculosis, septicemia, treponemal infections, protozoal infections, and bacterial endocarditis. In these instances, monocytes often assume functions of blood phagocytes. As such, they demonstrate voluminous cytoplasm containing multiple vacuoles. In keeping with their phagocytic function, monocytes in these conditions often exhibit evidence of erythrocytophagy. In all of these infectious disorders, monocytosis of the bone marrow can occur.

Monocytosis can also be found in disorders that may be neoplastic but not necessarily primary disorders of monocytes. These include monocytosis in association with Hodgkin's disease, multiple myeloma, and Di Guglielmo syndrome. In these disorders, monocytes usually appear normal. In some instances, particularly preleukemic refractory anemia, they can demonstrate abnormalities of nucleus and cytoplasm. These abnormalities raise the question of whether monocytes share in the panmyelotic disturbances, even though the morphologic abnormalities are not necessarily accompanied by pathologic monocytosis of the bone marrow.

In other neoplastic conditions, monocytosis of the blood is accompanied by pathologic monocytosis of the bone marrow. These disorders are the monocytic leukemias. They involve a spectrum of variants, some emphasizing granulocytic aberrations (myelomonocytic) and others emphasizing hemohistiocytic and hemohistioblastic abnormalities (histiomonocytic). In marrows and peripheral bloods of patients with monocytic leukemia, a wide variety of morphologic abnormalities of monocytes are found. These include aberrations in the size and configuration of the nucleus and in the caliber of chromatin strands, and cytoplasmic abnormalities that include pseudopodia and perinuclear clustering of nonspecific granules. While not diagnostic in themselves of neoplastic changes, when they occur in combination with each other and in a setting of pathologic monocytosis of the marrow, these nuclear and cytoplasmic abnormalities are highly suggestive of malignancy.

Nuclear Abnormalities

Giant monocytoid cells are usually found in monocytic leukemia (Fig. 4–4). In some of these cells, nuclear chromatin is delicate; in others, nuclear chromatin appears coarse and contains numerous large aggregates. Nuclei may show indentations, foldings, and convolutions.

Multiple Nuclear Lobulations. Neoplastic monocytes often exhibit multiple nuclear lobulations that seem to overlie one another. In some instances, they appear as fingerlike projections or protrusions of the nucleus (Fig. 4–5).

Monocytoid Cells With Large Prominent Nucleoli. In acute monocytic leukemia, abnormal monocytoid cells have large prominent nucleoli with perinucleolar condensations of chromatin. Cytoplasm is usually pale and may contain dustlike nonspecific granules (Fig. 4–6).

Figure 4–4   *Giant monocytes, monocytic leukemia. Cytoplasmic vacuoles are seen.*

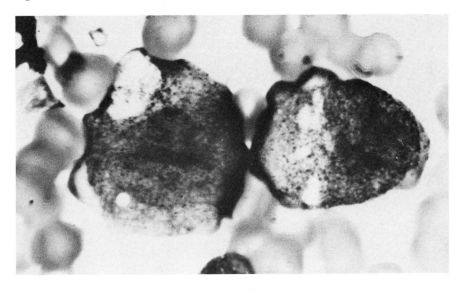

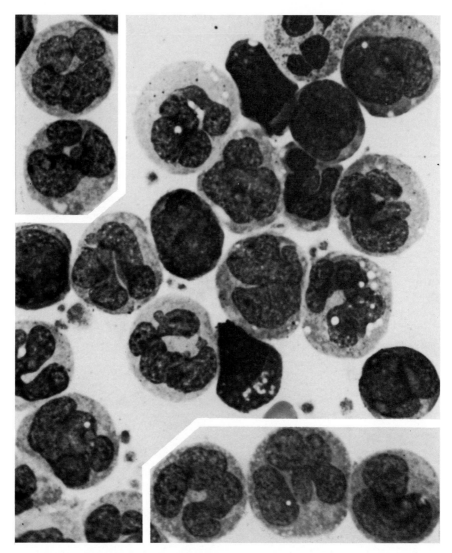

Figure 4–5   *Leukemic monocytes, monocytic leukemia, demonstrating multiple overlapping nuclear lobulations.*

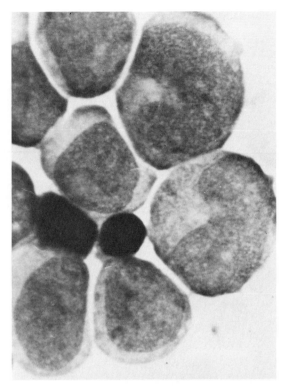

Figure 4–6   *Leukemic monocytes with prominent nucleoli and perinucleolar condensations of chromatin.*

Attenuation of Nuclear Chromatin. In contrast to coarse-appearing nuclear chromatin strands as found in normal monocytes, neoplastic monocytes can exhibit unusually delicate nuclear chromatin strands. Strands of chromatin are more numerous and more closely approximated than in normal monocytes (Fig. 4–7).

Monocytes With Prominent Chromatin Aggregates. Monocytes with prominent aggregates of chromatin are found in patients with heredofamilial Pelger-Huët anomaly. In these patients, similar-appearing chromatin is found in polymorphonuclear leukocytes (Fig. 4–8).

Monocytoid Cells With Numerous Large Aggregates of Chromatin. In some patients with monocytic leukemia, neoplastic monocytes have large aberrant-appearing nuclei that assume a "U" configuration (Fig. 4–9). Nuclear chromatin of these cells is often coarse appearing, with numerous large aggregates of chromatin connected to each other by thick-appearing strands of chromatin.

(Text continued on page 184)

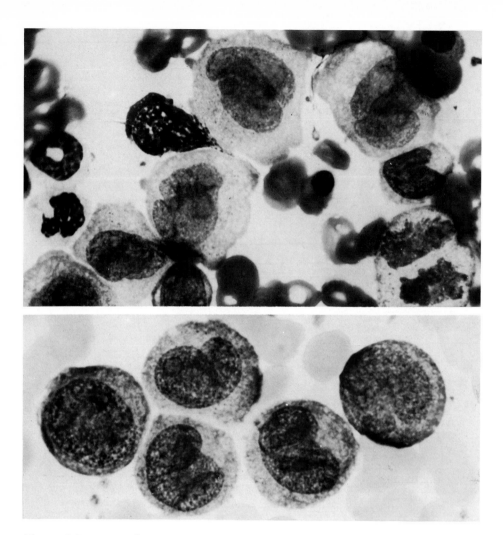

Figure 4–7   Leukemic monocytes, monocytic leukemia, showing delicate-appearing, finely attenuated nuclear chromatin.

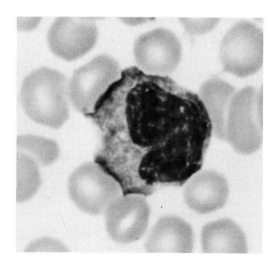

Figure 4–8
Blocklike aggregates of chromatin in a monocyte from a person with Pelger-Huët anomaly.

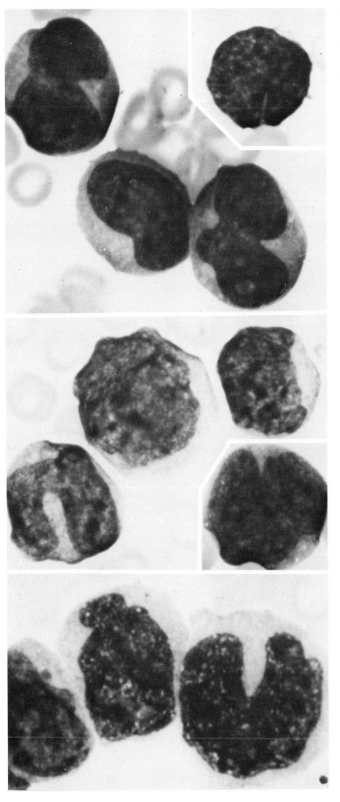

Figure 4–9
Giant monocytoid cells with dense
prominent aggregates of nuclear
chromatin and "U" shape of nucleus,
monocytic leukemia.

Monocytoid Changes in Granulocytic Cells. Particularly in the monocytic leukemias, cells of granulocytic origin such as promyelocytes, myelocytes, and metamyelocytes often demonstrate folding and lobulation of the nucleus as found in monocytes (Fig. 4–10). These cells also have specific neutrophilic or eosinophilic granules. In some instances, they may exhibit only nonspecific granulation as found in promyelocytes. Finding monocytic nuclear properties in a cell that is morphologically granulocytic suggests that in monocytic leukemias the neoplastic monocytes may share properties of granulocytes.

Monocytoid Changes in Primitive Cells. In monocytic leukemias, cells that have been regarded as primitive marrow cells such as hemohistiocytes, hemohistioblasts, and reticulum cells may exhibit monocytoid-type foldings, lobulations, and convolutions of the nucleus (Figs. 4–11 and 4–12). As in the case of monocytoid granulocytes, monocytic features in primitive marrow cells suggest that they have differentiated along monocytic lines in the monocytic leukemias.

Figure 4–10   *Monocytoid changes in nuclei of promyelocytes, monocytic leukemia.*

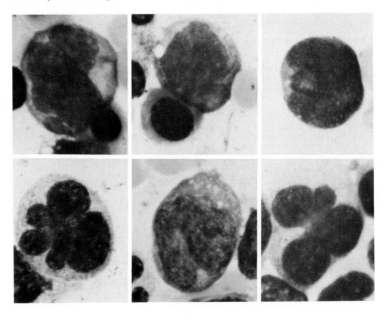

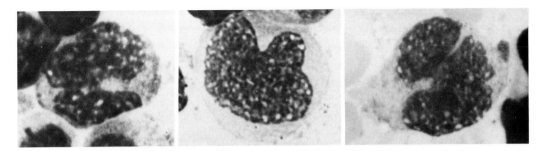

Figure 4–11   *Monocytoid-type convolutions and lobulations in hemohistiocytes and hemohistioblasts, monocytic leukemia. (Kass L: Preleukemic Disorders. Springfield, IL, Charles C Thomas, 1979)*

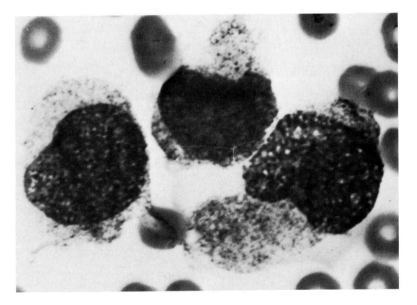

Figure 4–12   *Leukemic hemohistioblasts and hemohistiocytes with monocytoid nuclear convolutions.*

In some instances, monocytoid changes in these primitive cells are among the first recognizable morphologic changes prior to the emergence of overt leukemia and replacement of the marrow with neoplastic monocytes. These monocytoid hemohistiocytes, hemohistioblasts, and reticulum cells are often larger and more atypical than their normal counterparts and have prominent and multiple nucleoli with perinucleolar condensations of chromatin.

Cytoplasmic Abnormalities

Cytoplasmic Tail. Neoplastic monocytes often exhibit an elongation of clear cytoplasm in the form of a tail or protrusion (Fig. 4–13). This may indicate motility of the neoplastic monocyte or perhaps increased deformability of glass surfaces and fluidity of monocytic cytoplasm. In some instances, the monocytic tail contains numerous nonspecific granules arranged in a cluster.

Clear Cytoplasmic Pseudopodia. In neoplastic monocytes, numerous clear cytoplasmic pseudopodia can be found. They appear rounded and do not contain granules. These pseudopodia may reflect increased motility of the monocytes, as seen in phase-contrast preparations of living monocytes (Fig. 4–14).

Vacuolated Cytoplasm. Monocytes from patients with septicemia and from patients with monocytic leukemia often have multiple cytoplasmic vacuoles. These probably represent phagocytic structures (Fig. 4–15) or degenerative changes.

Perinuclear Clustering of Granules. Perinuclear clustering of nonspecific granules is often seen in neoplastic monocytes (Fig. 4–16).

Figure 4–13   *Leukemic monocytes with cytoplasmic "tail" containing granules.*

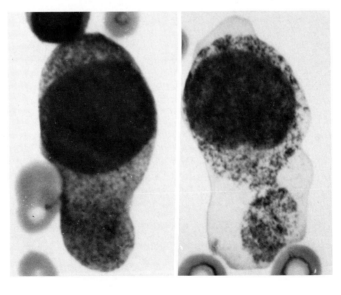

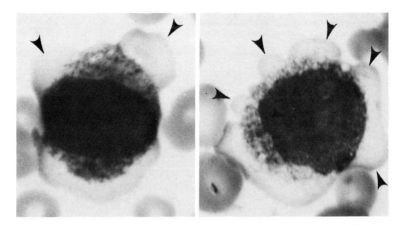

Figure 4–14 *Multiple clear cytoplasmic pseudopodia* (arrows) *in leukemic monocytes.*

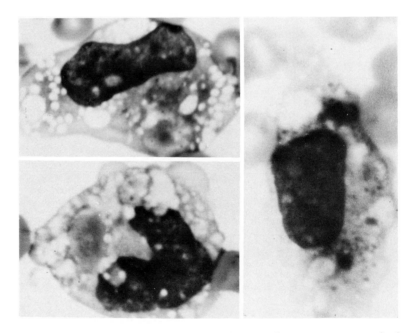

Figure 4–15 *Monocytes with voluminous vacuolated cytoplasm in monocytic leukemia* (left) *and septicemia* (right).

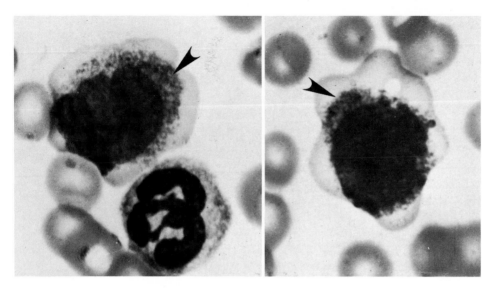

Figure 4–16   *Dense aggregates of nonspecific, darkly stained granules in perinuclear distribution (arrows) in the cytoplasm of leukemic monocytes.*

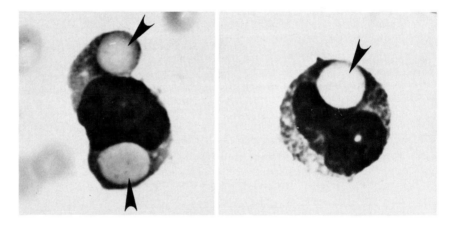

Figure 4–17   *Erythrocytophagy (arrows) by monocytes in cold agglutinin disease.*

Erythrocytophagy by Monocytes. In patients with septicemia and cold agglutinin disease, monocytes can show erythrocytophagy (Fig. 4–17). Monocytes possess receptors for immunoglobulins on their cell membranes, facilitating the process of phagocytosis of erythrocytes coated with immunoglobulins in autoimmune hemolytic anemia. Similar erythrocytophagy can be found in leukemic monocytes, although in this instance the mechanism is not necessarily an immune one.

Monocytic Leukemia

Monocytic leukemia represents a spectrum of variants, all of which are probably monocytoid representations of myeloblastic leukemia. Within the spectrum of monocytic leukemia, several morphologic types have been identified. In some cases, these types differ in clinical course and manifestations.

Subacute Myelomonocytic Leukemia

Subacute myelomonocytic leukemia is indolent, and the time from diagnosis of the disease to death in untreated cases is 6 months to 1 year. Patients usually demonstrate monocytosis, macrocytic anemia, hepatomegaly, splenomegaly, soft tissue infections, and hemorrhagic manifestations. In all likelihood, subacute myelomonocytic leukemia is closely related to, if not identical with, chronic myelomonocytic leukemia, a disorder that has been included in the current definition of myelodysplastic syndromes.

Marrows from patients with subacute myelomonocytic leukemia are hypercellular (Fig. 4–18). Monocytes and/or monocytoid cells comprise up to 20% of the marrow cells in a differential cell count (Figs. 4–18 and 4–19). Monocytes are often atypical, with multiple nuclear lobulations, attenuated chromatin strands, nucleoli, and granulocytic-type granulations (Figs. 4–18 through 4–20). Monocytoid changes are often observed in primitive marrow cells such as hemohistiocytes and hemohistioblasts. Increased numbers of reticulum cells are also found.

Erythropoiesis is increased, and many erythroblasts show megaloblastoid nuclear chromatin patterns (Figs. 4–19 and 4–21). Some erythroblasts are multinuclear (Fig. 4–22). Proerythroblasts are often increased in number. In some late intermediate erythroblasts, coarse basophilic stippling and multiple Howell-Jolly bodies are observed.

Megakaryocytes are normal, increased, or decreased in number. They demonstrate numerous nonspecific nuclear and cytoplasmic abnormalities, including gigantism, vacuolation of the cytoplasm, hypergranularity, hypogranularity, and unusual coarseness of nuclear chromatin strands. Micromegakaryocytes contain a single unlobulated nucleus or a nucleus with only one lobulation and abundant hypergranular cytoplasm.

(Text continued on page 194)

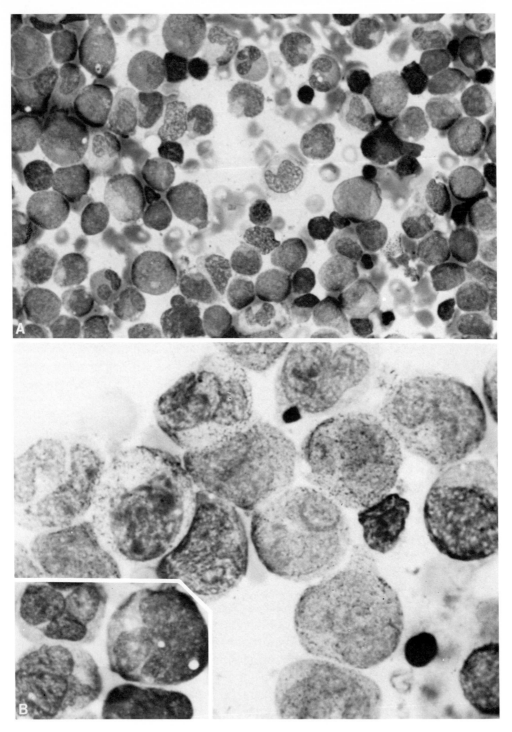

Figure 4–18   *Marrow, subacute myelomonocytic leukemia. (A) Low-power view demonstrating hypercellularity and increased numbers of monocytoid cells and promyelocytes. (B) Increased numbers of leukemic monocytes having multiple nuclear lobulations (inset). (Kass L: Preleukemic Disorders. Springfield, IL, Charles C Thomas, 1979)*

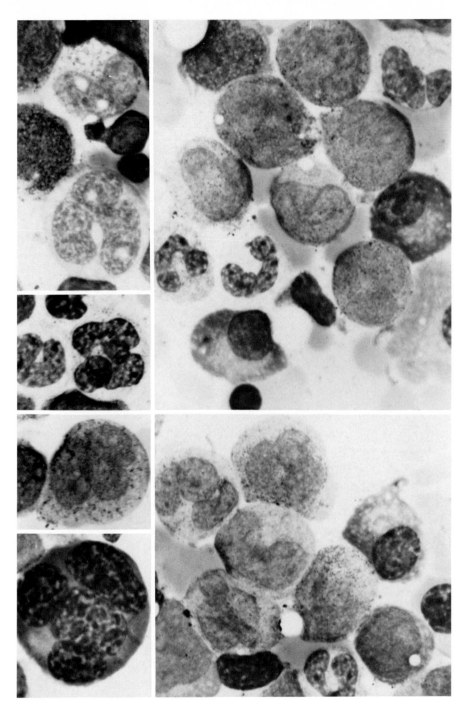

Figure 4–19   *Marrow, subacute myelomonocytic leukemia, demonstrating bizarre-appearing monocytoid cells and increased numbers of plasma cells. Insets, left, top to bottom, depict monocytoid-appearing nuclei in giant metamyelocytes, hypersegmented polymorphonuclear leukocyte, monocytoid nucleus in promyelocyte, and giant multinuclear erythroblast with a megaloblastoid nuclear chromatin pattern.*

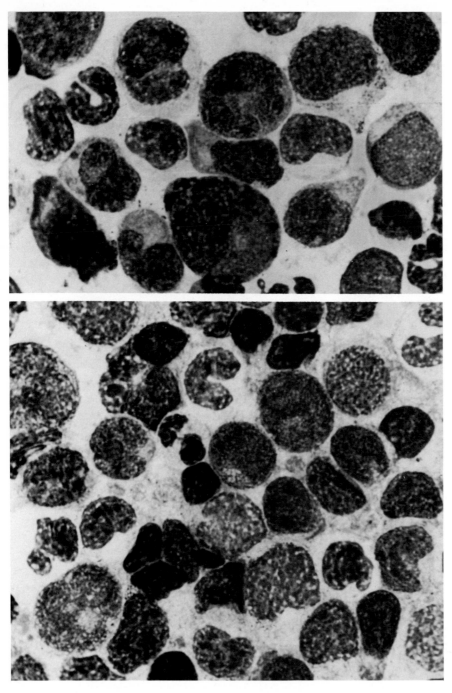

Figure 4–20   *Subacute myelomonocytic leukemia, illustrating aberrant-appearing monocytes and granulocytic cells with atypical nuclei.*

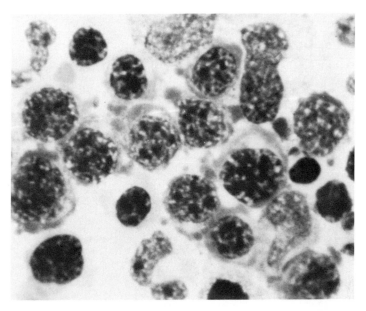

Figure 4–21   *Increased numbers of megaloblastoid intermediate macronormoblasts, subacute myelomonocytic leukemia.*

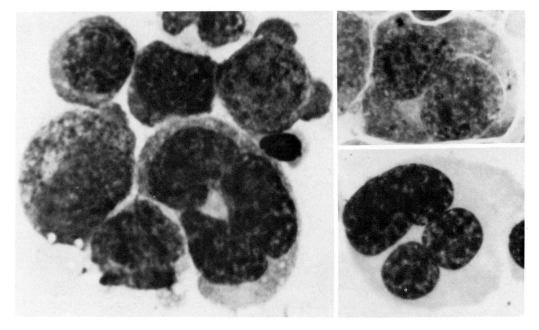

Figure 4–22   *Bizarre-appearing multinuclear erythroblasts, subacute myelomonocytic leukemia.*

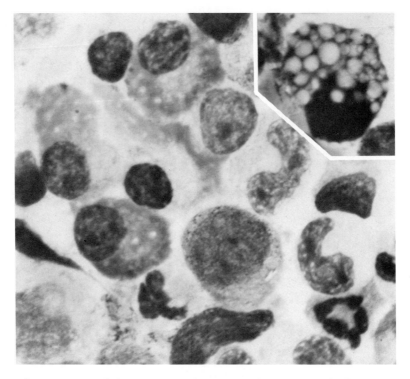

Figure 4–23   *Plasmacytosis of the marrow, subacute myelomonocytic leukemia, with plasma cell showing multiple large cytoplasmic vacuoles* (inset).

Increased numbers of mature-appearing plasma cells (Fig. 4–23) and eosinophils are observed frequently (Fig. 4–24). Occasionally, erythrocytophagy of erythroblasts and mature eythrocytes by monocytoid cells is observed.

On H and E section, marrows in subacute myelomonocytic leukemia are hypercellular and show increased numbers of erythroblasts and large cells with monocytic-type lobulations of the nucleus (Fig. 4–25).

Acute Monocytic Leukemia

Once thought to be sharply demarcated into myelomonocytic and histiomonocytic types, monocytic leukemia is more properly regarded at this time as a broad disorder in which some variants demonstrate more abnormalities referable to cells of granulocytic origin (M4 variant), as shown in Figure 4–26. Other variants reflect abnormalities primarily of primitive cells such as hemohistiocytes,

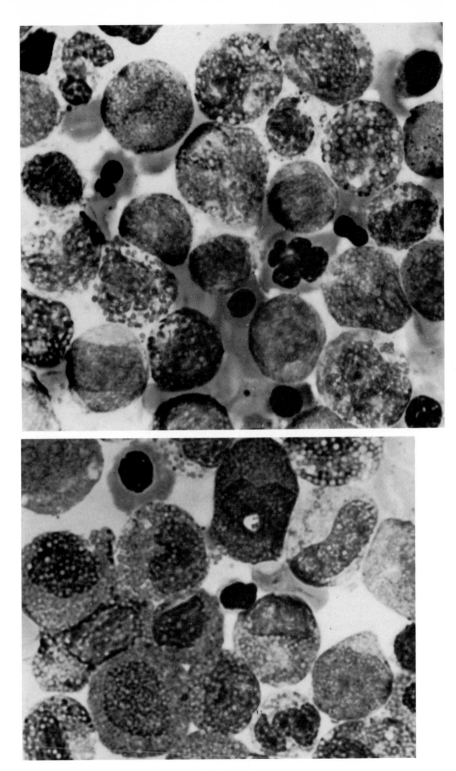

Figure 4–24   *Eosinophilia of the marrow, subacute myelomonocytic leukemia. Leukemic monocytes are also seen.*

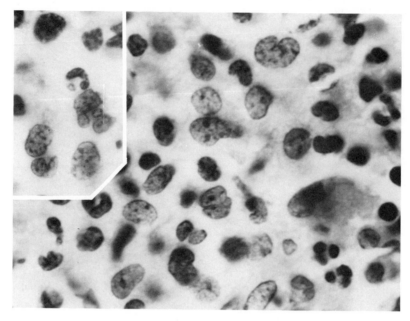

Figure 4–25   *H and E section of marrow biopsy, subacute myelomonocytic leukemia, demonstrating nuclear convolutions in monocytoid cells (inset).*

hemohistioblasts, and reticulum cells (M5 variant), as depicted in Figure 4–27. In all instances of monocytic leukemia, it is possible to demonstrate granulocytic properties of cells under proper cytochemical conditions. Accordingly, it may be more appropriate to regard all monocytic leukemias as morphologic variants of myeloblastic leukemia.

Marrows from patients with monocytic leukemia are hypercellular and composed primarily of neoplastic monocytes (see Figs. 4–26 and 4–27). These are large pleomorphic cells that have multiple nuclear lobulations and convolutions, delicate-looking nuclear chromatin strands that appear closely approximated, and cytoplasmic tails and pseudopodia. Granules may be clustered around the nucleus or dispersed throughout the cytoplasm. Erythrocytophagy of erythrocytes and erythroblasts by atypical monocytoid cells and/or histiocytes is observed frequently.

In some instances, abnormal monocytoid cells may be gigantic, with prominent aggregates of chromatin and prominent nucleoli having perinucleolar condensations of chromatin.

Megakaryocytes are greatly reduced in number and show cytologic features similar to those in subacute myelomonocytic leukemia. Erythropoiesis is greatly decreased and may be megaloblastoid in type.

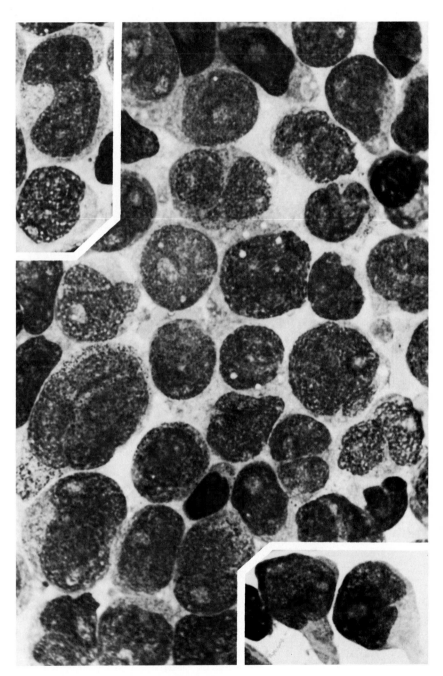

Figure 4–26   *M4 variant of acute myeloblastic leukemia (acute myelomonocytic leukemia). Bizarre-appearing monocytoid cells are shown. Some have aberrant nuclear configurations (figure and upper left inset), nonspecific azurophilic granulation, and a cytoplasmic "tail" (lower right inset).*

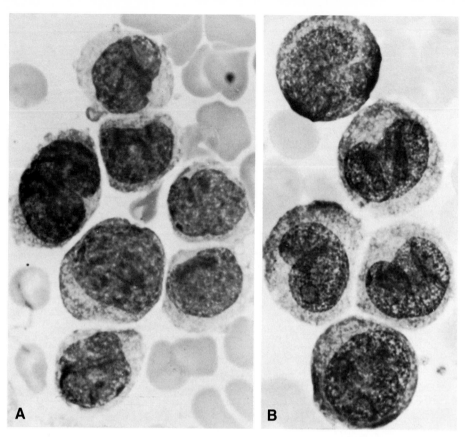

Figure 4–27   *Leukemic monocytes, acute monocytic leukemia (M5 variant). A and B represent monocytes from two different patients. Nuclear chromatin appears coarse in A and delicate in B. Nuclei show lobulations and foldings, and cytoplasm is abundant.*

Monocytoid changes of the nuclei of primitive cells such as hemohistiocytes, hemohistioblasts, and reticulum cells are observed frequently. In some cases the number of these cells may be substantially greater than in other cases. These atypical primitive cells may have numerous, tiny, nonspecific granules in the cytoplasm. Some of them exhibit erythrocytophagy. Granulopoiesis is substantially reduced and in severe cases may be virtually absent. Immature granulocytes such as promyelocytes and myelocytes predominate. Marked atypicality of nuclear configurations can be found in metamyelocytes and bands. Loopings, twistings, and convolutions of the nucleus may be found in these cells (Fig. 4–28).

On H and E section, marrows from patients with acute monocytic leukemia show large pleomorphic cells with convolutions and lobulations of the nuclei and prominent nucleoli (Fig. 4–29). Cytoplasm is abundant and stains deeply eosinophilic.

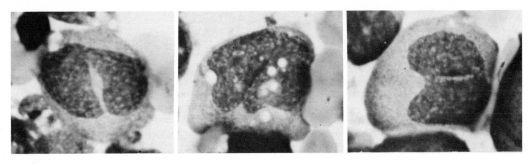

Figure 4–28   *Monocytoid changes in the nuclei of granulocytic cells, monocytic leukemia. Nuclear "bridging" is seen in the cell on the right. (Kass L: Preleukemic Disorders. Springfield, IL, Charles C Thomas, 1979)*

Figure 4–29   *Acute monocytic leukemia. Low-power view (A) shows hypercellular marrow, and higher-power view (B) shows large leukemic monocytes with nuclear twistings and convolutions.*

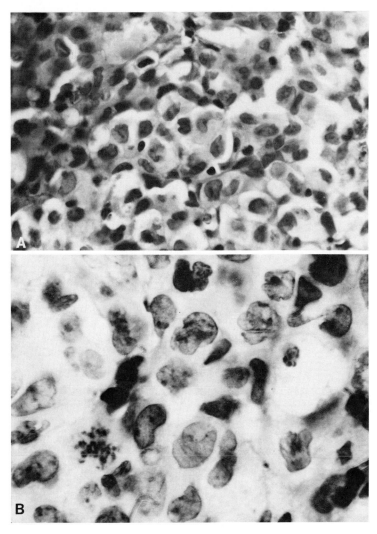

Cytochemistry of Monocytic Leukemias

In leukemic blasts from patients with monocytic leukemia, *PAS* stain shows faint diffuse positivity. *Sudan black B, oil red O,* and *peroxidase* stains detect granulocytic properties of cells, and these cytochemical reactions in neoplastic monocytes are faintly positive.

Cytochemical reactions designed to demonstrate *esterase* enzymes have attained importance in the cytochemistry of acute leukemias. Particularly in the identification of monocytic leukemias, specific and nonspecific esterases have been especially valuable in distinguishing monocytic leukemias from other types of acute leukemia. *Nonspecific esterase,* demonstrable with alpha naphthyl acetate or alpha naphthyl butyrate as substrate, is a cytoplasmic enzyme. Nonspecific esterase activity that can be inhibited or obliterated by sodium fluoride is believed to be characteristic of cells of monocytic origin. In monocytic leukemias, nonspecific esterase activity is intense in neoplastic monocytes and is inhibited by sodium fluoride (Fig. 4–30*A* and *B*). Enzymatic activity can vary in different cells. Some cells show intense activity, whereas others show weaker activity. Weak activity often seems to be a property of immature monocytoid cells, whereas intense activity is observed more frequently in neoplastic monocytes that appear typical and mature.

Figure 4–30
(opposite)

(A) *Nonspecific esterase activity in leukemic monocytes, subacute myelomonocytic leukemia, alpha naphthyl acetate and pararosaniline.* (B) *Higher-power view of intense nonspecific esterase activity in leukemic monocytes, alpha naphthyl acetate and pararosaniline. Enzymatic activity appears more intense in monocytes that look mature, as judged by the extent of nuclear lobulations.*

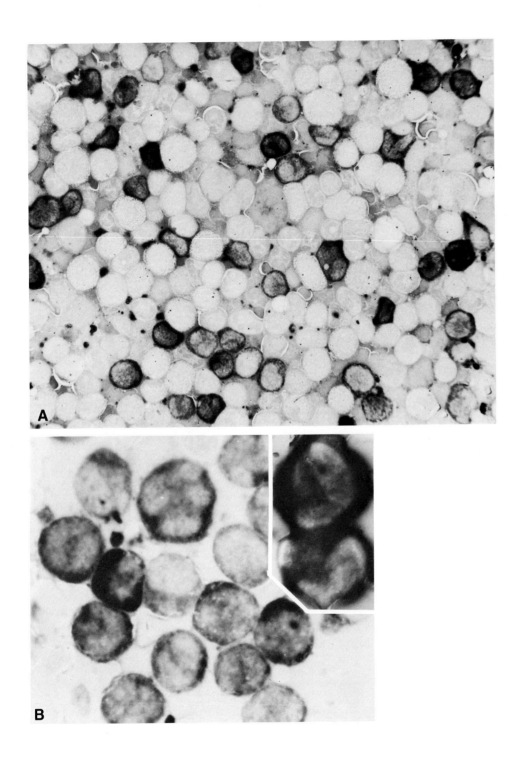

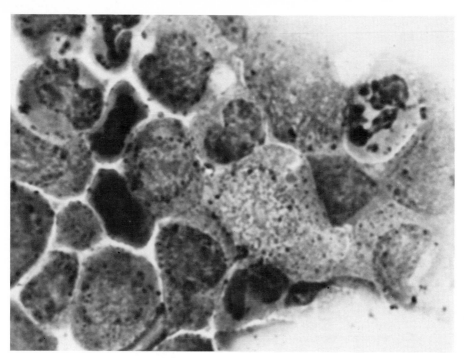

Figure 4–31   *Black punctate specific esterase activity in leukemic monocytes, naphthol ASD-chloroacetate and fast blue BBN.*

Specific esterase activity is demonstrable with the use of naphthol ASD-chloroacetate as substrate. This is a lysosomal enzyme and consequently is a valuable marker for cells of granulocytic origin and for the identification of granulocytic properties of cells. In monocytic leukemia, reaction for specific esterase activity is positive in neoplastic monocytes and in monocytoid-appearing granulocytic cells (Fig. 4–31). With the use of appropriate dye indicators such as fast garnet GBC, it is possible to identify specific esterase activity on the basis of reaction products that are not apparent when other dye couplers such as fast blue BBN are used. This dependency of the visualization and detection of the specific esterase activity on the dye coupler used in the cytochemical reaction explains in part the lack of enzymatic activity in those cases that have been called "pure" monocytic leukemia or so-called histiomonocytic leukemia. With the use of appropriate dye couplers, it is now possible to demonstrate properties of granulocytic cells in the form of specific esterase activity in atypical monocytoid cells from virtually all variants of monocytic leukemia.

Using the dis-azo dye Biebrich scarlet, *lysozyme* (muramidase) can be detected in the cytoplasm of leukemic monocytes. Pretreatment of the leukemic blasts with oligosaccharides causes binding of oligosaccharides to the lysozyme molecule and prevents staining of lysozyme with Biebrich scarlet. Accordingly, abolition of Biebrich scarlet stainability of the cytoplasm with oligosaccharide pretreatment is believed to indicate the presence of lysozyme in the cells. Increased content of cytoplasmic lysozyme is found in leukemic monocytes but not in lymphoblasts or myeloblasts.

Other Primitive Marrow Cells in the Monocyte Spectrum

Reticulum cells, hemohistioblasts, and hemohistiocytes are poorly defined primitive-appearing marrow cells that have been topics of controversy for many years. Nomenclature for this group of cells has shown considerable ambiguity. In all likelihood, reticulum cells, hemohistiocytes, and hemohistioblasts belong to a single class of primitive-appearing cells that can assume various morphologic appearances corresponding to different functional states. As yet it is not known whether reticulum cells are progenitor cells for hemohistiocytes and hemohistioblasts. According to some authors, hemohistiocytes and hemohistioblasts do not exist as such, but rather represent artifacts of spreading and fixation of disrupted promyelocytes and myelocytes. Presently, the role of hemohistiocytes and hemohistioblasts in normal hematopoiesis is unknown, and it has been suggested that under abnormal conditions such as leukemia they function as stem cells.

In the case of reticulum cells, names that have been given to different forms of these cells correspond to alterations in their cytoplasm. For example, phagocytes may be reticulum cells that have assumed phagocytic capacities and in which the cytoplasm contains cellular debris. Similarly, "histiocytes" may represent reticulum cells in which the cytoplasm has become voluminous and contains numerous vacuoles. Since these vacuoles are usually phagocytic vacuoles, phagocytes and histiocytes are probably the same cell, and it may be impossible to distinguish between them.

Reticulum Cells. These cells have an oval nucleus with delicate, poorly defined chromatin strands and a single indistinct nucleolus. Cytoplasm of reticulum cells is abundant and often stellate in configuration. It stains pale gray, is usually devoid of inclusions, and often contains vacuoles (Figs. 4–32 and 4–33).

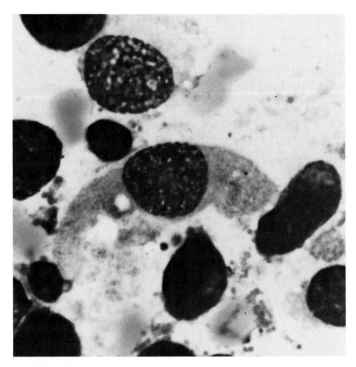

Figure 4–32   *Normal reticulum cell.*

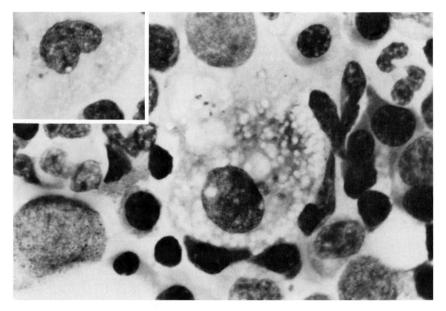

Figure 4–33   *Normal reticulum cells.*

Phagocytes. These cells are also called macrophages. They have a delicately fenestrated oval-shaped nucleus like a reticulum cell and abundant vacuolated cytoplasm that frequently contains cytoplasmic and nuclear debris of ingested cells (Figs. 4–34 through 4–36).

In some phagocytes, particularly in untreated deficiency of vitamin B_{12} or folate, Di Guglielmo syndrome, monocytic leukemia, malignant histiocytosis, and thrombotic thrombocytopenic purpura, phagocytosis of mature erythrocytes and degenerating erythroblasts is often prominent (Fig. 4–37). Increased numbers of phagocytes are also found in angioimmunoblastic lymphadenopathy (Fig. 4–38) and in Burkitt's lymphoma (Fig. 4–39).

(Text continued on page 208)

Figure 4–34   *Phagocytes containing debris, septicemia.*

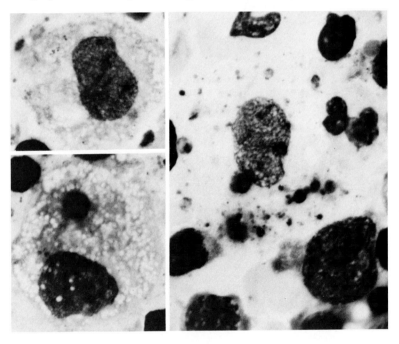

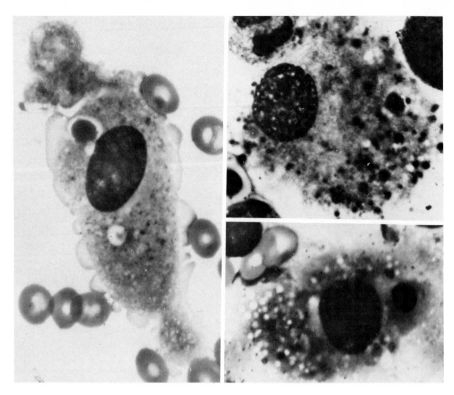

Figure 4–35 *Large phagocytes from patients with monocytic leukemia. Some show erythrocytophagy.*

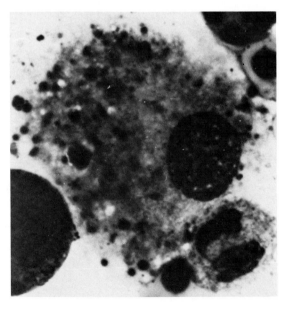

Figure 4–36 *Large phagocyte containing debris, septicemia.*

206

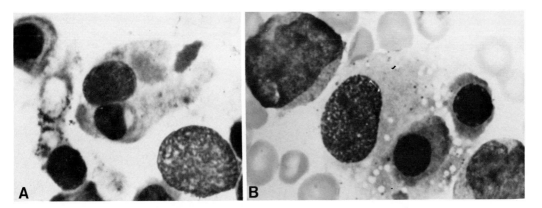

Figure 4–37   *Erythrocytophagy of mature erythrocytes and erythroblasts in pernicious anemia* (A) *and in monocytic leukemia* (B).

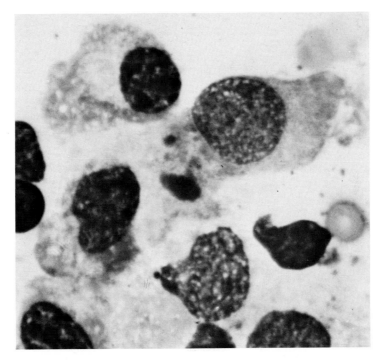

Figure 4–38   *Reticulum cell, angioimmunoblastic lymphadenopathy.*

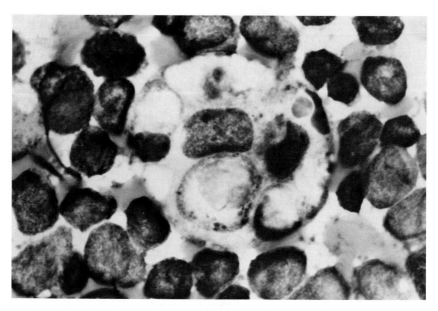

Figure 4–39   *Large phagocyte containing nuclear and cytoplasmic debris, Burkitt's lymphoma.*

Hemohistioblasts. Hemohistioblasts are large cells that have coarse magenta-staining nuclear chromatin strands. One of two light blue–staining nucleoli are found, and the cytoplasm is basophilic and devoid of inclusions (Fig. 4–40). Increased numbers of hemohistioblasts are found in marrows of patients with Di Guglielmo syndrome (Fig. 4–41) and in acute lymphoblastic and nonlymphoblastic leukemia.

Hemohistiocytes. These primitive cells have elongated or oval nuclei with the nuclear characteristics of hemohistioblasts. Cytoplasm is richly abundant with stellate configurations and contains numerous nonspecific granules and fibrillar structures of unknown type (Fig. 4–42). Increased numbers of hemohistioblasts, hemohistiocytes, reticulum cells, and phagocytes are seen in a wide variety of disorders such as septicemia (Fig. 4–43), chronic anemias, chronic renal failure, mycobacterial infections, thrombotic thrombocytopenic purpura, and especially acute leukemias. Using esterase reactions, specific esterase activity has been detected in hemohistiocytes and hemohistioblasts, suggesting that they may be cells of granulocytic origin (Fig. 4–44). In nonlymphoblastic leukemias, proliferation of

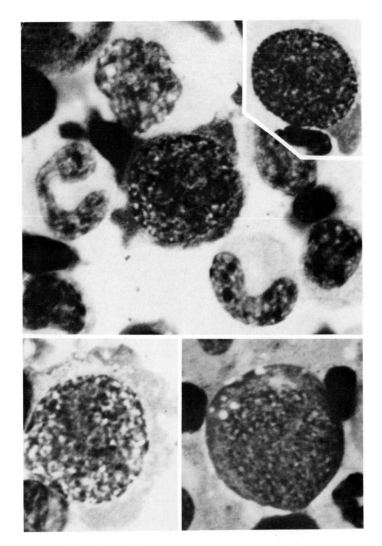

Figure 4–40   *Normal hemohistioblasts.*

these primitive cells is substantially greater than that seen in lymphoblastic leukemias. In monocytic leukemia and its variants, proliferation of these primitive marrow cells is often striking.

Sometimes in myeloproliferative disorders and myelomonocytic leukemia, hemohistiocytes demonstrate eosinophilic or neutrophilic granulation (Fig. 4–45). These granules are large and stain intensely. Specific granules in these presumed primitive cells suggest that they have differentiated along specific cell lines.

(Text continued on page 212)

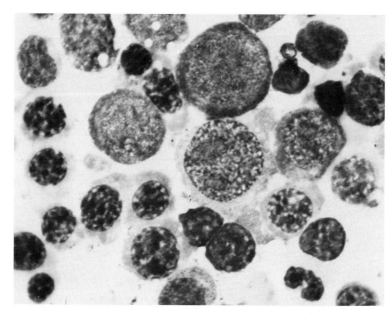

Figure 4–41   *Large hemohistioblast in the marrow of a patient with autoimmune hemolytic anemia. Increased numbers of normoblasts and proerythroblasts are shown.*

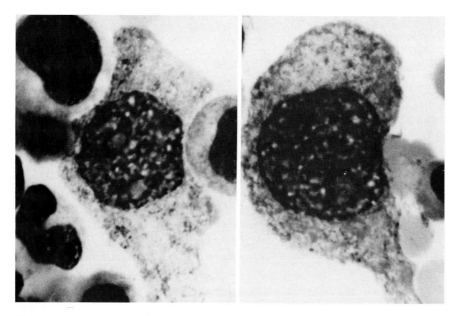

Figure 4–42   *Normal hemohistiocytes.*

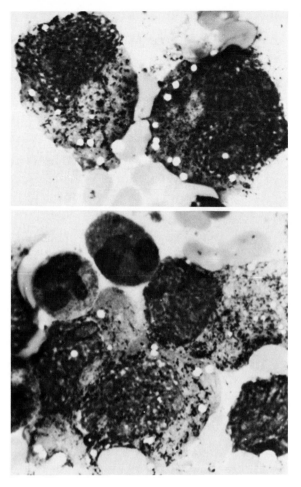

Figure 4–43   *Increased numbers of hemohistiocytes in septicemia.*

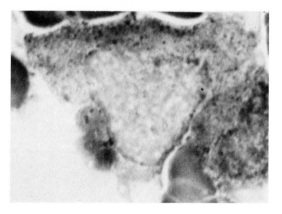

Figure 4–44   *Black punctate specific esterase activity in normal hemohistiocyte, naphthol ASD-chloroacetate and fast blue BBN.*

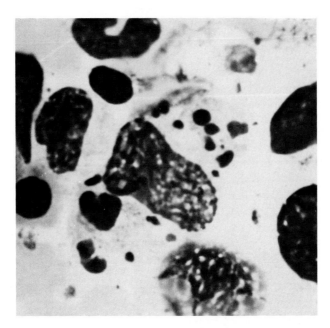

Figure 4–45   *Hemohistiocyte containing large prominent basophilic and eosinophilic granules, monocytic leukemia.*

Disorders of Histiocytic Cells

Malignant Histiocytosis. Malignant histiocytosis is characterized by hepatosplenomegaly, lymphadenopathy, fever, and proliferation of neoplastic histiocytes in lymph nodes and visceral organs. Marrow involvement by malignant histiocytes is rare. Typically, histiocytes have irregular nuclear membranes with prominent nucleoli and show phagocytosis of mature erythrocytes. Erythrocytophagy is believed to be an important diagnostic feature and helps to distinguish malignant histiocytosis from histiocytosis X in which phagocytes appear typical and do not demonstrate erythrocytophagy. Proliferation of histiocytes is usually within sinusoids of lymph nodes and red pulp and sinusoids of the spleen. In advanced stages, lymph node architecture is obliterated by histiocytic proliferation.

Histiocytosis X. A spectrum of histiocytic disorders, histiocytosis X includes Letterer-Siwe disease, Hand-Schüller-Christian disease, and eosinophilic granuloma. More recently, these closely related entities have been united under the term *histiocytosis X*, since it is often difficult to distinguish between them on pathologic grounds. Marrows from patients with histiocytosis X show proliferation of benign-appearing histiocytes (Fig. 4–46). Some of these cells are multinuclear and gigantic (Fig. 4–47). Erythrocytophagy is usually not observed. Eosinophils are increased in number and in some instances form dense aggregates (Fig. 4–47).

Figure 4–46   *Histiocytosis X. (A) Low-power view of marrow, demonstrating eosinophilia and increased numbers of histiocytes. (B) Similar cells are shown in the higher-power view.*

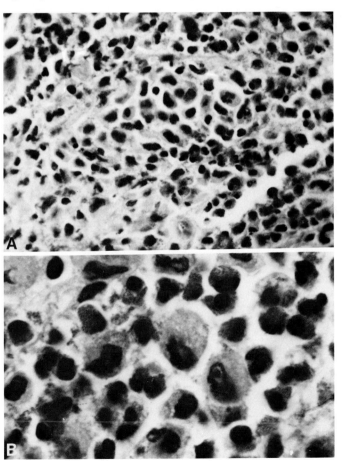

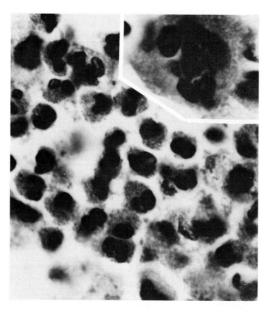

Figure 4–47   *Histiocytosis X, showing increased numbers of eosinophils and giant multinuclear histiocyte* (inset).

Gaucher's Disease. Gaucher's disease is an inherited disorder in which deficiency of lysosomal glucocerebrosidase leads to accumulation of glucocerebroside. Clinically, hepatomegaly and splenomegaly are found. Hematologically, pancytopenia usually occurs. In Gaucher's disease, marrows contain increased numbers of histiocytes filled with glucocerebroside. These histiocytes may occur singly or in clusters and in some instances replace most of the normal marrow cells. Gaucher cells have an eccentric nucleus with an irregular nuclear membrane. Cytoplasm shows a typical crinkled appearance, as though the cell were filled with needlelike structures (Fig. 4–48*A*). With panoptic stains, Gaucher cells stain light blue. Cells that are morphologically indistinguishable from Gaucher cells have been identified in the marrows taken from patients with thalassemia and chronic granulocytic leukemia (Fig. 4–48*B*). In H and E–stained sections of bone marrow biopsies, Gaucher cells have abundant pale cytoplasm and a single nucleus. As in a Wright's-stained aspirate, Gaucher cells in a biopsy section have a fibrillar-appearing cytoplasm (Fig. 4–49).

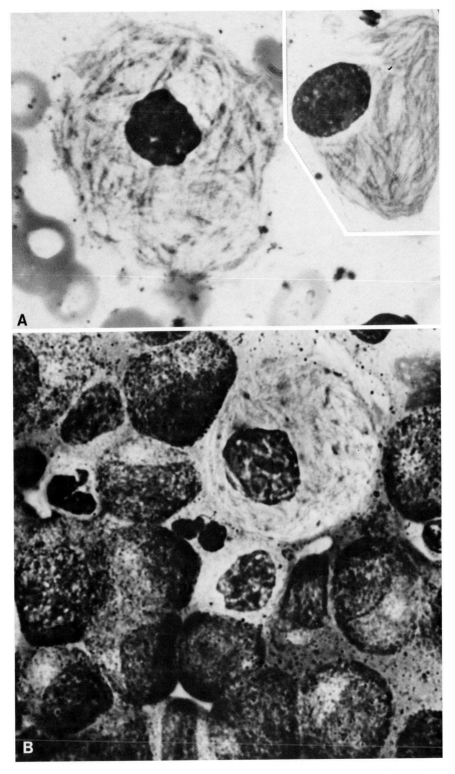

Figure 4–48   (A) *Gaucher cells from a patient with Gaucher's disease.* (B) *Gaucher-type cell in marrow from a patient with chronic granulocytic leukemia.*

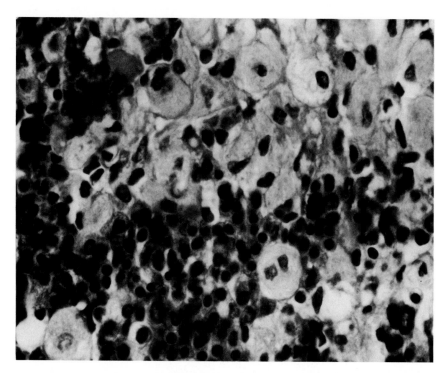

Figure 4–49   *H and E section of Gaucher cells in bone marrow biopsy.*

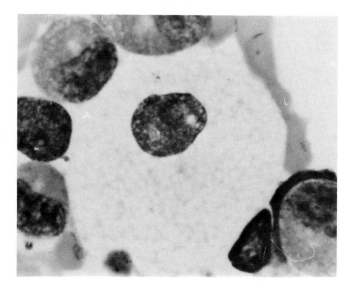

Figure 4–50   *Niemann-Pick cell.*

Niemann-Pick Disease. Niemann-Pick disease is an inherited disorder characterized by hepatomegaly, splenomegaly, mental retardation, and the occurrence in the bone marrow and visceral organs of large numbers of histiocytes filled with sphingomyelin. Niemann-Pick cells show multiple small vacuoles in the cytoplasm (Fig. 4–50). These vacuoles contain the characteristic sphingomyelin.

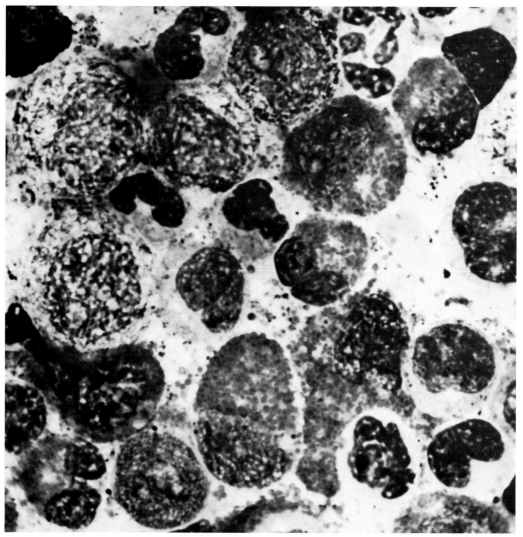

Increased numbers of eosinophil myelocytes, mature eosinophils, and promyelocytes with splinter-shaped granules from a patient with chronic granulocytic leukemia.

5   *Granulocytosis*

Granulocytic cells comprise approximately 50% to 60% of normal marrow cells. On the basis of characteristic staining properties, they have been classified into neutrophilic, eosinophilic, and basophilic types. Normally, maturation of granulocytes follows an orderly sequence, beginning with the myeloblast and culminating in the mature granulocyte. In all likelihood, granulocytic maturation is a continuum, and the names given to the various stages, such as promyelocyte and myelocyte, are probably arbitrary. Within this framework, one or more cell types representing different stages of maturation of granulocytes, such as myelocytes, metamyelocytes, or promyelocytes, can be increased with a corresponding decrease in cells at other stages of granulocytic maturation. Similarly, one or more cell types representing different aspects of granulocytic differentiation, such as eosinophils, basophils, or neutrophils, can be increased. In some instances, both the stage of maturation and the cell type are abnormal, as found in marrows that show increased numbers of basophilic myelocytes or eosinophilic metamyelocytes.

Myeloblast. The myeloblast is the earliest, recognizable granulocytic precursor (Fig. 5–1). In normal marrows it is a small cell, comprising less than 1% of the normal marrow differential cell count. Nuclear chromatin is finely attenuated, and chromatin strands are closely approximated. Nuclear striped chromatin patterns seen in lymphoid cells and leukemic lymphoblasts are not observed in normal or leukemic myeloblasts. Chromatin aggregates are rare in myeloblasts, and they are small when they do occur. Several inconspicuous

Figure 5–1   *Normal myeloblast.*

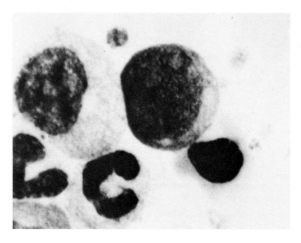

nucleoli are present in normal myeloblasts, and cytoplasm is scant, basophilic, and devoid of inclusions.

Promyelocyte. The promyelocyte is a large granulocyte. It contains a large nucleus that usually has one or more prominent nucleoli with perinucleolar condensation of chromatin (Fig. 5–2). Cytoplasm is lightly basophilic in some cells and deeply basophilic in others. Granulation is nonspecific and stains magenta to purple. Granules are usually small and round and may be numerous or sparse. Some promyelocytes have monocytoid foldings and convolutions of the

Figure 5–2   *Normal promyelocytes.*

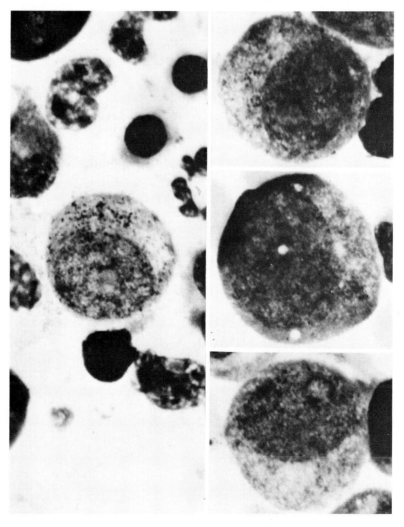

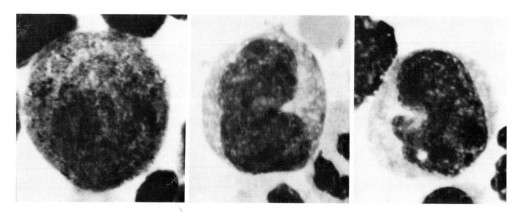

Figure 5–3   *Monocytoid changes in the nuclei of promyelocytes.*

nucleus (Fig. 5–3). These cells may be progenitors of monocytes in the bone marrow.

Myelocyte. In the myelocytic stage of granulocytic development, the nucleus occupies approximately half of the volume of the cell. Nuclear chromatin shows numerous aggregates that are connected to each other by thin and coarse strands of chromatin (Fig. 5–4). Cytoplasm is lightly eosinophilic, and granules have attained specificity of neutrophilic, eosinophilic, or basophilic types.

Figure 5–4   *Normal myelocytes.*

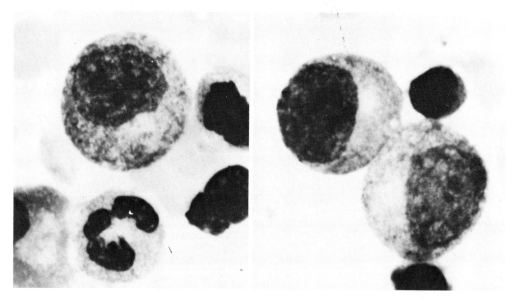

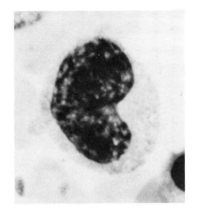

Figure 5–5 *Normal metamyelocyte.*

Metamyelocyte. The nucleus of a metamyelocyte shows indentation and occupies approximately one third of the cell (Fig. 5–5). Granules show specificity according to cell type.

Band (Stab) Cell. The nucleus occupies approximately one fourth of the band cell (Fig. 5–6).

Figure 5–6 *Normal band (stab) forms.*

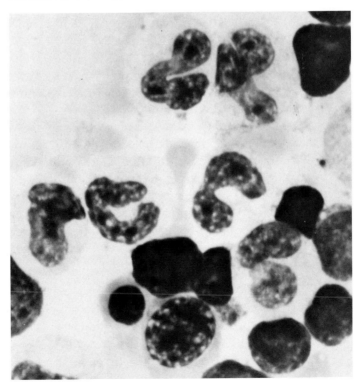

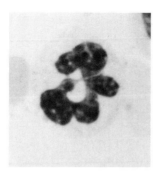

Figure 5–7   *Normal polymorphonuclear leukocyte.*

Segmented Mature Granulocyte. Segments of the nuclei of polymorphonuclear leukocytes, eosinophils, and basophils are connected by thin, single filaments of chromatin in normal circumstances. Usually, eosinophils and basophils have two nuclear lobes. Neutrophils have two to four nuclear lobes (Fig. 5–7).

Granulocytic Hyperplasia

Neutrophilic Granulocytic Hyperplasia. Increased numbers of neutrophilic granulocytes are seen in a variety of disorders. Increased numbers of promyelocytes are observed in patients who have infections, leukemoid reactions (Fig. 5–8), carcinoma, septicemia, and partial interference with further granulocytic maturation as a result of exposure to various drugs (Fig. 5–9). Increased numbers of myelocytes are observed in the same conditions (Fig. 5–10). Increased numbers of metamyelocytes also occur in deficiency of vitamin B_{12} or folate, in septicemia, and as a result of drug administration.

Characteristically, increased numbers of myelocytes and metamyelocytes and relatively few bands and mature segmented granulocytes are found in disorders in which there is an impediment to further maturation of the granulocytes. Typically, this hyperplasia of cell types up to and including the metamyelocyte-band stage of development is seen in Felty's syndrome and after exposure to various medications (Fig. 5–11). Increased numbers of band forms and mature segmented granulocytes are seen in septicemia and leukemoid reactions due to various causes (Fig. 5–12).

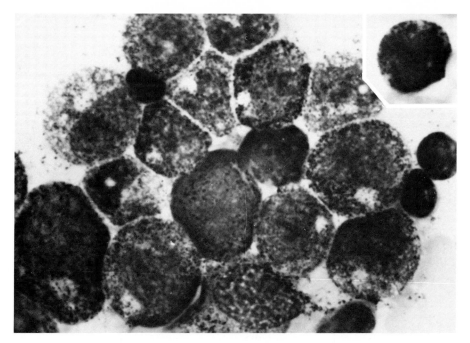

Figure 5–8   *Increased numbers of promyelocytes, leukemoid reaction. These cells show intensely staining or toxic-type granules. Inset shows large basophil.*

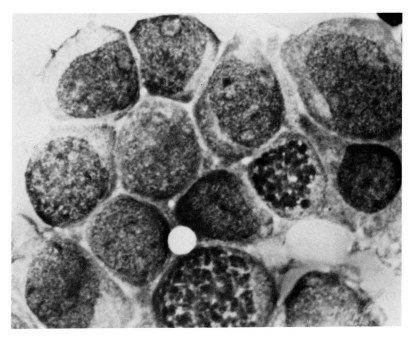

Figure 5–9   *Increased numbers of promyelocytes, drug sensitivity. There is little if any maturation beyond the promyelocyte stage.*

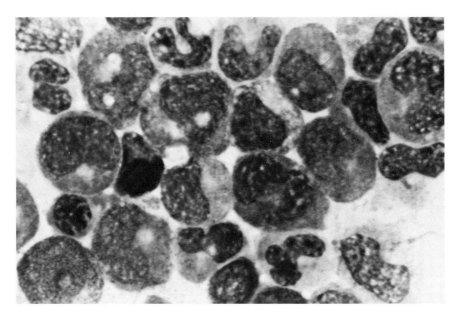

Figure 5–10   *Increased numbers of myelocytes, leukemoid reaction.*

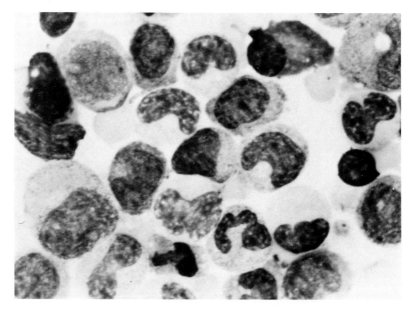

Figure 5–11   *Increased numbers of myelocytes and metamyelocytes with few mature polymorphonuclear leukocytes, Felty's syndrome.*

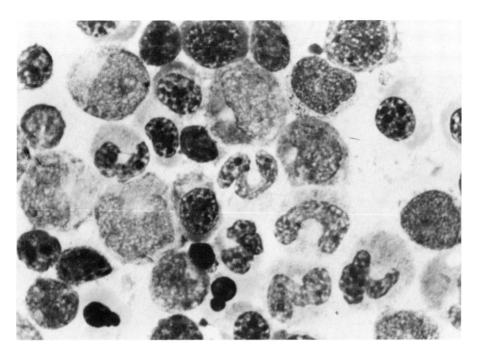

Figure 5–12 *Increased numbers of myelocytes, metamyelocytes, and band forms, leukemoid reaction due to septicemia.*

Eosinophila. Increased numbers of eosinophils, particularly myelocytes, metamyelocytes, and mature eosinophils, are found in numerous disorders. They include the hypereosinophilic syndromes comprising Löffler's syndrome (Fig. 5–13), eosinophilic collagenosis and eosinophilic variant of chronic granulocytic leukemia, Hodgkin's disease, lymphocytic lymphoma, pernicious anemia, refractory anemia with excess blasts (Fig. 5–14), agnogenic myeloid metaplasia, myeloproliferative disorders including Di Guglielmo syndrome, chronic granulocytic leukemia, polycythemia vera, acute myeloblastic and myelomonocytic leukemia (Fig. 5–15A), parasitic infestations, Addison's disease, allergic disorders, collagen diseases such as polyarteritis nodosa (Fig. 5–15B), subacute myelomonocytic leukemia (Fig. 5–16), and after exposure to various medications such as semisynthetic penicillins.

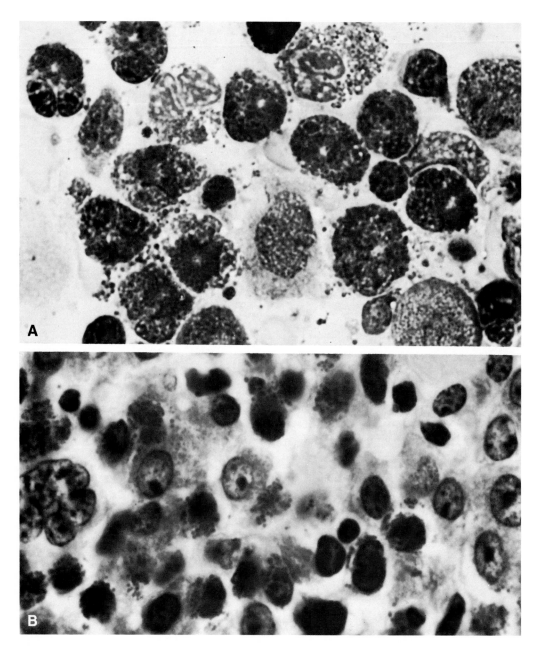

Figure 5–13   *Eosinophilia of marrow, Löffler's syndrome. (A) Wright's-stained marrow aspirate. (B) H- and E-stained section of marrow biopsy.*

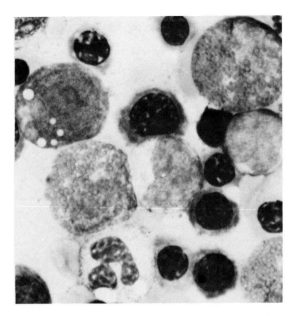

Figure 5–14   *Eosinophilia of marrow, refractory anemia with excess blasts.*

In rare patients with increased eosinophils in the marrow, typical Charcot-Leyden crystals can be found in macrophages in the marrow. These needlelike crystals are believed to be composed of degenerative products of eosinophil granules (Fig. 5–17). Cytochemically, the granules of eosinophils contain peroxidase activity that is resistant to inhibition by cyanide.

Basophilia. Increased numbers of basophils are found in myeloproliferative disorders such as agnogenic myeloid metaplasia, chronic granulocytic leukemia, myelodysplastic disorders such as "preleukemia" and refractory anemia with excess blasts, and polycythemia vera. Basophils are also increased in bone marrows from patients with Di Guglielmo syndrome and in patients with basophilic leukemia (see Fig. 5–53; Plate 3D). In erythroleukemia and in the M4 variant of acute myeloblastic leukemia in which increased numbers of eosinophils occur, large atypical-appearing myelocytes can contain both eosinophilic and basophilic granulation in the same cell, reflecting its disordered maturation. Cytochemically, basophils are peroxidase negative and stain metachromatically with toluidine blue and alcian blue.

(Text continued on page 233)

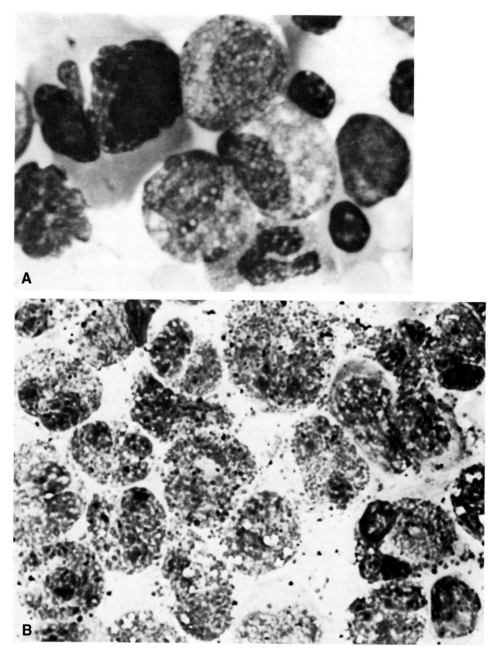

Figure 5–15   (A) *Eosinophilia of marrow, acute myelomonocytic leukemia.* (B) *Increased numbers of eosinophils from bone marrow of a patient with polyarteritis nodosa.*

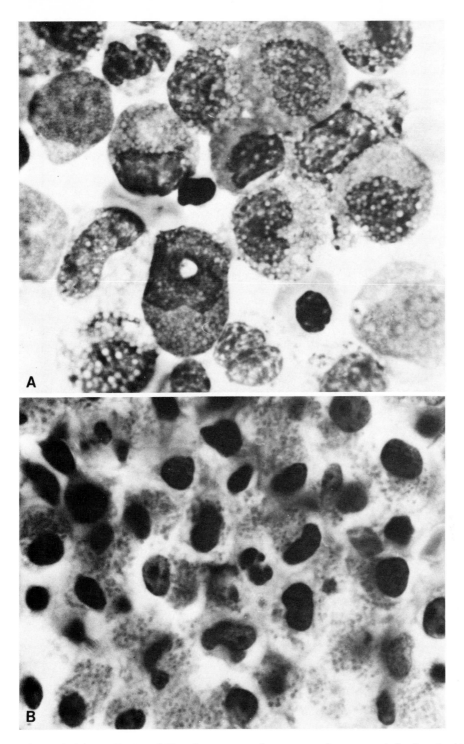

Figure 5–16   *Eosinophilia of marrow, subacute myelomonocytic leukemia. (A) Increased numbers of eosinophil myelocytes. (B) Increased numbers of eosinophils in H and E section of biopsy.*

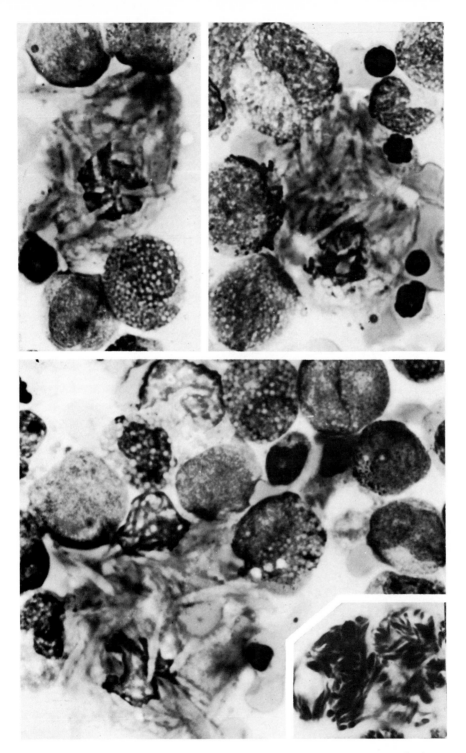

Figure 5–17   Charcot-Leyden crystals in macrophages, monocytic leukemia. Increased numbers of eosinophils are also depicted. Presumably, the crystals arise from degradation products of eosinophil granules. Bottom right inset shows Charcot-Leyden crystals stained with methenamine silver.

Mastocytosis. Increased numbers of mast cells are found in patients with systemic mast cell disease. In these patients, levels of circulating histamine are elevated. Presumably, histamine originates in granules of mast cells and basophils. Granules of mast cells stain metachromatically with toluidine blue, probably indicating their content of highly charged compounds like heparin. With the use of routine aqueous fixatives, granules of basophils and mast cells undergo dissolution. Consequently, for optimal demonstration with Giemsa stain or with toluidine blue, mast cells must be fixed in organic fixatives such as formalin for brief periods of time prior to staining. Increased numbers of mast cells along with increased numbers of lymphocytes and plasma cells are found in marrows of some patients with aplastic anemia and in patients with Waldenström's macroglobulinemia.

Abnormalities of Granulocytic Cells

Various types of nuclear and cytoplasmic abnormalities have been described in cells of granulocytic origin. In many instances, these abnormalities in conjunction with abnormalities in other cell lines have been of diagnostic importance.

Nuclear Abnormalities

Leukemic Myeloblast. Leukemic myeloblasts are of two morphologic types. Large leukemic myeloblasts have delicate chromatin strands that are closely approximated, and chromatin aggregates are rare (Fig. 5–18). Nucleoli are often multiple and prominent in leukemic myeloblasts and demonstrate perinucleolar condensation of chromatin. Nuclei are usually round. In some leukemic myeloblasts, nuclei have folds and indentations (Fig. 5–19). Small leukemic myeloblasts demonstrate chromatin aggregates that are larger and more numerous than in large leukemic myeloblasts. Small myeloblasts are believed to be in a dormant or nonproliferating phase and are found more often in smoldering acute leukemia than in acute myeloblastic leukemia. Superficially, small myeloblasts resemble intermediate-sized lymphocytes. Accordingly, assessment of the morphologic type of acute leukemia should be based on cells that are large, well spread, well fixed, and well stained to minimize confusion.

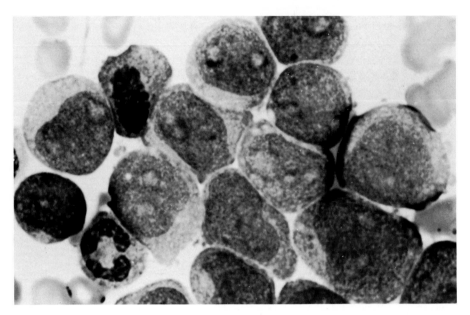

Figure 5–18   *Leukemic myeloblasts, acute myeloblastic leukemia.*

Hyposegmentation of the Nucleus (Pelger-Huët Anomaly). In mature polymorphonuclear leukocytes in the Pelger-Huët anomaly, nuclear segmentation fails to occur to the same extent as in normal polymorphonuclear leukocytes. In Pelger-Huët cells, nuclear lobulations usually do not number more than two and are connected by a thin filament of chromatin. In some of these cells, the nuclei fail to show any segmentation. Nuclear chromatin also demonstrates increased number and size of chromatin aggregates. Similar abnormalities of nuclear chromatin in the form of blocklike aggregates are also found in monocytes in the Pelger-Huët anomaly.

Cells resembling those in the Pelger-Huët anomaly are found in patients who have myeloproliferative disorders such as agnogenic myeloid metaplasia, polycythemia vera, myeloblastic and myelomonocytic leukemia, and preleukemic disorders including Di Guglielmo syndrome and refractory anemia with excess blasts (Fig. 5–20). In these circumstances, the nuclear anomaly has been called pseudo Pelger-Huët to distinguish it from the heredofamilial variety. In patients with refractory macrocytic anemia (Di Guglielmo syndrome) who have the pseudo Pelger-Huët anomaly, the likelihood of evolution of the anemia into acute leukemia is believed to be especially high.

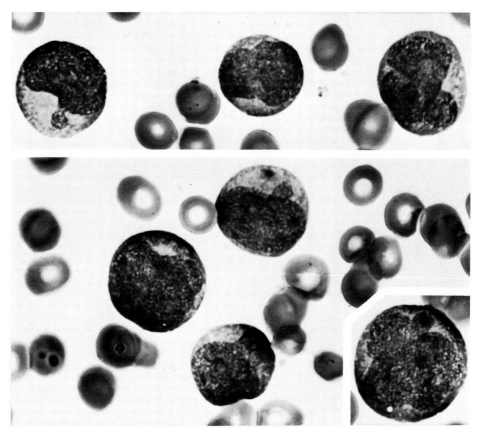

Figure 5–19   *Leukemic myeloblasts, showing irregular nuclear contours and nuclear folding.*

Figure 5–20   *Pseudo Pelger-Huët anomaly in a neutrophil, refractory anemia with excess blasts.*

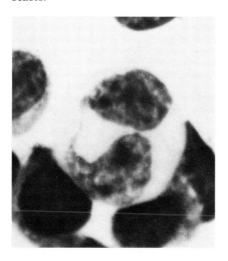

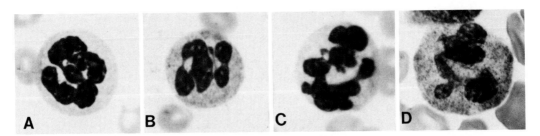

Figure 5–21   *Hypersegmented polymorphonuclear leukocytes from patients with myelomonocytic leukemia (A and B) and pernicious anemia (C and D).*

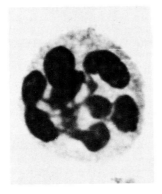

Figure 5–22   *Giant hypersegmented polymorphonuclear leukocyte with multiple connections between nuclear lobulations, pernicious anemia.*

Hypersegmentation of the Nucleus. Increased numbers of nuclear lobulations, especially greater than four lobules connected by thin filaments of chromatin, occur in untreated deficiency of vitamin B_{12} or folate and in myeloproliferative disorders, especially myeloblastic or myelomonocytic leukemia (Fig. 5–21). In untreated deficiency of vitamin B_{12} or folate, adjacent nuclear lobulations are often connected by multiple delicate filaments of chromatin (Fig. 5–22).

Gigantism. Giant granulocytic cells are found particularly in untreated deficiency of vitamin B_{12} and/or folate and in myeloproliferative disorders (Fig. 5–23). Gigantism is especially noticeable in the metamyelocyte stage of development and is also found in band and mature granulocytic stages. Giant promyelocytes and myelocytes are seen in myeloproliferative disorders including acute non-lymphoblastic leukemia and preleukemia.

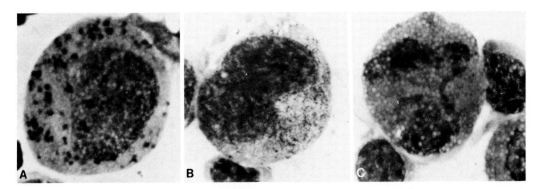

Figure 5–23   *Giant, bizarre-appearing promyelocytes with prominent granulation. (A) Erythroleukemia. (B) Promyelocytic leukemia. (C) Monocytic leukemia.*

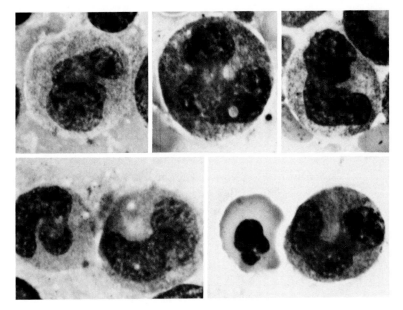

Figure 5–24   *Bulbous nuclear ends in metamyelocytes, pernicious anemia.*

Bulbous Ends of Nucleus. In metamyelocytes from patients with untreated deficiency of vitamin B_{12} and/or folate, and to a lesser degree in myeloproliferative disorders, nuclei of metamyelocytes may have prominent bulbous ends of the nucleus (Fig. 5–24). In some of these cells, one end of the nucleus exhibits a large bulbous configuration, whereas the other end of the nucleus appears smaller and less bulbous. In some instances, there are focal constrictions between the ends of the nucleus. These constrictions usually occur in the middle of the nucleus but can also occur at the base of the bulbous end of the nucleus.

Nucleus With Squared Corners and Focal Constrictions at Right-Angle Bends of the Nucleus. In metamyelocytes from patients with untreated deficiency of vitamin B_{12} or folate, nuclei appear square shaped along their inner curvature, and there are focal constrictions at the right-angle bends of the nucleus (Fig. 5–25).

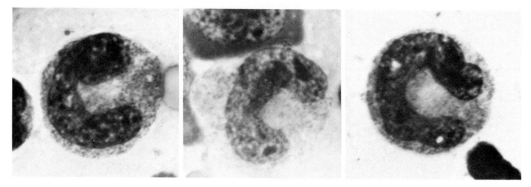

Figure 5–25   *Square-appearing inner curvature of the nucleus with focal constrictions at right-angle bends, metamyelocytes, pernicious anemia.*

Sigma- or "E"-Shaped Nucleus. In patients with deficiency of vitamin B_{12} and/or folate, and to a lesser extent in myeloproliferative disorders, some giant metamyelocytes demonstrate nuclear configurations in the shape of a sigma or letter E (Fig. 5–26). In this configuration, the central portion of the nucleus contains a fingerlike protrusion, imparting the appearance of the letter E to the nucleus.

Serpentine Nucleus. Nuclei with multiple convolutions, twistings, and loopings are seen in metamyelocytes and bands from patients with deficiency of vitamin B_{12} and/or folate and in some patients with myeloproliferative disorders (Fig. 5–27).

Monocytoid Changes. Lobulations of the nucleus resembling those seen in cells of monocytic origin and in monocytes are also observed in granulocytic cells, primarily in promyelocytes, myelocytes, and metamyelocytes, from patients with myeloproliferative disorders (Fig. 5–28). They are especially prominent in myelomonocytic leukemia and in preleukemic disorders, suggesting intimate relationships between monocytic and granulocytic cells in these conditions.

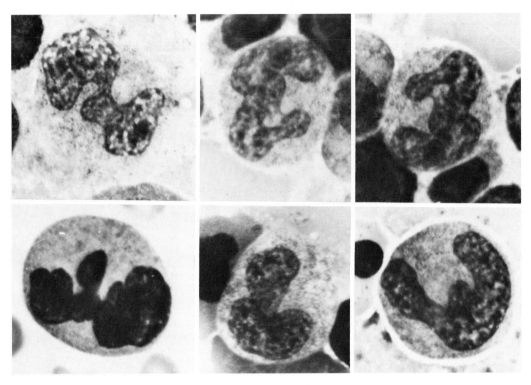

Figure 5–26   *Sigma- or "E"-shaped nucleus in metamyelocytes, pernicious anemia.*

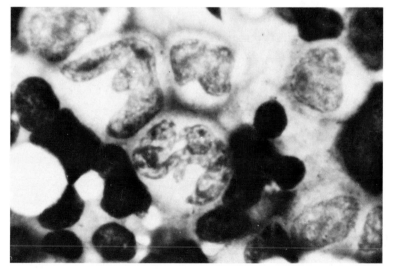

Figure 5–27   *Serpentine nucleus in metamyelocyte, pernicious anemia.*

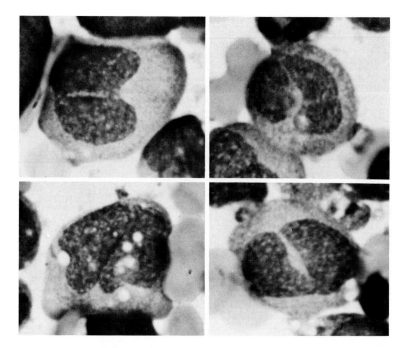

Figure 5–28   *Aberrant monocytoid-appearing nuclei in granulocytic cells from a patient with monocytic leukemia.*

Doughnut Hole. In this nuclear abnormality, a large hole or small multiple holes seem to occupy the central portion of the nucleus, imparting an open appearance to it (Fig. 5–29). Cells of this type are particularly frequent in myeloproliferative disorders such as myeloblastic leukemia.

Aberrant Mitotic Figures in Granulocytic Precursors. Unusual-appearing mitotic figures in early granulocytic cells are found in myeloproliferative disorders and in myeloblastic and myelomonocytic leukemia (Fig. 5–30). They constitute morphologic expressions of abnormalities of cellular division in neoplastic granulocytes.

Cytoplasmic Abnormalities

Auer Rod. Cytoplasm of leukemic myeloblasts may contain the distinctive Auer rod (Fig. 5–31). This brightly eosinophilic-staining inclusion is found in leukemic myeloblasts and never in leukemic lymphoblasts, making the structure a valuable marker for blasts of granulocytic origin. It is found in neoplastic monocytes from

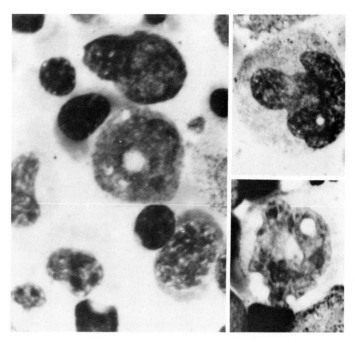

Figure 5–29   *Granulocytic percursors in monocytic leukemia and in pernicious anemia (insets), showing nuclear "hole."*

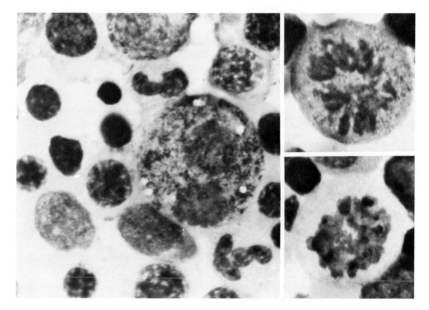

Figure 5–30   *Aberrant nitotic figures in granulocytic precursors, preleukemia.*

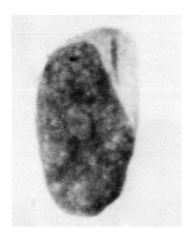

Figure 5–31   *Auer rod in leukemic myeloblast, acute myeloblastic leukemia.*

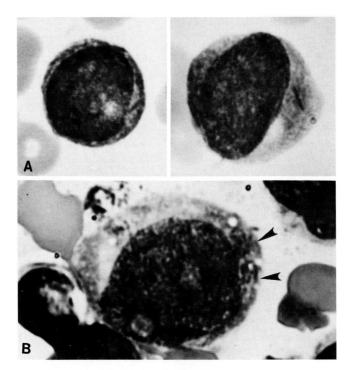

Figure 5–32   (A) *Leukemic blasts with prominent Auer rods in monocytic leukemia.* (B) *Leukemic myeloblast containing eosinophilic-staining structures in a concentric, laminated pattern* (arrows). *These may be precursors of Auer rods.*

patients with monocytic leukemia (Fig. 5–32*A*) and has also been described in leukemic promyelocytes and in neoplastic megakaryocytes. In some leukemic myeloblasts, thin orange-staining structures appear in a concentric laminated pattern (Fig. 5–32). These structures may be precursors of Auer rods. Multiple Auer rods can be found in the same cell. Auer rods are believed to be formed from coalescence of lysosomal membranes. In keeping with a lysosomal origin, Auer rods contain activities of peroxidase, acid phosphatase, and specific esterase.

Hypogranularity. Decreased numbers of granules in the cytoplasm of mature neutrophils are seen in patients with myeloproliferative disorders and particularly in preleukemic disorders of erythropoiesis such as Di Guglielmo syndrome, preleukemia, refractory anemia with excess blasts, and in myeloperoxidase deficiency. Decreased granularity leads to pale-appearing cytoplasm and reflects aberrations in the development and maturation of the cells (Fig. 5–33*A*).

Eosinophils from patients who have hypereosinophilic syndromes and from patients with myeloproliferative disorders often contain fewer granules than normal eosinophils (Fig. 5–33*B*). Also, granules in these abnormal eosinophils appear smaller and stain lighter than normal eosinophil granules (Fig. 5–33*B, lower left inset*). Cytochemically, granules in these cells contain cyanide-resistant peroxidase activity, as do normal eosinophils. Unlike normal eosinophils, granules in the abnormal cells often possess specific esterase activity (Fig. 5–33*B, lower right inset*).

Hypergranularity. Increased number and size of granules are observed in myeloproliferative disorders, acute infections and septicemia, and nonlymphoblastic leukemia (Fig. 5–34). When using panoptic stains, these prominent granules may also stain intensely, presumably due to their high content of alkaline phosphatase. In the Chédiak-Higashi syndrome, granules are unusually large and bizarre appearing. In the Alder-Reilly anomaly as seen in gargoylism, granules in leukocytes stain intensely and are numerous in the cytoplasm of cells.

Figure 5–33
(A) *Polymorphonuclear leukocytes with pale, hypogranular cytoplasm, refractory anemia with excess blasts. Inset shows neutrophil with pseudo Pelger-Huët abnormality and hypogranular cytoplasm. (B) Hypogranular eosinophils in marrow and peripheral blood (lower left inset) of patient with hypereosinophilic syndrome. Lower right inset shows specific esterase activity in these abnormal eosinophils, using naphthol ASD-chloroacetate and fast blue BBN.*

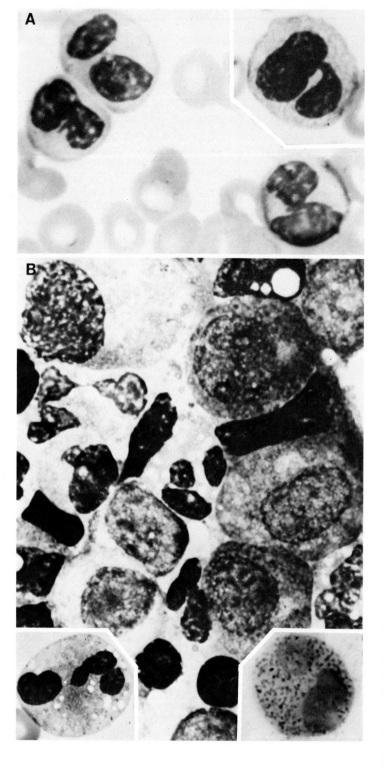

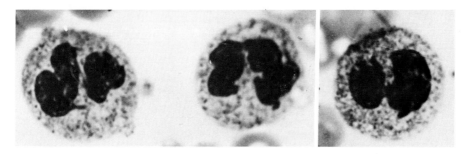

Figure 5–34 *Polymorphonuclear leukocytes with prominent (basophilic) granulation, septicemia.*

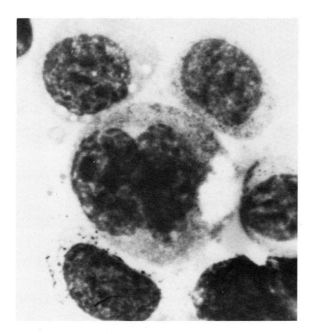

Figure 5–35 *Promyelocyte with large cytoplasmic vacuole.*

Cytoplasmic Vacuoles. Vacuolation of the cytoplasm of mature and immature granulocytic cells is seen in nonlymphoblastic leukemias and in toxic and metabolic disorders such as septicemia and ketoacidosis (Fig. 5–35). Presumably, vacuoles represent degenerative changes. In septicemia they also represent phagocytic structures. Some myeloblasts in myeloblastic leukemia also contain numerous cytoplasmic vacuoles.

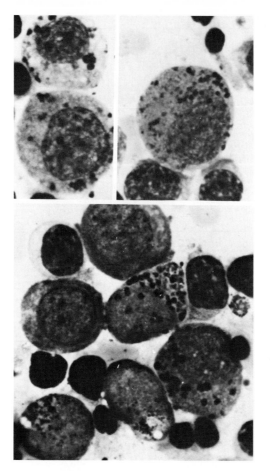

Figure 5–36   *Myelocytes and promyelocytes containing eosinophilic and basophilic granules, erythroleukemia.*

Disturbances in Granule Differentiation. Particularly in myeloproliferative disorders, promyelocytes, myelocytes, metamyelocytes, and hemohistiocytes contain both eosinophilic and basophilic granules within the same cell (Fig. 5–36). In these apparent hybridizations of two-cell types, granulation is usually intense and granules are unusually large. Cells of this type indicate disturbances in differentiation of granulocytic cells. They are found in monocytic leukemia and erythroleukemia as well as in myeloblastic leukemia and agnogenic myeloid metaplasia. Recently, myelocytes containing both eosinophilic and basophilic granules have been identified in bone marrows from patients with a variant form of acute myelomonocytic leukemia (M4), in conjunction with increased numbers of eosinophils and abnormalities of chromosome 16.

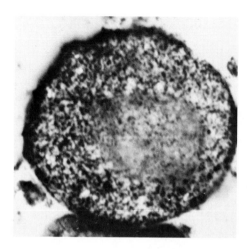

Figure 5–37   *Giant promyelocyte with large splinter-shaped granules, promyelocytic leukemia.*

Large Splinter-Shaped Granules. Large granules in splinter shape may be found in leukemic promyelocytes in myeloproliferative disorders and particularly in the promyelocytic variant of acute myeloblastic leukemia (Fig. 5–37).

Granulocytic Hyperplasia in Megaloblastic Anemia

In marrows from patients with untreated deficiency of vitamin B_{12} or folate, increased numbers of aberrant-appearing metamyelocytes and band forms occur. These cells are often gigantic, with unusual nuclear configurations (Fig. 5–38). Increased numbers of aberrant-appearing granulocytes can be found in patients who have minimal degrees of anemia. With increasing severity of the anemia, the number of metamyelocytes decreases and the number of proerythroblasts and megaloblasts increases. Gigantic metamyelocytes and bands resembling those found in untreated deficiency of vitamin B_{12} or folate can also occur in marrows from patients with untreated acute lymphoblastic or myeloblastic leukemia.

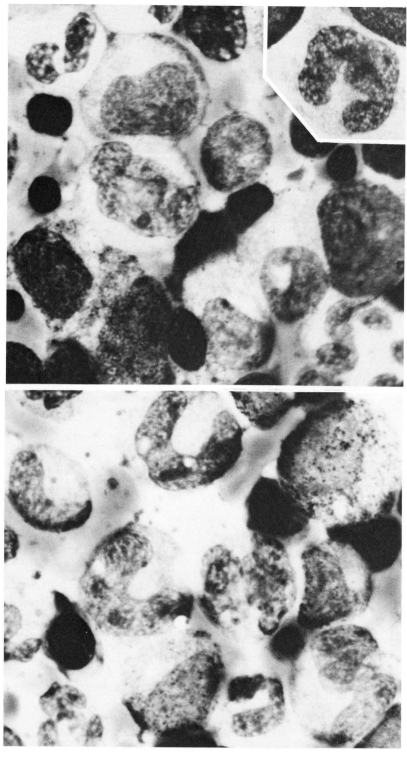

Figure 5–38 *Increased numbers of giant aberrant-appearing metamyelocytes, untreated pernicious anemia.*

Neoplastic Disorders of Granulocytes

Polycythemia Vera. Marrows from patients with polycythemia vera are hypercellular with increased numbers of granulocytic precursors, especially immature granulocytes, and increased numbers of erythroblasts and megakaryocytes. Increased numbers of erythroblasts help to distinguish this disorder from chronic granulocytic leukemia, in which hyperplasia of granulocytic cells predominates (Fig. 5–39).

Chronic Granulocytic Leukemia. Marrows from patients with chronic granulocytic leukemia are hypercellular with increased numbers of granulocytic cells and megakaryocytes (Fig. 5–*40A* and *B*). On H and E biopsy section, promyelocytes and myelocytes are increased (Fig. 5–41). Granulocytic development is normal, proceeding to the mature polymorphonuclear stage. Increased numbers of eosinophils and basophils are also seen (see Fig. 5–*40A* and Fig. 5–*41A*).

Erythropoiesis is usually decreased, and increased numbers of megakaryocytes are found (Fig. 5–41*B*). Megakaryocytes vary in size and shape. Some are large and contain multiple nuclear lobulations and richly granular cytoplasm, whereas others are small and appear as micromegakaryocytes.

It may be difficult to distinguish marrows from patients with leukemoid reactions due to septicemia and/or carcinoma from marrows from patients who have chronic granulocytic leukemia. In chronic granulocytic leukemia, megakaryocytic hyperplasia is prominent. Evaluation of the presence or absence of the Ph[1] chromosome and assessment of leukocyte alkaline phosphatase are useful in helping to distinguish between the two conditions.

Agnogenic Myeloid Metaplasia. In early stages, agnogenic myeloid metaplasia may have cellular phases alternating in some instances with hypoplasia. In the cellular areas, increased numbers of promyelocytes, myelocytes, and metamyelocytes are found, as well as increased numbers of megakaryocytes (Fig. 5–42). Megakaryocytic hyperplasia is often intense, and megakaryocytes are often of the micromegakaryocytic variety with abundant cytoplasmic granularity and few or no lobulations of the nucleus (Fig. 5–42). In many instances, these megakaryocytes occur in clusters and are particularly numerous in the central area of the marrow particle. In later stages, increased numbers of fibroblasts and dense bands of fibrous connective tissue replace the usual cellular composition of the bone marrow.

On H and E sections of biopsies from patients with agnogenic myeloid metaplasia, areas of hypercellularity often alternate with areas of dense fibrosis and megakaryocytic hyperplasia (Fig. 5–43). Areas of hypercellularity are composed largely of immature granulocytes such as promyelocytes (Fig. 5–43). In some instances, hypercellular areas represent proliferation of erythroblasts within marrow sinuses (Fig. 5–44). In many patients with agnogenic myeloid metaplasia, routine aspiration of bone marrow yields a dilute specimen containing only small clusters of erythroblasts and reticulum cells. Presumably, these cells have been dislodged from marrow sinuses during the process of marrow aspiration.

Megakaryocytes vary in size and shape. Some are large and multilobulated and others are small and contain few or no lobulations of the nucleus (Fig. 5–45). Cytoplasm is abundant and pink staining. Fibroblasts with elongated and oval nuclei show alignment along trabeculae of bone and along the sides of megakaryocytes. Areas of fibroblastic proliferation and collagen deposition are often most prominent in areas of megakaryocytic proliferation (see Figs. 5–43 and 5–45). With the use of reticulin stains, numerous reticulin fibers may be found in the marrows of patients with agnogenic myeloid metaplasia and to a lesser degree in marrows of patients with polycythemia vera. Collagen bands are numerous and dense in areas of fibrosis (Fig. 5–46).

(Text continued on page 261)

Figure 5–39   *Marrow, polycythemia vera. (A) Increased numbers of myelocytes,*
(opposite)   *metamyelocytes, and normoblasts. (B) H and E section of marrow biopsy,*
demonstrating large nuclei of granulocytic precursors and smaller, darkly
stained nuclei of normoblasts.

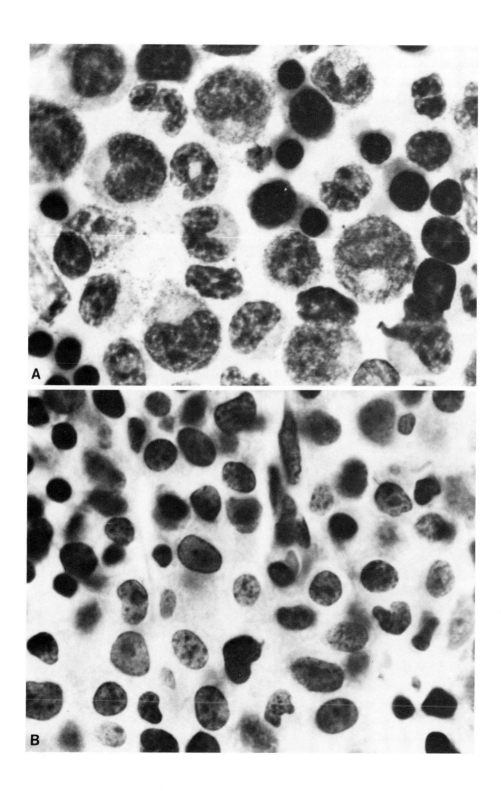

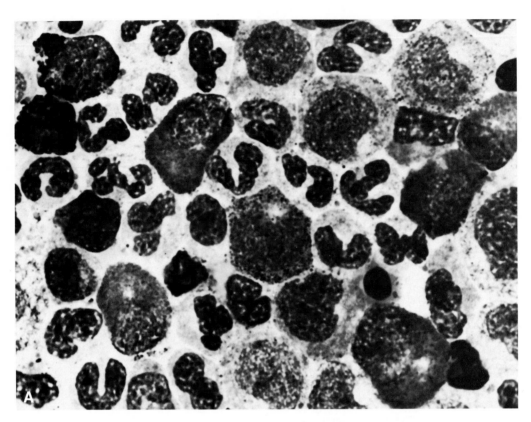

Figure 5–40
(opposite
and above)

(A) *Chronic granulocytic leukemia, demonstrating increased numbers of granulocytic cells at all maturational ages and increased numbers of eosinophils and basophils (upper left).* (B) *Chronic granulocytic leukemia, depicting increased numbers of eosinophils and basophils and promyelocytes with prominent granules. Upper left inset illustrates Gaucher-type cell as found in some cases of chronic granulocytic leukemia. Lower right inset shows two micromegakaryocytes with a single nucleus containing few or no lobulations and richly granular cytoplasm (megakaryocyte near bottom).*

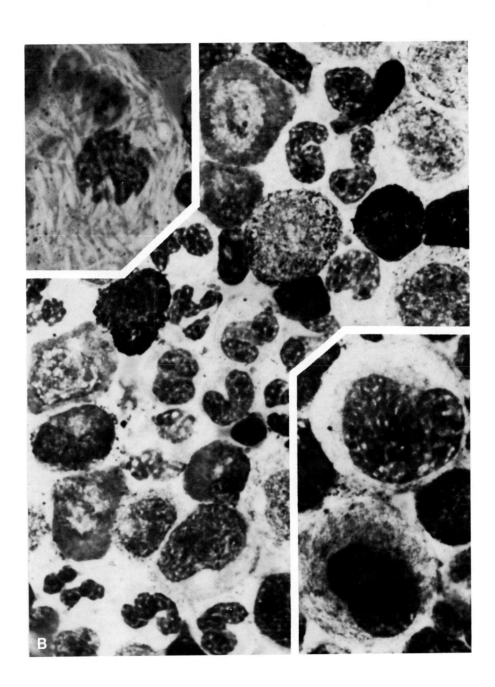

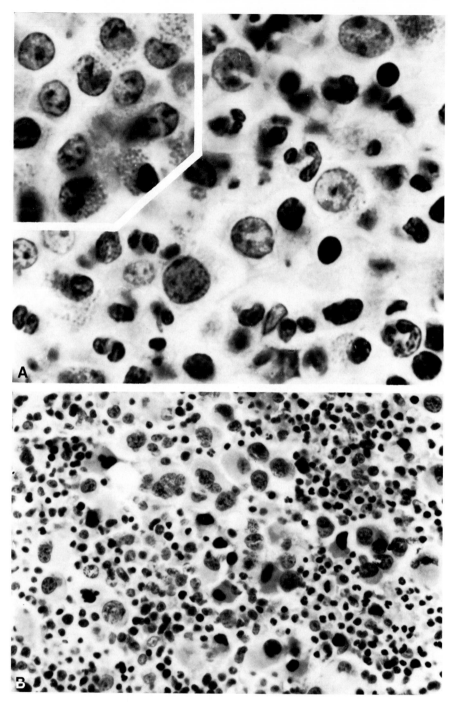

Figure 5–41   *Chronic granulocytic leukemia, H and E-stained section of marrow biopsy.*
(A) Large nuclei of promyelocytes are seen along with darkly stained nuclei
of erythroblasts. Inset at upper left shows increased numbers of eosinophils.
(B) Lower power view of bone marrow depicting a striking increase in
megakaryocytes of varying size and shape.

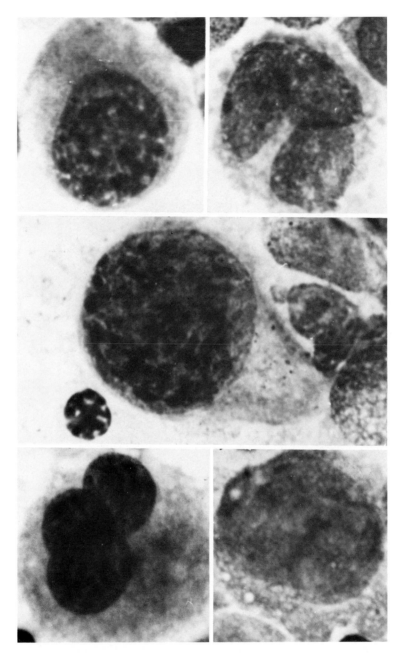

Figure 5–42   *Aberrant-appearing megakaryocytes with hypergranular cytoplasm,*
agnogenic myeloid metaplasia.

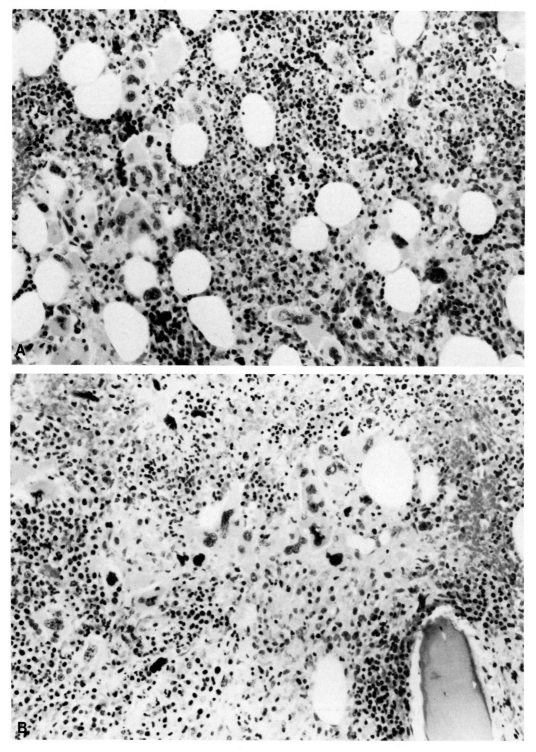

Figure 5–43   *Agnogenic myeloid metaplasia, demonstrating early or proliferative phase with megakaryocytosis and hypercellularity of the bone marrow (A) and later phase characterized by focal areas of megakaryocytes and fibrosis (B).*

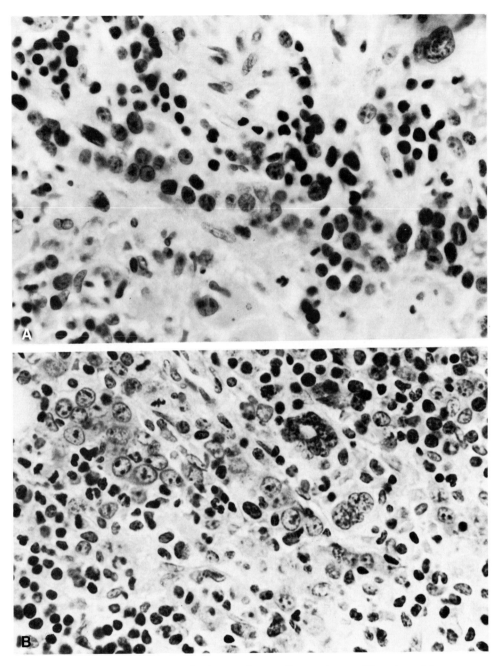

Figure 5–44 *Agnogenic myeloid metaplasia, illustrating proliferation of late intermediate normoblasts within the sinusoid (A) and sinusoidal proliferation of proerythroblasts (B).*

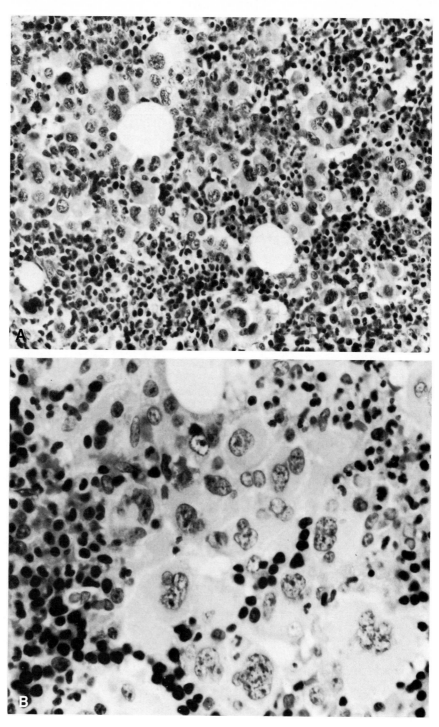

Figure 5–45 *Agnogenic myeloid metaplasia, demonstrating striking megakaryocytosis in a low-power view of the bone marrow H and E biopsy (A) and in a higher-power view (B). Megakaryocytes vary in size and shape and in the number of nuclear lobulations. In agnogenic myeloid metaplasia, megakaryocytes frequently occur in clusters.*

258

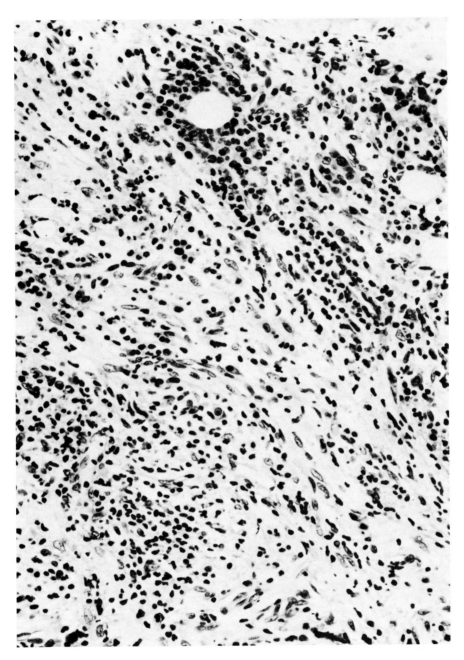

Figure 5–46   *Agnogenic myeloid metaplasia, demonstrating intense fibrosis of the bone marrow, numerous fibroblasts, and few focal areas of erythroblast proliferation.*

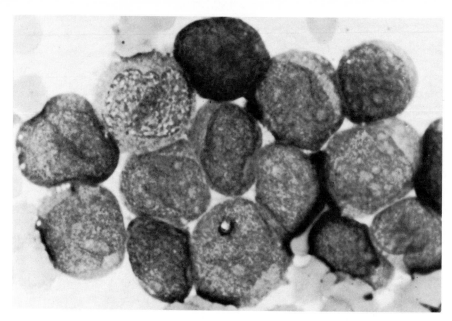

Figure 5–47   *Myeloblasts, acute myeloblastic leukemia, M1 variant. These cells are uniform in size and have one or more small nucleoli with perinucleolar condensation of chromatin and delicate-appearing chromatin strands that appear closely approximated. Cytoplasm in basophilic and devoid of granularity. There is little if any maturation beyond the myeloblast stage.*

Figure 5–48   *Acute myeloblastic leukemia, M1 variant, illustrating increased numbers of myeloblasts and foci of megaloblastoid intermediate macronormoblasts. Inset depicts a large, bizarre-appearing multinuclear erythroblast.*

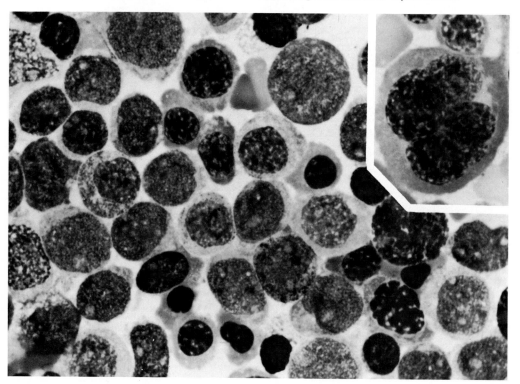

Acute Nonlymphoblastic Leukemia

Using the FAB (French-American-British) classification for the acute leukemias, acute myeloblastic leukemia is believed to occur in six forms. In the M1 form, myeloblasts are small, are uniform in size, and have a delicate nuclear chromatin pattern and small nucleoli. Cytoplasm is basophilic and contains a few granules that may be peroxidase positive (Figs. 5–47 and 5–48). In the M2 variant, differentiation beyond the promyelocyte stage can be observed. Leukemic myeloblasts in this variant show considerable pleomorphism, and some of the promyelocytes and metamyelocytes demonstrate abnormalities of nuclear size and shape. Nucleoli are prominent, and there may be perinucleolar condensations of chromatin. Cytoplasm of most of the immature cells is deeply basophilic, and the cytoplasm frequently contains peroxidase-positive granules (Fig. 5–49).

Figure 5–49   *Myeloblasts, acute myeloblastic leukemia, M2 variant. The marrow is hypercellular and contains large and small myeloblasts, as well as aberrant-appearing metamyelocytes with unusual nuclear configurations.*

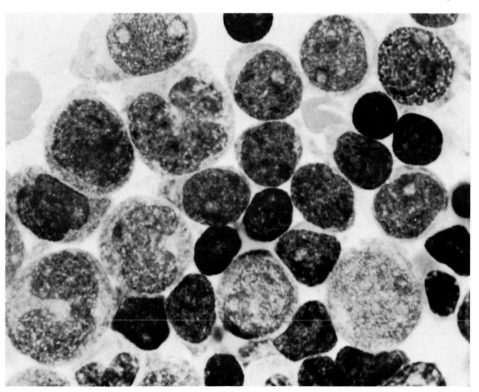

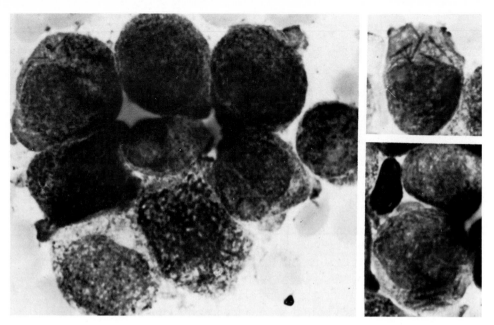

Figure 5–50   *Acute promyelocytic leukemia, M3 variant, showing leukemic promyelocytes containing one or more Auer rods. Sometimes, Auer rods are multiple and their configuration resembles a "stack of twigs" or a "bundle of hay."*

The M3 variant corresponds to promyelocytic leukemia (Fig. 5–50). Leukemic promyelocytes show round to oval nuclei, prominent nucleoli, and basophilic cytoplasm containing many coarse-appearing azurophilic granules. Often, multiple Auer rods in a "stack of twigs" configuration are seen. Some leukemic promyelocytes are gigantic. Hemorrhagic diathesis due to disseminated intravascular coagulation is thought to occur more frequently in the promyelocytic variant than in other variants of nonlymphoblastic leukemia. Presumably, profibrinolysin (plasminogen) is present in high concentrations in the granules of the leukemic promyelocytes. During treatment, disruption of these cells occurs, and with liberation of plasminogen, a hemorrhagic disorder may ensue.

As a subtype of the M3 variant, a microgranular promyelocytic leukemia has been described. Leukemic blasts in this condition demonstrate unusual nuclear convolutions and indentations, superficially resembling those found in monocytic leukemias. Blasts in the microgranular variant may contain numerous cytoplasmic granules, but multiple Auer rods as found in the typical promyelocytic variant are rare (Fig. 5–51 and Plate 3*B*).

Cytochemically, it is possible to distinguish the microgranular promyelocytic variant of acute promyelocytic leukemia from a more typical acute myelomonocytic leukemia. In microgranular promyelocytic leukemia, the peroxidase reaction is strongly positive and the

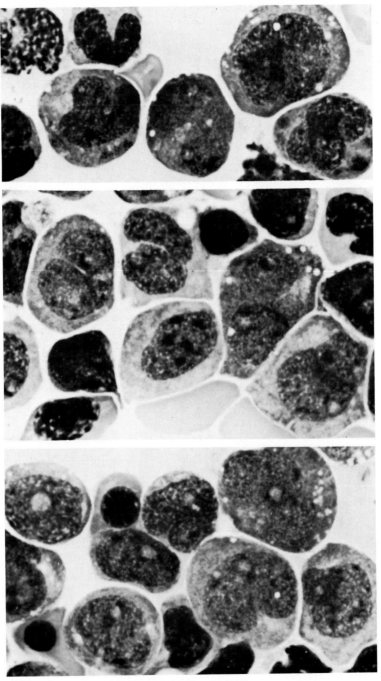

Figure 5–51   *Microgranular promyelocytic leukemia, depicting leukemic promyelocytes with monocytoid-appearing nuclei and abundant cytoplasm containing a few prominent granules and vacuoles. Although these cells may resemble leukemic monocytes superficially, they do not contain fluoride-sensitive nonspecific esterase as do monocytes. Furthermore, these cells exhibit activities of myeloperoxidase and specific esterase, indicating that they are of myeloblastic origin.*

reaction for nonspecific esterase activity is usually negative. In myelomonocytic leukemia, leukemic blasts are peroxidase negative and show strong activity of fluoride-sensitive nonspecific esterase. Because of the increased incidence of hemorrhagic complications in promyelocytic leukemia, it is important to identify the microgranular variant prior to treatment with antileukemic agents so that a hemorrhagic diathesis can be anticipated and treated accordingly if it should occur.

The M4 variant represents acute myelomonocytic leukemia (see Fig. 4–26). As a subtype of the M4 category, a myelomonocytic leukemia with increased numbers of eosinophils has been described (Fig. 5–52 and Plate 3C). This type of leukemia can be associated with abnormalities of chromosome 16. The M5 variant represents acute monocytic leukemia (see Fig. 4–27), or what may have been called acute histiomonocytic leukemia in older terminology. The M6 variant represents erythroleukemia (see Figs. 2–88 and 2–89).

In recent years, it has become appreciated that acute myeloblastic leukemia or its variants can occur as a terminal event in other hematologic disorders. These include paroxysmal nocturnal hemoglobinuria, agnogenic myeloid metaplasia with myelofibrosis, chronic granulocytic leukemia, Fanconi's syndrome, polycythemia vera, and multiple myeloma. In some instances, it appears that acute leukemia evolves terminally as a natural course of the disorder. In other instances, particularly multiple myeloma and Hodgkin's disease, leukemic transformation may be related in part to chemotherapy with alkylating agents.

Chemotherapy-related acute leukemia has been seen with increasing frequency in recent years. Generally, the drugs implicated most often as provoking agents in leukemic transformation include procarbazine, the nitrosureas, and alkylating agents. In patients with ovarian cancer treated with alkylating agents and in patients with Hodgkin's disease treated with chemotherapy and particularly with the combination of chemotherapy and radiation therapy, the likelihood of leukemic transformation as a terminal event is strikingly increased.

Morphologically, leukemic blasts from these acute leukemias that have evolved from a setting of another disorder treated with chemotherapy and/or radiation therapy have few if any morphologic criteria that distinguish them from acute myeloblastic or monocytic leukemia that seems to arise *de novo* (see Fig. 5–69). Cytochemically, leukemic blasts in these treatment-related acute leukemias usually contain little if any activities of the enzymes used traditionally to classify the acute leukemias. Accordingly, it may be difficult

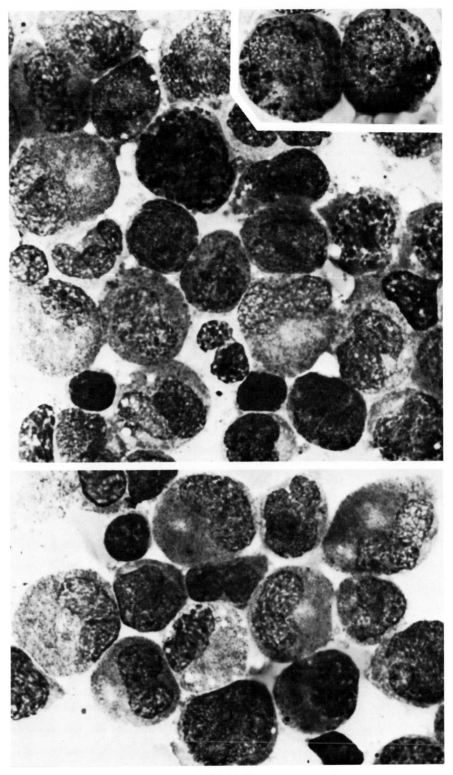

Figure 5–52   *Myelomonocytic leukemia, M4 variant, with increased eosinophils. Increased numbers of leukemic blasts and eosinophils are seen. Top and inset also illustrate leukemic cells containing both eosinophilic and basophilic granulation in the same cell.*

to classify these leukemias either morphologically or cytochemically. Clinically, acute leukemia arising as a secondary malignancy is usually resistant to the treatments available at the present time.

In most patients with chronic granulocytic leukemia who do not die of the disease or during treatment, a terminal leukemic blast phase ensues. Although this may be indolent in onset, in many persons it is heralded by fever, the appearance of immature cells in the blood, rising white blood cell count, and clinical deterioration. In some of these persons, cytogenetic studies of the marrow at the time of acute leukemic evolution reveal an abrupt chromosomal change, consistent with population of the marrow by a clone of neoplastic cells.

For many patients with chronic granulocytic leukemia, the terminal blast phase will be myeloblastic leukemia. In these instances, it may be indistinguishable from acute myeloblastic leukemia that seems to develop *de novo.* However, in some of these cases, the Philadelphia chromosome has been detected. This suggests that some patients with what seems to be *de novo* acute myeloblastic leukemia may have actually had undiagnosed chronic granulocytic leukemia for a brief period before the emergence of acute leukemia.

In other patients with chronic granulocytic leukemia, the leukemic blast phase may assume other morphologic forms. Some may have an erythroleukemic blast phase, in which the marrow shows typical erythroleukemia. In atypical cases of the erythroleukemic phase of chronic granulocytic leukemia, leukemic blasts may lack the usual morphologic and cytochemical features of erythroblasts. In these cases it may be possible to identify some "primitive"-appearing leukemic blasts as actually erythroblasts with the use of antibodies to glycophorin A, a membrane protein specific for erythroblasts. Some patients with chronic granulocytic leukemia may have a promyelocytic phase, in which the marrow is composed largely of leukemic promyelocytes. Others have a megakaryoblastic phase, in which the marrow is populated with immature megakarocytes and the peripheral blood contains numerous dwarf megakaryocytes. Identification of megakaryoblasts in this disorder has been achieved with immunologic techniques using antiplatelet peroxidase. Other immunologic reagents, such as antibodies to factor VIII and to β-thromboglobulin have also been used. Cytochemically, megakaryoblasts in this disorder contain weak activity of nonspecific esterase and focal activity of acid phosphatase.

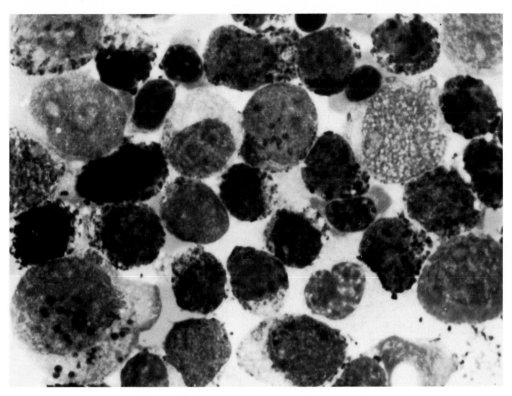

Figure 5–53   *Basophilic leukemia, terminal phase, in a patient who previously had chronic granulocytic leukemia. Leukemic blasts vary in size and shape. They have delicate nuclear chromatin patterns and few small nucleoli. Most of the blasts contain metachromatically staining granules as found in typical basophils.*

In other patients, a myelomonocytic terminal blast phase occurs. In some patients, a terminal phase may be eosinophilic leukemia or basophilic leukemia (Fig. 5–53 and Plate 3D). Still other patients have what has been identified by morphologic, cytochemical, and enzymatic criteria as a lymphoblastic terminal blast phase. In these patients, leukemic blasts may possess terminal deoxynucleotidyl transferase (TdT) activity, a property believed to be distinctive for cells of lymphoid origin.

Although activity of this enzyme is found more frequently in cells of lymphoid origin compared to other types of cells, it is not as highly specific as once thought. Apparently, 10% to 15% of Auer rod–positive leukemic myeloblasts may also contain activity of TdT, as a result of a derepression of the genome for TdT by the leukemic blasts. A mixed lymphoblastic-myeloblastic leukemia has also been described.

Preleukemic Disorders

In recent years, a number of panmyelopathic disorders preceding the development of acute myeloblastic or monocytic leukemia have been identified and described. Some of these disorders have been given different names by different authors, but they probably represent the same or closely related entities. Recently, the term *myelodysplastic syndrome* has been suggested as a general term embracing refractory anemia, refractory anemia with ringed sideroblasts, refractory anemia with excess blasts, refractory anemia with excess blasts "in transformation," and chronic myelomonocytic leukemia. The word myelodysplastic describes the panmyelopathic involvement of the bone marrow in these disorders, as well as the generalized disturbance of cellular maturation found in all cell lines.

In many patients with preleukemic panmyelopathic disorders, clinical courses are indolent and patients die of complications of pancytopenia, including infection and/or hemorrhage. In other instances, patients with preleukemic panmyelopathic disorders show evolution into acute leukemia. Soft agar tissue culture studies of marrow have indicated that colony growth of marrows from patients with "preleukemia" shows features similar to marrow from patients with acute leukemia. Also, marrows from patients with "preleukemia" often display cytogenetic abnormalities that are identical to those found in the acute leukemia phase that evolves later. These findings support the belief that "preleukemia" actually represents acute leukemia in a slowly developing or indolent form. However, at present it is not possible to predict with certainty which patients with one of the preleukemic disorders will develop acute leukemia and when leukemic evolution will occur. The occurrence of a new chromosomal abnormality such as aneuploidy or polyploidy that was not present earlier or a change in growth characteristics of marrow in tissue culture may precede the development of acute leukemia by weeks to months.

Preleukemia

Preleukemia is a controversial disorder characterized by refractory macrocytic anemia, monocytosis, and normoblastemia. Most likely, "preleukemia" fits within the spectrum of myelodysplastic disorders. In preleukemia, marrows are hypercellular and show panmyelosis with increased numbers of promyelocytes, myelocytes, and metamyelocytes (Figs. 5–54 and 5–55), as well as increased numbers of micromegakaryocytes (Fig. 5–56 and Plate 2*B*), plasma cells, and eosinophils (Fig. 5–57). Erythropoiesis is abundant, and proerythroblasts are increased (Fig. 5–58). Some proerythroblasts contain multiple cytoplasmic pseudopodia (Fig. 5–58, *top*). Erythroblastic gigantism also occurs, and nuclear chromatin patterns in erythroblasts are usually of the megaloblastoid type (Fig. 5–59). Sometimes, small clusters of myeloblasts are found and constitute less than 20% of the differential cell count (Fig. 5–59). In addition to megaloblastoid-type erythropoiesis, several other types of morphologic abnormalities can be found in erythroblasts from patients with preleukemia.

(Text continued on page 275)

Figure 5–54   *Preleukemia, demonstrating increased numbers of metamyelocytes and bands, many of which have unusual nuclear configurations.*

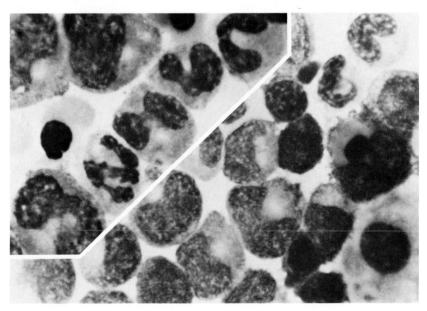

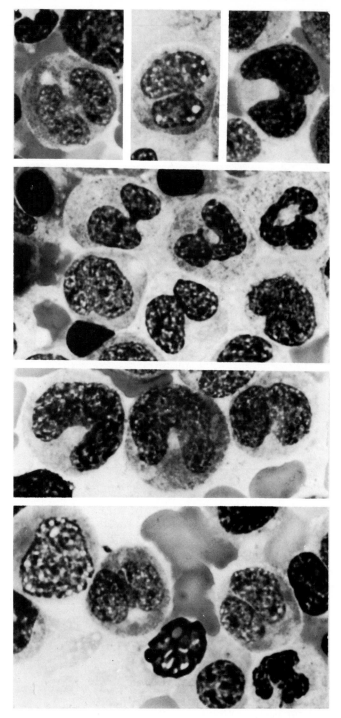

Figure 5–55   *Preleukemia, showing bands and metamyelocytes with pseudo Pelger-Huët anomaly. Nuclear abnormalities of this type are found frequently in bands and metamyelocytes from patients with preleukemia and other types of preleukemic disorders. Along with the other morphologic abnormalities found in preleukemia, the pseudo Pelger-Huët anomaly is believed to represent an increased likelihood of evolution into acute leukemia.*

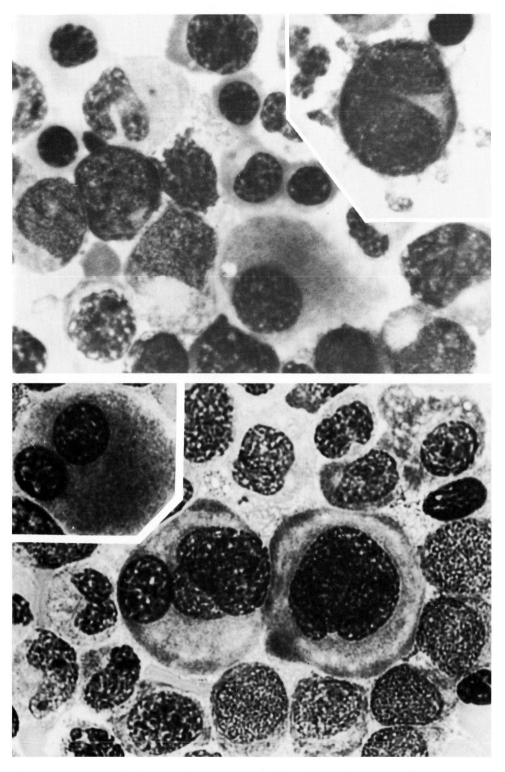

Figure 5–56   *Preleukemia, showing increased numbers of micromegakaryocytes.*

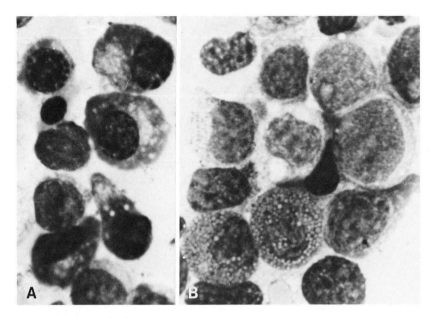

Figure 5–57   *Preleukemia. (A) Plasmacytosis. (B) Eosinophilia.*

Figure 5–58
(opposite)   *Marrow from a patient with preleukemia, illustrating increased numbers of aberrant-appearing metamyelocytes and increased numbers of megaloblastoid intermediate macronormoblasts. Cytoplasmic pseudopodia are seen in proerythroblasts (top).*

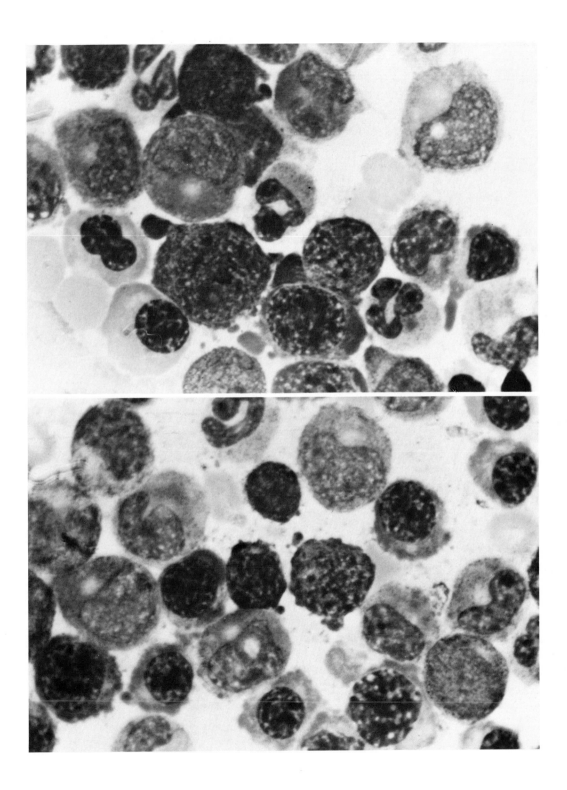

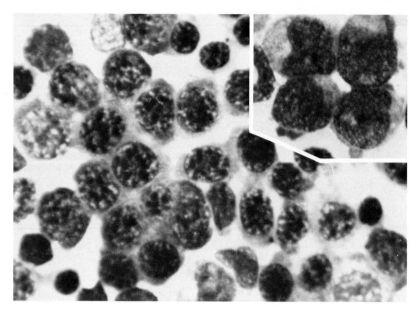

Figure 5–59 *Increased numbers of megaloblastoid intermediate macronormoblasts and small cluster of myeloblasts (inset) from marrow of a patient with preleukemia.*

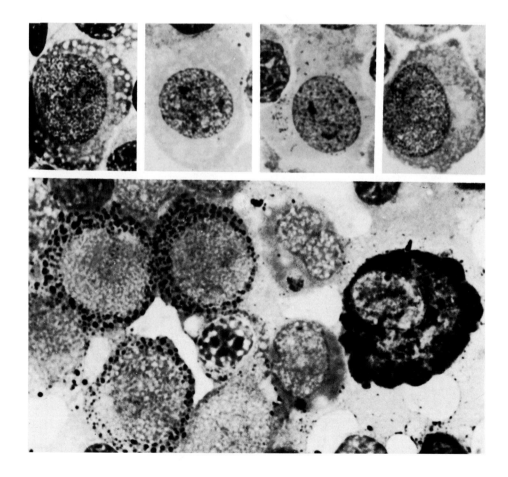

In one type of abnormality, as shown in Figure 5–60, atypical megalo-blasts are found. These cells exhibit a fried egg appearance of the nucleus. Nuclear chromatin is usually attenuated, and few small aggregates of nuclear chromatin are observed. Nucleocytoplasmic asynchronism is seen often. With the PAS stain, these atypical megaloblasts show intense and diffuse cytoplasmic staining, indicating a high content of glycogen that is dispersed evenly throughout the cytoplasm.

In a second type of erythroblastic abnormality, shown in Figure 5–61, erythroblasts have attenuated-appearing nuclear chromatin, few small aggregates of chromatin, and abundant cytoplasm containing many large and small vacuoles. When stained with the PAS reagent, these vacuoles contain glycogen that appears as large block-like aggregates. Usually, erythroblasts such as these constitute less than 1% of the differential cell count of marrows from patients with preleukemia. However, their presence may constitute an additional morphologic clue to the diagnosis of a preleukemic disorder.

Increased numbers of hemohistiocytes and hemohistioblasts are also found. In some immature granulocytes and hemohistioblasts (Fig. 5–62), aberrations such as monocytoid convolutions and lobulations occur, raising the possibility that preleukemia may not exist as such but may be monocytic leukemia in an early, indolent phase. As the leukemic process accelerates, marrows from patients with pre-leukemia become more heavily populated with typical myeloblasts or with blasts having monocytoid nuclei. As leukemic evolution is completed, the marrow is virtually replaced by leukemic blasts (Figs. 5–63 and 5–64).

On H and E section, biopsies from patients with preleukemia show pale vesicular nucleli of promyelocytes and proerythroblasts and more darkly stained nuclei of intermediate macronormoblasts (Fig. 5–65).

Figure 5–60
(opposite)

Atypical erythroblasts in preleukemia. Cells across the top of the figure are megaloblasts as found in patients with preleukemia. As in erythroleukemia, these atypical megaloblasts exhibit unusually attenuated nuclear chromatin with few small aggregates, a fried egg appearance of the nucleus, and evidence of nucleocytoplasmic asynchronism. The bottom half of the figure illustrates the PAS stain applied to these atypical megaloblasts. As shown in the darkly stained cell to the right, these atypical megaloblasts stain diffusely and intensely positive for glycogen. Cells in the upper left portion of the bottom figure are proerythroblasts containing blocklike aggregates of glycogen demonstrated by the PAS stain.

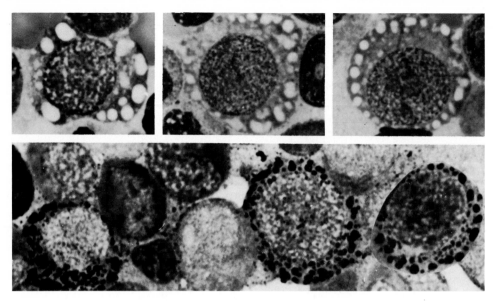

Figure 5–61   *Atypical erythroblasts in preleukemia. In this type of erythroblast, the nucleus contains delicate-appearing nuclear chromatin with few aggregates. Cytoplasm contains many large vacuoles, some of which appear confluent. As shown in the bottom half of the figure, the PAS stain reveals that these vacuoles contain glycogen, and the staining pattern demonstrates large chunklike aggregates of PAS-positive material.*

Figure 5–62   *Monocytoid changes of nuclei of primitive cells such as hemohistiocytes and hemohistioblasts. Several myeloblasts are also included in the field.*

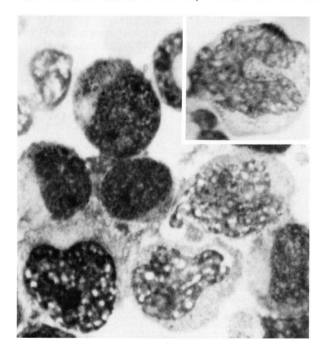

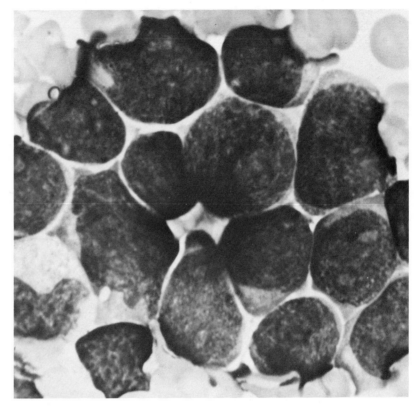

Figure 5–63 *Myeloblasts from a patient with acute leukemia that had evolved from preleukemia.*

In some patients it may be possible to trace leukemic evolution in marrow specimens from findings consistent with preleukemia through the development of acute leukemia. In patients with primary acquired refractory anemia, early signs of granulocytic abnormalities and possible leukemic changes include gigantism of metamyelocytes with aberrant nuclear configurations, including doughnut-hole nuclei and hypersegmentation of the nuclei. At this stage, few or no myeloblasts can be identified in the marrow. With acceleration of the leukemic process, myeloblasts can be identified in greater numbers. Factors controlling myeloblastic proliferation, accelerating in some instances and impeding in others, are unknown.

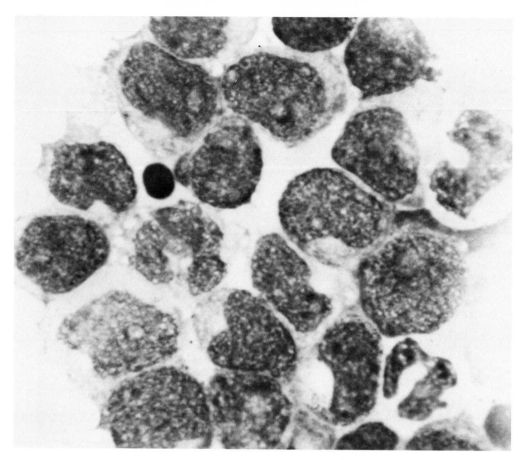

Figure 5–64   *Acute monocytic leukemia that evolved from preleukemia.*

Figure 5–65   *H and E section of marrow from a patient with preleukemia, showing increased numbers of granulocytic precursors and immature erythroblasts (inset).*

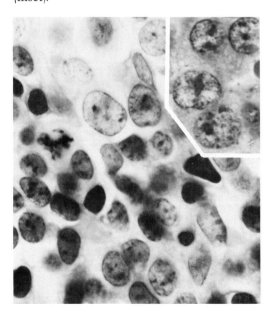

Cytochemistry of Acute Nonlymphoblastic Leukemias

With the advent of differing forms of therapy for lymphoblastic leukemias and nonlymphoblastic leukemias, it is essential to distinguish leukemic blasts of lymphoid origin from those of granulocytic origin. A number of cytochemical reactions have been applied to leukemic blasts in an effort to amplify morphologic assessments and aid in making these distinctions. These cytochemical tests are designed to detect granulocytic properties of the leukemic blasts.

Using *oil red O*, lipids can be identified in leukemic blasts. These lipids are found more frequently in myeloblasts than in lymphoblasts.

With the use of the *Sudan black B* stain, substances with affinity for this dye occur in cells of granulocytic origin such as myeloblasts and do not occur in lymphoblasts (Fig. 5–66). Substances in granulocytic cells having affinity for the dye are most likely lipids contained in granules. Although valuable for distinguishing cells of granulocytic origin, Sudan black B may not be a specific stain for cells of this type.

Other cytochemical tests detect enzymes that are present in lysosomes. Since these lysosomal enzymes are typical of cells of granulocytic origin, cytochemical tests designed to detect them may be of value in the assessment of the morphologic type of leukemic blast. *Myeloperoxidase* is a lysosomal enzyme typical of cells of

Figure 5–66   *Sudan black B–positive material in a leukemic myeloblast.*

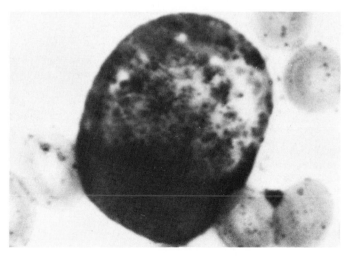

granulocytic origin. It is demonstarted with the use of benzidine, O-tolidine (Fig. 5–67), or a variety of other chromogens that have been described as alternatives to benzidine. Benzidine is not used widely at present because of its reputed carcinogenicity. Erythroblasts from patients with acute erythremic myelosis and erythroleukemia have peroxidase activity, indicating that these abnormal cells have differentiated along both erythroblastic and granulocytic lines.

Specific esterase is a lysosomal enzyme believed to be a highly characteristic marker for cells of granulocytic origin (Fig. 5–68). This enzyme is detected with the use of naphthol ASD-chloroacetate as substrate. In myeloblasts from patients with myeloblastic leukemia (Fig. 5–69), as well as in leukemic blasts from patients with mono-

Figure 5–67   (A) *Peroxidase activity (gray and black) in leukemic myeloblasts, using O-tolidine as a stain. (B) Peroxidase activity (black punctate) in leukemic myeloblasts, using benzidine. Immature granulocytic cells, such as myeloblasts, contain less peroxidase activity than more mature granulocytic cells, such as promyelocytes and myelocytes.*

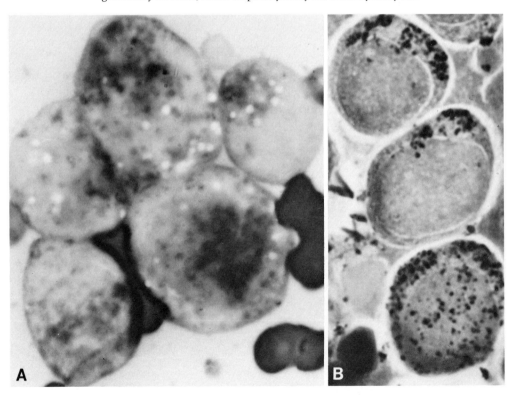

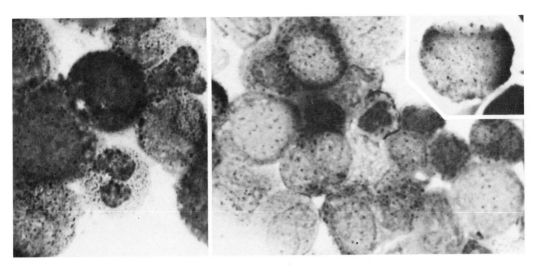

Figure 5–68 *Specific esterase activity (black punctate) in mature and immature granulocytes, using naphthol ASD-chloroacetate and fast blue BBN, normal bone marrow.*

cytic leukemia and erythroblasts from patients with acute erythremic myelosis and erythroleukemia, specific esterase activity can be detected in the cytoplasm. As noted earlier, cytochemical detection of small amounts of specific esterase activity is facilitated with the use of highly sensitive dye couplers such as fast garnet GBC.

Leukocyte alkaline phosphatase is an enzyme demonstrable with a variety of techniques. Alkaline phosphatase activity is found in secondary or specific granules. Demonstration of alkaline phosphatase activity is particularly valuable in the assessment of marrows thought to be consistent with the diagnosis of chronic granulocytic leukemia and in distinguishing these marrows from those believed to represent a leukemoid reaction. In chronic granulocytic leukemia, leukocyte alkaline phosphatase activity is low. In leukemoid reactions and in the hypercellular phase of agnogenic myeloid metaplasia, leukocyte alkaline phosphatase activity is normal or elevated. Low leukocyte alkaline phosphatase activity is not pathognomonic for chronic granulocytic leukemia. It can be low in other disorders such as acute myeloblastic leukemia, paroxysmal nocturnal hemoglobinuria, and congenital hypophosphatasia.

PAS reaction is usually weak and diffuse in leukemic myeloblasts. In some instances, myeloblasts are PAS negative.

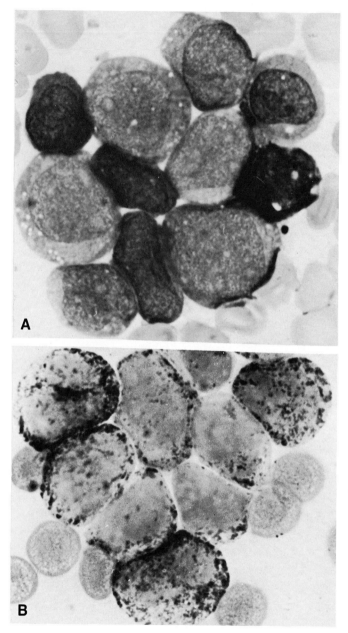

Figure 5–69   *Leukemic myeloblasts from a patient with acute myeloblastic leukemia that had evolved after prolonged treatment with alkylating agents for carcinoma of the ovary (A). In B, specific esterase activity can be demonstrated in the leukemic myeloblasts using naphthol ASD-chloroacetate as substrate.*

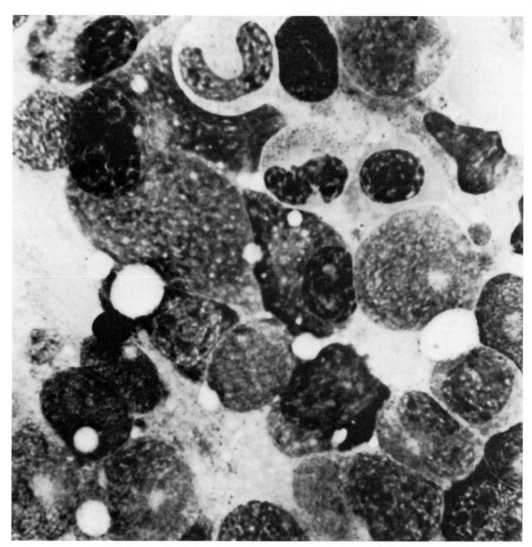
Plasmacytosis of the marrow in a patient with the myelodyplastic syndrome.

6   *Plasmacytosis*

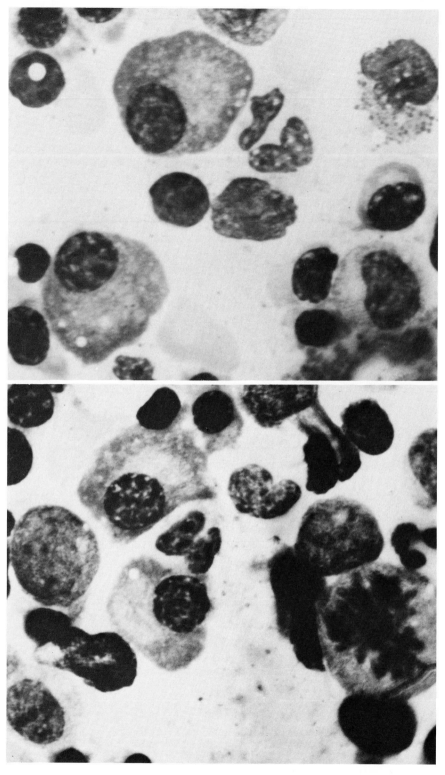

Figure 6–1   *Plasma cells, normal marrow.*

In normal marrows, plasma cells usually do not constitute greater than 10% of the differential cell count.

Normal Plasma Cell. The normal plasma cell has an eccentric nucleus with prominent aggregates of chromatin arranged in a concentric fashion around the nuclear membrane (Fig. 6–1). Nucleoli are indistinct or absent. Cytoplasm is deeply basophilic due to the high content of ribosomal RNA, and frequently there are numerous small vacuoles. A perinuclear pale area may be found and probably represents the Golgi region. Superficially, plasma cells resemble osteoblasts (Fig. 6–2). These large cells with abundant basophilic cytoplasm usually occur in clusters and are found in pediatric marrow specimens.

Plasmacytosis of the Marrow. Increased numbers of normal-appearing plasma cells are found in a variety of disorders. In benign plasmacytosis, the numbers of plasma cells do not usually exceed 10% of the marrow differential count. Disorders in which increased numbers of plasma cells are found include acute and chronic infections, acquired immune deficiency syndrome (AIDS) as shown in Figure 6–3, Hodgkin's disease (Fig. 6–4), cirrhosis of the liver, collagen disease, autoimmune hemolytic anemia (Fig. 6–5), infectious mononucleosis, angioimmunoblastic lymphadenopathy, monocytic leukemia (Fig. 6–6), mycobacterial infections, lymphocytic lymphoma, multiple myeloma, and Waldenström's macroglobulinemia.

(Text continued on page 289)

Figure 6–2   *Osteoblasts, normal marrow.*

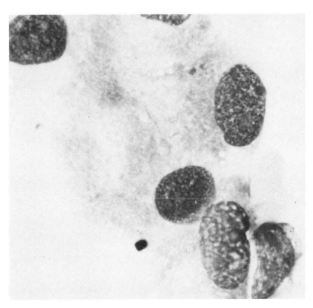

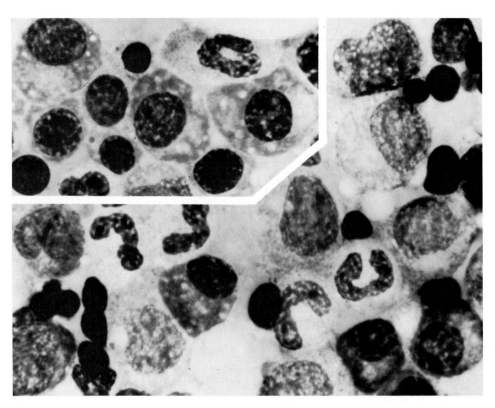

Figure 6–3   *Acquired immune deficiency syndrome (AIDS), showing increased numbers of mature-appearing plasma cells.*

Figure 6–4
(opposite)

Eosinophilia and plasmacytosis (inset, left) of the marrow, Hodgkin's disease. In this disorder, increased numbers of eosinophils and plasma cells in the bone marrow are not necessarily associated with advanced disease. Eosinophilia and plasmacytosis are also found in bone marrow specimens from patients with cirrhosis of the liver, also rheumatoid arthritis, and chronic infections.

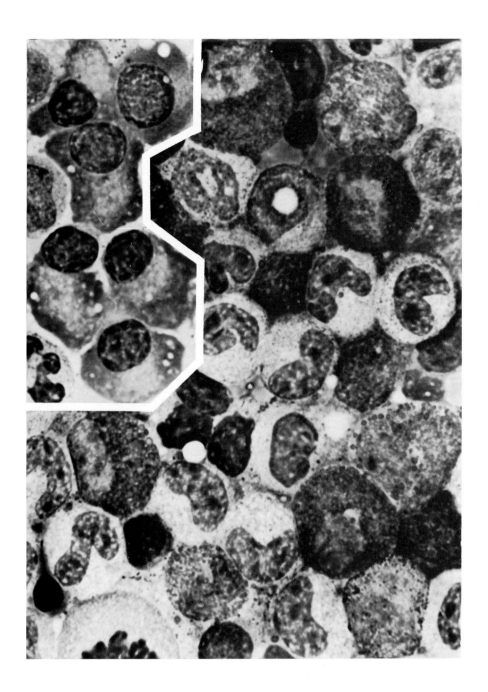

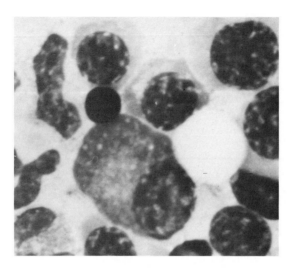

Figure 6–5   *Plasmacytosis of the marrow, autoimmune hemolytic anemia.*

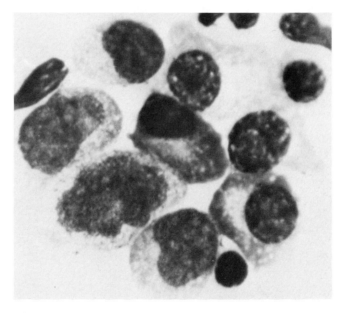

Figure 6–6   *Plasmacytosis of the marrow, monocytic leukemia.*

Nuclear Abnormalities

Binuclearity. Plasma cells containing two separate nuclei can be found in normal marrows as well as in pathologic specimens, particularly in dysproteinemias and in monocytic leukemia (Figs. 6–7 and 6–8).

Figure 6–7
Binuclear plasma cell, normal bone marrow.

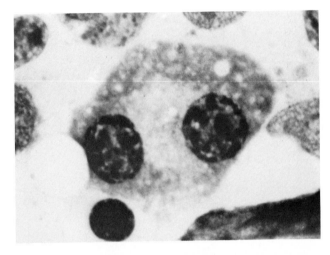

Figure 6–8
Binuclear plasma cells, normal bone marrow aspirate. A binuclear plasma cell (center) and other typical-appearing plasma cells are seen in an H and E section of bone marrow from a patient with chronic infection.

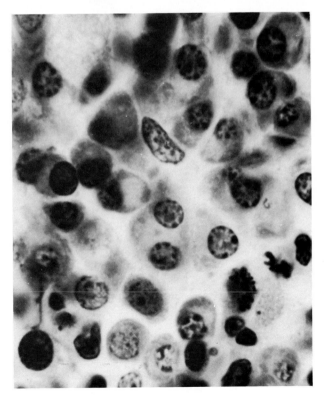

Multinuclearity. More than two separate nuclei may be found in pathologic plasma cells, particularly in the dysproteinemias. These multinuclear plasma cells are often gigantic (Fig. 6–9).

Figure 6–9   *Giant, multinuclear plasma cells from two different patients with multiple myeloma.*

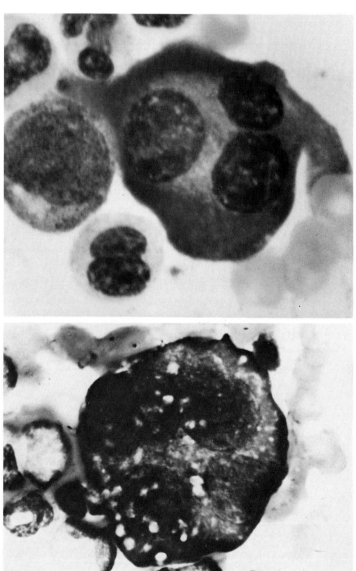

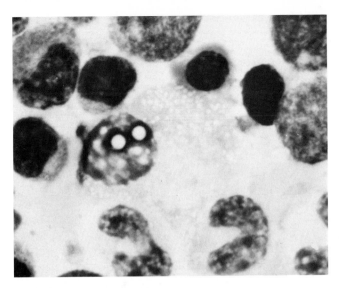

Figure 6–10   *Plasma cell with nuclear vacuoles, multiple myeloma.*

Nuclear Vacuoles. In nuclei of plasma cells from patients with dys-proteinemias, particularly macroglobulinemia, one or two prominent vacuoles may be found (Fig. 6–10). When stained with the PAS reagent, these vacuoles contain glycogen or glycoprotein. They have been called Dutcher bodies.

Nucleolus. Neoplastic plasma cells may have one or more prominent nucleoli with perinucleolar condensation of chromatin (Fig. 6–11).

Figure 6–11   *Myeloma cells with prominent nucleoli and perinucleolar condensations of chromatin.*

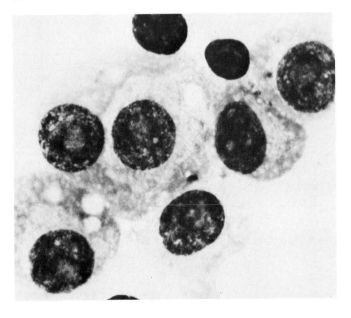

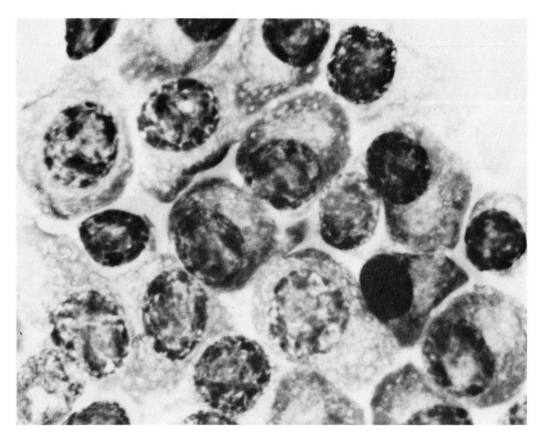

Figure 6–12   *Myeloma cells, showing prominent aggregates of nuclear chromatin.*

Hyperaggregated Chromatin. In some neoplastic plasma cells from patients with dysproteinemias, nuclear chromatin can show unusually prominent aggregates that are larger and more numerous than in normal plasma cells (Fig. 6–12). It has been postulated that plasma cells possessing these nuclear characteristics are more highly differentiated than those that do not possess these features.

Cytoplasmic Abnormalities

Cytoplasmic Vacuoles. Plasma cells may demonstrate numerous large cytoplasmic vacuoles (Fig. 6–13). At times, these vacuoles may fill the cell (Mott or mulberry cell). Presumably, these cells are actively involved in the biosynthesis of immunoglobulins. Cells of

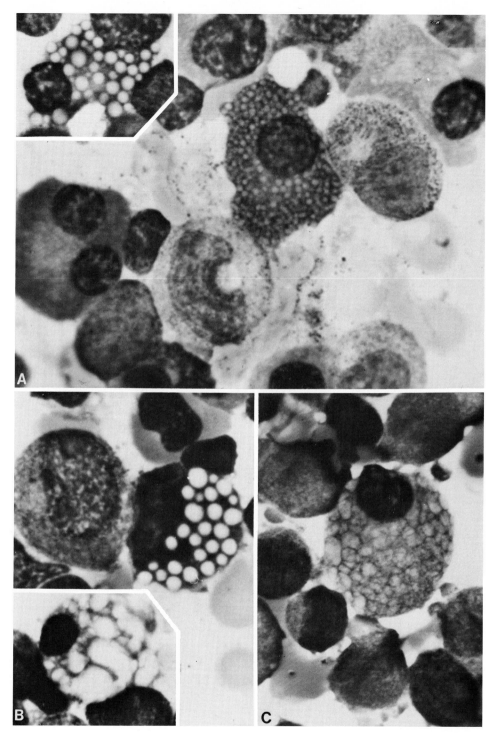

Figure 6–13   *Vacuolated plasma cells. (A) Subacute myelomonocytic leukemia; inset shows multiple myeloma. (B) Untreated pernicious anemia. (C) Myeloblastic leukemia. Vacuoles vary in size, shape, and number.*

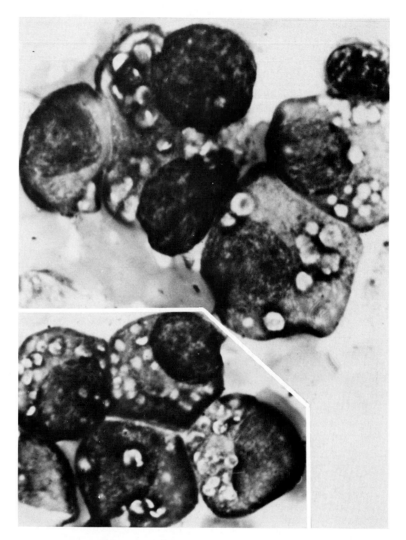

Figure 6–14   *Plasma cells, multiple myeloma, containing numerous Russell's bodies.*

this type are found in patients with untreated pernicious anemia, multiple myeloma and macroglobulinemia, chronic lymphocytic leukemia in which there is a concomitant hypergammaglobulinemia, and monocytic leukemia. Vacuolated plasma cells may also be seen in acute lymphoblastic leukemia.

Russell's Bodies. Russell's bodies are globular-shaped eosinophilic-staining inclusions that represent deposits of immunoglobulin (Fig. 6–14). They are found in neoplastic plasma cells in the dysproteinemias and occasionally in normal plasma cells. Russell's bodies are often surrounded by a clear zone as though the immunoglobulin precipitate had retracted from the vacuole as a result of fixation.

Snapper-Schneid Granules. Snapper-Schneid granules are coccoid-shaped or bacillary shaped basophilic-staining inclusions that represent precipitates of immunoglobulin (Fig. 6–15A). They are observed most frequently in dysproteinemias.

Cytoplasmic Crystals. Rarely, ovoid- or angular-shaped crystals can be found in normal plasma cells and in myeloma cells. These crystals contain immunoglobulins and vary in color from pale green to red (Fig. 6–15B).

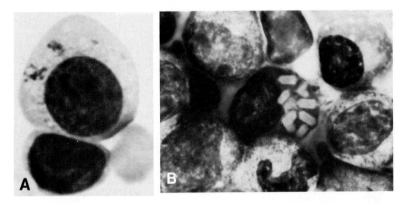

Figure 6–15   (A) *Azurophilic inclusions (Snapper-Schneid granules) in the cytoplasm of myeloma cell.* (B) *Large, pale-staining crystals in plasma cell.*

Multiple Myeloma

Multiple myeloma is a disorder of neoplastic plasma cells that is associated with plasmacytosis of the marrow and often with abnormalities of serum and urinary proteins and lytic lesions of bones.

Plasma Cells in Multiple Myeloma. In most instances, marrows from patients with multiple myeloma contain large numbers of neoplastic plasma cells at the time of diagnosis (Fig. 6–16). Nuclear features of plasma cells in multiple myeloma are highly variable. Some plasma cells have small nuclei with either attenuated chromatin strands or multiple dense aggregates of chromatin in radial configuration along the inner surface of the nuclear membrane (Fig. 6–17A).

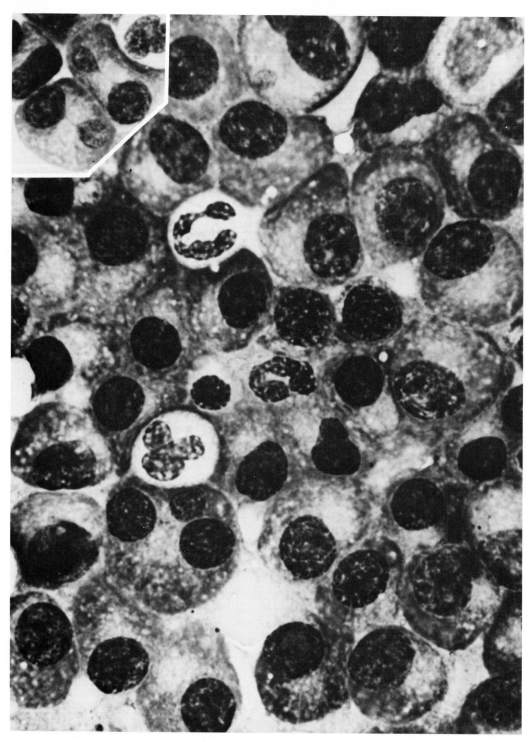

Figure 6–16　*Marrow, multiple myeloma, demonstrating large numbers of neoplastic plasma cells. Nuclei of these cells show prominent chromatin aggregates. Cell at top, center, contains a small polar body. Some polar bodies are connected to a larger nucleus by a thin strand of chromatin (inset).*

Other plasma cells have unusually large nuclei with attenuated nuclear chromatin strands that appear widely separated and few aggregates of chromatin (Fig. 6–17*B*). In some myeloma cells, nucleoli can be gigantic, with perinucleolar condensations of chromatin (Fig. 6–17*C* and *D*).

Cytoplasmic features of myeloma cells are also variable. Some myeloma cells exhibit deep basophilia, as do normal plasma cells. More often, myeloma cells demonstrate pale blue to blue gray cytoplasmic staining that is lighter than that found in normal plasma cells. Other cells have multiple vacuoles of various sizes. In many neoplastic plasma cells, cytoplasmic pseudopodia may be found, and fragments of cytoplasm are noted in marrow preparations. Cytoplasmic shedding of this type is found in macroglobulinemia and multiple myeloma. In some neoplastic plasma cells, cytoplasm stains brightly eosinophilic. Other cells have eosinophilic-staining cytoplasmic borders whereas the rest of the cytoplasm is pale blue gray. Plasma cells that show affinity for eosin have been called "flame cells." Eosinophilia is thought to reflect increased amounts of glycoprotein, as found in plasma cells from patients with IgA myeloma. However, flame cells can be found in all types of dysproteinemias.

Marrows from patients with multiple myeloma contain greater than 10% plasma cells and may be normocellular, hypocellular, or hypercellular. In those patients with minimal plasmacytosis, it is possible to ascertain marrow involvement with myeloma cells if plasma cells show the cytologic abnormalities listed above. Involvement of marrow with myeloma cells may be focal but is often diffuse with extensive proliferation of cells and reduction of normal marrow elements. Often, myeloma cells form large sheets of cells that have indistinct cellular borders, resembling a syncytium.

H and E–stained sections of marrow from patients with multiple myeloma contain large numbers of cells with eccentric nuclei, large nucleoli, prominent aggregates of chromatin that often appear in a "spoke-of-the-wheel" configuration, and abundant cytoplasm (Fig. 6–17*D*). When these myeloma cells are unusually pleomorphic, they can be confused with anaplastic carcinoma cells, myeloblasts in granulocytic sarcoma (chloroma), histiocytic lymphoma cells, and neoplastic cells in amelanotic melanoma. Cytochemical tests for specific esterase and melanin may help to identify these disorders. Marrows from patients with plasma cell leukemia are indistinguishable from marrows of patients with multiple myeloma.

(Text continued on page 300)

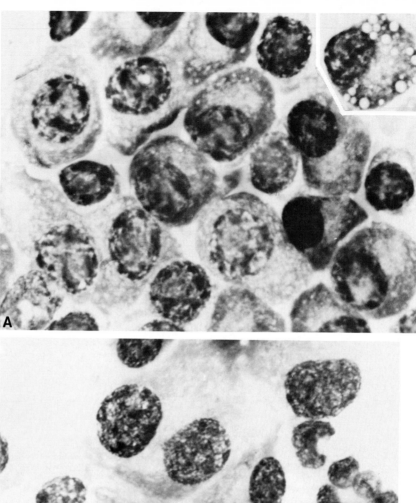

Figure 6–17
*(above and
opposite)*

(A) *Multiple myeloma, showing increased numbers of plasma cells having prominent aggregates of nuclear chromatin and large nucleoli. Inset shows plasma cell with large cytoplasmic vacuoles.* (B) *Multiple myeloma, demonstrating large neoplastic plasma cells with voluminous cytoplasm, indistinct cellular borders, and a finely reticular nuclear chromatin pattern with few aggregates of chromatin.* (C) *Myeloma cells illustrating unusually large nucleoli with perinucleolar condensation of chromatin and pleomorphism.* (D) *On H and E section of bone marrow biopsy, myeloma cells show large nuclei with prominent aggregates of nuclear chromatin arranged in a circumferential pattern on the inner surface of the nuclear membrane. The nuclei are often positioned eccentrically in the cell. Nucleoli are large and darkly stained.*

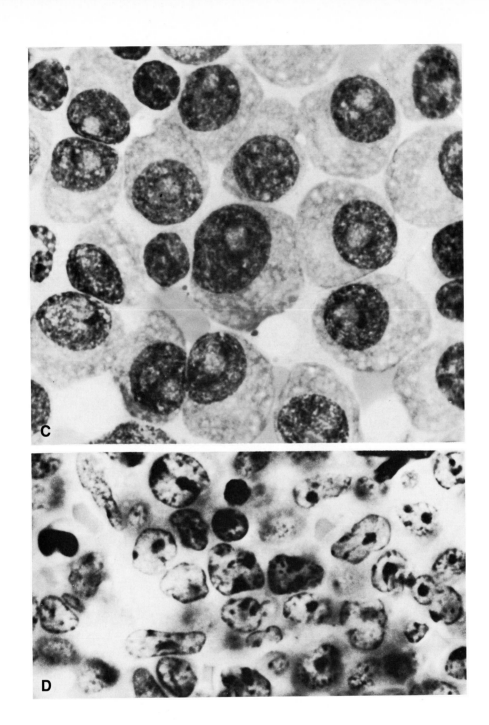

Cytochemically, myeloma cells contain intense activity of non-specific esterase and acid phosphatase that appear as multiple localized sites of enzymatic activity in the cytoplasm (Fig. 6–18A). In normal plasma cells, activities of these enzymes have a similar distribution. Myeloma cells also demonstrate diffuse PAS positivity of the cytoplasm (Fig. 6–18B). Using the methyl green-pyronine stain, myeloma cells show intense pyroninophilia, representing areas of high concentration of ribosomal RNA (Fig. 6–18C).

Figure 6–18   (A) *Intense nonspecific esterase activity (black areas) in myeloma cells, alpha naphthyl acetate and hexazotized pararosaniline.* (B) *PAS-positive material representing glycogen and/or glycoprotein in myeloma cell.* (C) *Intense pyroninophilia of cytoplasm of nyeloma cells (gray and black), methyl green-pyronine.*

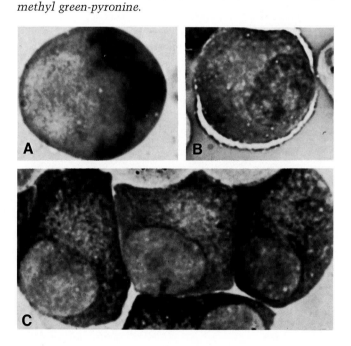

Macroglobulinemia. Waldenström's macroglobulinemia is a disorder of neoplastic lymphoid cells and plasma cells associated with elevations of IgM. Cytologically, marrows from patients with macroglobulinemia are hypercellular. They are composed of intermediate-sized lymphocytes, plasma cells and cells that have nuclear characteristics of plasma cells, and cytoplasmic features of lymphocytes. These cells have been called "lymphocytoid plasma cells" (Fig. 6–19) and are believed to be hybridizations of lymphoid and plasma cells in the sense that they share morphologic features of each cell type. Increased numbers of tissue mast cells and reticulum cells are found (Fig. 6–20). Cytochemically, the cytoplasm of plasma cells in macroglobulinemia often contains PAS-positive material representing glycoprotein. Nuclear vacuoles in plasma cells (Dutcher bodies) also contain glycoprotein.

Figure 6–19   *Lymphocytoid plasma cells in macroglobulinemia. Typically, these cells have a centrally located nucleus.*

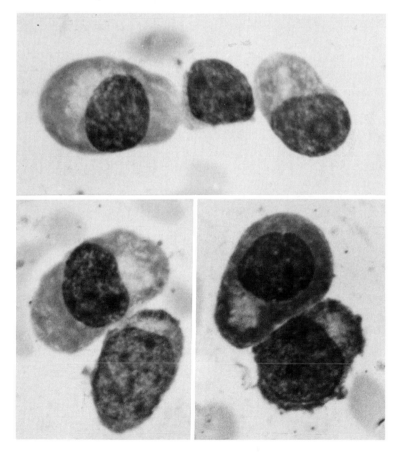

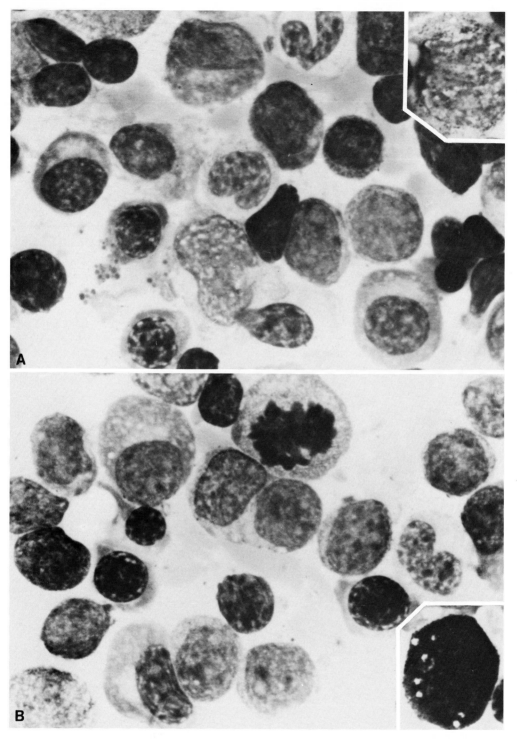

Figure 6–20 *Bone marrow, macroglobulinemia. Increased numbers of plasma cells, plasmacytoid lymphocytes, and lymphocytes are shown. Insets show hemohistiocyte* (A) *and mast cell* (B).

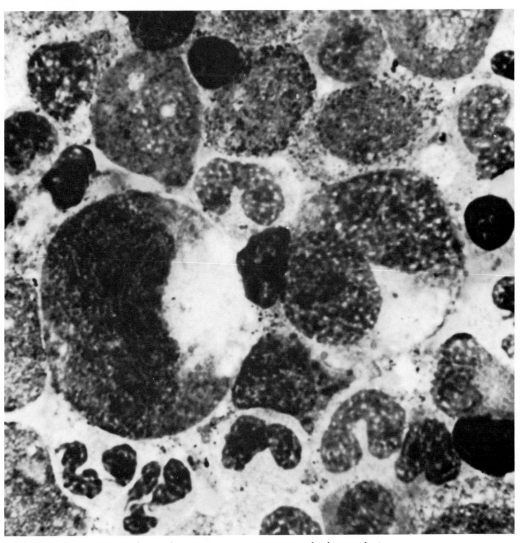

Atypical megakaryocytes in agnogenic myeloid metaplasia.

7 *Megakaryocytosis*

In normal bone marrows, megakaryocytes constitute less than 1% of the differential cell count. Megakaryocytes are the cells from which platelets originate.

Normal Megakaryocytes

Megakaryoblast. Earliest recognizable megakaryocytes are cells approximately as large as promyelocytes. They often have few or no nuclear lobulations, and nuclear chromatin patterns show either diffuse or dense chromatin strands and few large chromatin aggregates (Fig. 7–1). Cytoplasm is usually deeply basophilic and may contain hypergranular cytoplasmic excrescences that have been interpreted as "platelet budding."

In other early megakaryocytes, nuclear configurations resemble those in reticulum cells. Some of these megakaryocytes are binuclear or have two lobulations of the nucleus. Nuclear chromatin is reticular in appearance with attenuated chromatin strands and few or no aggregates. Cytoplasm stains pale blue to blue gray. In some instances hypergranular cytoplasmic excrescences resembling platelets may be found.

Mature Megakaryocytes. Mature megakaryocytes are giant cells having multiple nuclear lobulations (Figs. 7–2 and 7–3). Rarely, mitotic figures are seen in megakaryocytes in normal marrow. In some of

Figure 7–1   *Megakaryoblasts, normal bone marrow. These are small megakaryocytes with a large nucleus, reticular-appearing nuclear chromatin, and scant hypogranular cytoplasm that may show excrescences resembling platelets.*

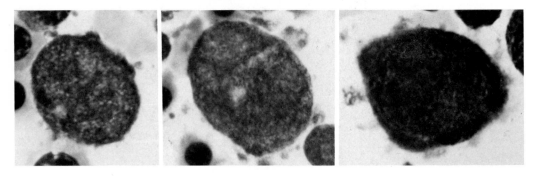

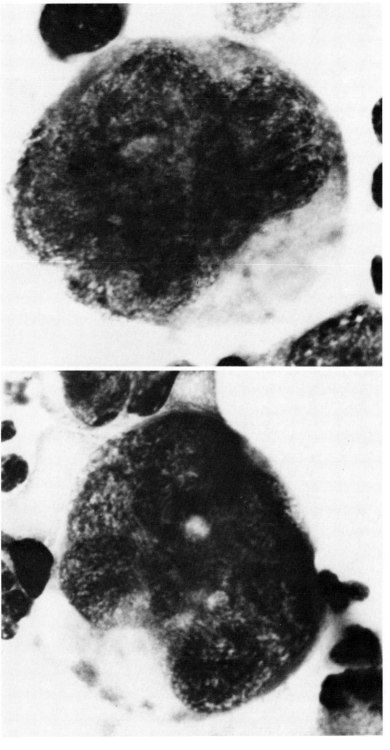

Figure 7–2   *Normal megakaryocytes, showing increased nuclear size compared to volume of cytoplasm, reticular-appearing nuclear chromatin, and relatively hypogranular cytoplasm.*

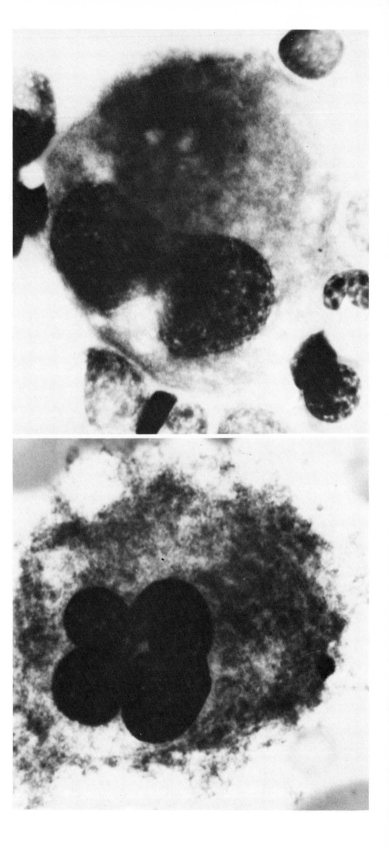

Figure 7–3
*Normal mature megakaryocytes
with lobulated nuclei (*top *and*
bottom) *and intensely granular
cytoplasm containing
sequestrations of granular
material (*bottom).

these cells nuclear chromatin is diffuse; in others it appears spongy and coarse. Aggregates of chromatin are seen frequently, and some of them are large. Strands of chromatin connect adjacent aggregates. Nucleoli are usually not observed.

Cytoplasm of mature megakaryocytes is usually hypergranular and contains many blue and dark pink granules, some of which form aggregates as found in platelets (Figs. 7–3 and 7–4). Cytoplasmic borders are usually distinct and sometimes show platelet excrescences. In normal bone marrow, fragments of megakaryocytes may be observed. Some of these appear as isolated nuclei with small clusters of platelets or hypergranular cytoplasm adherent to them. Other disrupted megakaryocytes appear as large masses of hypergranular cytoplasm with a few large platelets adherent to the periphery of the cytoplasmic mass.

Figure 7–4   *Mature megakaryocyte with hypergranular cytoplasm and nucleus containing dense nuclear chromatin.*

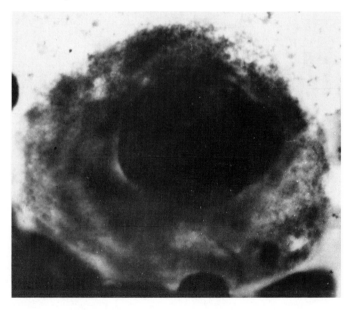

Mature megakaryocytes can be confused with Sternberg-Reed cells (Fig. 7–5*A* and *B*). Sternberg-Reed cells exhibit multilobularity or multinuclearity. Usually, they have large and prominent oval nucleoli that stain bright blue with panoptic stains, indicating a high content of RNA in the nucleolus. Strands of chromatin connect the prominent nucleolus to the nuclear membrane, and the nuclear chromatin appears disorderly, with strands crossing each other at irregular intervals. The cytoplasm is lightly basophilic with indistinct cellular margins and little or no granularity.

Mature megakaryocytes can also be confused with osteoclasts (Fig. 7–5*C*). Osteoclasts are giant cells involved in the resorption and remodeling of bone. They are found in pediatric marrow specimens, in bone marrows from patients with Paget's disease, and in hyperparathyroidism. In contrast to megakaryocytes, osteoclasts are multinuclear rather than multilobular. Generally, nuclei of osteoclasts are small and similar in size and shape, compared with the lobulations of megakaryocyte nuclei that vary considerably in size and shape and in delicacy of connections between lobulations. Also, the cytoplasm of osteoclasts is diffusely basophilic and does not exhibit the coarse granularity that is found in megakaryocytes.

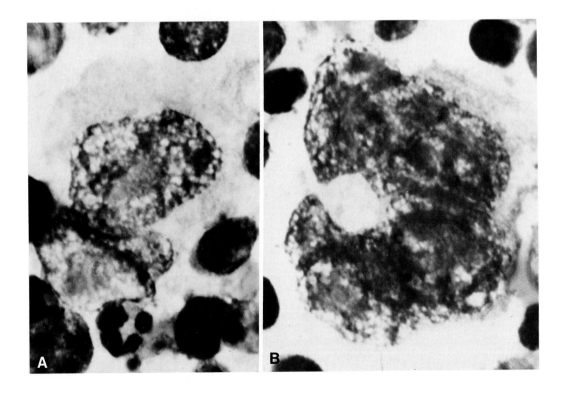

Figure 7–5
(opposite
and below)

(A *and* B) *Sternberg-Reed cells from the marrow of a patient with Hodgkin's disease.* (C) *Osteoclasts in H and E section of bone marrow biopsy from a patient with Paget's disease. Osteoclasts are multinuclear, in contrast to normal megakaryocytes, which show multilobularity of the nucleus. Osteoclasts are often found in close proximity to bone.*

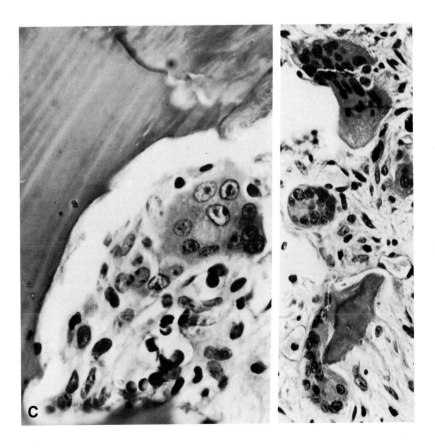

Megakaryocytosis

Increased numbers of mature megakaryocytes can be found in a variety of benign and neoplastic disorders, such as iron deficiency anemia, thalassemia, collagen disorders such as rheumatoid arthritis, and carcinomatosis of the marrow. Sometimes these disorders are associated with thrombocytosis, and platelet counts as high as 1 million/cu mm occur. Although they are responsible for increased numbers of platelets in the blood, megakaryocytes in these disorders are regarded as benign. They appear normal and are believed to respond normally to the negative feedback mechanism by which elevations of the platelet count suppress the size and number of nuclear lobulations of the megakaryocyte.

Increased numbers of abnormally large megakaryocytes occur in marrows of patients with essential thrombocythemia. This myeloproliferative disorder is characterized by megakaryocytes that have voluminous, hypergranular cytoplasm and multiple nuclear lobulations. Megakaryocytes in essential thrombocythemia are regarded as autonomous. Apparently they do not respond to the normal negative feedback mechanism in which fluctuations in platelet count control the size and number of nuclear lobulations of megakaryocytes. In essential thrombocythemia, thrombocytosis is associated with megakaryocytosis, but megakaryocyte proliferation, size, and nuclear lobulations are independent of peripheral platelet counts. By similar mechanisms, increased numbers of abnormal-appearing megakaryocytes are associated with thrombocytosis in some patients with chronic granulocytic leukemia, erythroleukemia, agnogenic myeloid metaplasia, and preleukemic disorders such as chronic erythremic myelosis.

Increased numbers of megakaryocytes are associated with thrombocytopenia in disorders that are believed to be characterized by peripheral destruction of platelets and/or impediment to normal maturation of megakaryocytes. These disorders include immune thrombocytopenic purpura, thrombotic thrombocytopenic purpura, conditions in which there is hypersplenism with hypercellular bone marrow as in Felty's syndrome, and the giant platelet disorders such as May-Hegglin anomaly and Bernard-Soulier syndrome. Sometimes increased numbers of megakaryocytes are found in marrows from patients with untreated deficiencies of vitamin B_{12} and/or folate. In these disorders, thrombocytopenia is believed to be the result of "ineffective thrombopoiesis," characterized by intramedullary destruction of effete megakaryocytes and decreased production of platelets by these megakaryocytes.

Decreased numbers of megakaryocytes occur in acute leukemias, preleukemic disorders, nutritional megaloblastic anemias, after exposure to a wide variety of different kinds of medication, and in hypoplastic anemias, some of which can be precursors of acute leukemia. In these conditions, peripheral thrombocytopenia is attributed to decreased numbers of platelet-producing megakaryocytes in the bone marrow.

Nuclear Abnormalities

Micromegakaryocyte. Micromegakaryocyte is a tiny megakaryocyte frequently found in marrows of patients with myeloproliferative disorders and in preleukemic disorders such as smoldering acute leukemia, preleukemia, and Di Guglielmo syndrome. It is a small cell approximately the size of a metamyelocyte and has few or no nuclear lobulations, a reticular-appearing nuclear chromatin pattern, and richly granular cytoplasm (Fig. 7–6 and Plate 2*B*). Rarely, two separate nuclei are seen (Fig. 7–7).

Figure 7–6   *Typical-appearing micromegakaryocytes, agnogenic myeloid metaplasia.*

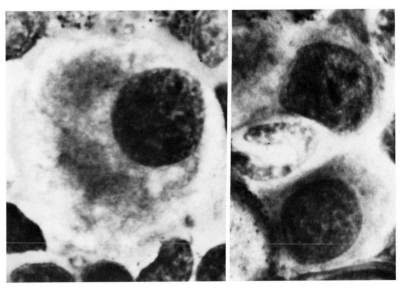

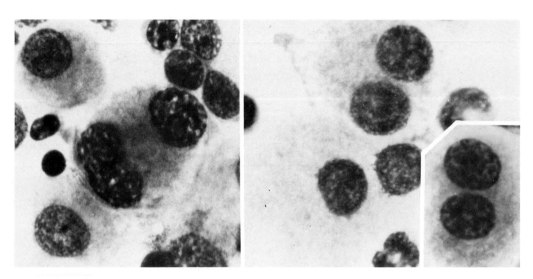

Figure 7–7   *Micromegakaryocytes, most of which are binuclear.*

Megakaryocytes With Two Nuclear Lobulations. Some small megakaryocytes have small nuclei with two lobulations that seem to have a tenuous connection (Fig. 7–8). Sometimes they are binuclear. These megakaryocytes have indistinct or small nucleoli, somewhat coarse reticular-appearing nuclear chromatin, and hypogranular cytoplasm. They are found in myeloproliferative disorders.

Megakaryocytes With Multiple Disconnected Nuclear Lobulations.
In some large megakaryocytes, multiple nuclear lobulations of varying sizes are disconnected or may be connected to each other by thin filaments of chromatin. The nuclear chromatin pattern in nuclear lobulations is finely reticular. Cytoplasm is often hypergranular. Megakaryocytes like these are found in patients with untreated deficiency of vitamin B_{12} or folate (Fig. 7–9).

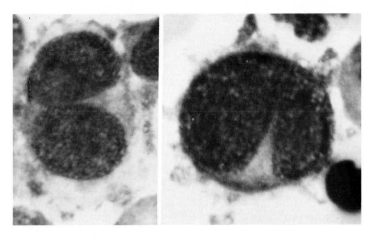

Figure 7–8   *Binuclear micromegakaryocytes with reticular-appearing nuclear chromatin and cytoplasmic excrescences that may represent platelets.*

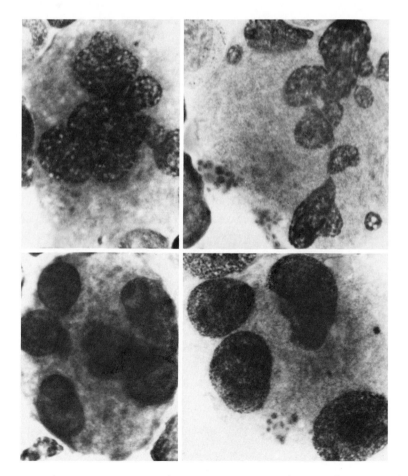

Figure 7–9   *Megakaryocytes, untreated pernicious anemia, showing disconnected nuclear lobulations of varying sizes and shapes and finely attenuated nuclear chromatin.*

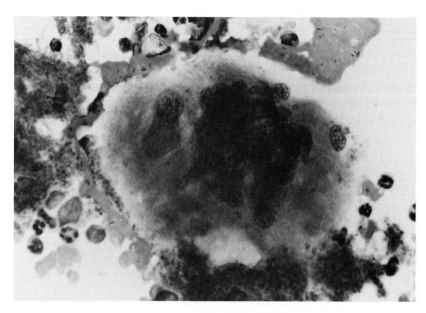

Figure 7–10   *Giant megakaryocyte with multiple nuclear lobulations and voluminous hypergranular cytoplasm, essential thrombocythemia.*

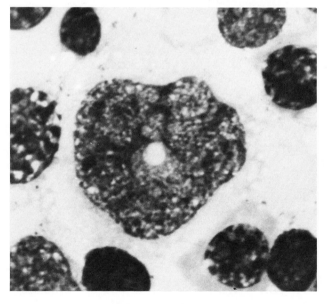

Figure 7–11   *Megakaryocyte with "hole" in nucleus.*

***Unusually Large Megakaryocytes With Multiple Nuclear
Lobulations.*** Giant megakaryocytes with many nuclear lobulations
often demonstrate richly granular cytoplasm showing sequestrations
of granular material (Fig. 7–10). They are found most frequently in
marrows of patients with essential thrombocythemia.

Megakaryocytes With "Hole" in Nucleus. Cells with a nuclear hole
are found in patients with immune thrombocytopenic purpura and
thrombotic thrombocytopenic purpura (Fig. 7–11).

Megakaryocytes With Finely Reticular Nuclear Chromatin. In some
types of megakaryocytes, nuclear chromatin strands are unusually
attenuated in appearance and are closely approximated (Fig. 7–12).
Chromatin aggregates are infrequent. Megakaryocytes like these can
be found in marrows of patients with myeloproliferative disorders
and in thrombotic thrombocytopenic purpura.

Figure 7–12   *Megakaryocytes with finely reticular attenuated strands of nuclear
chromatin.*

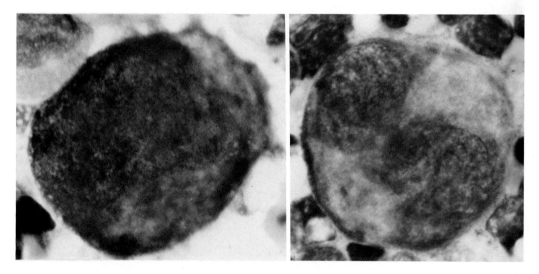

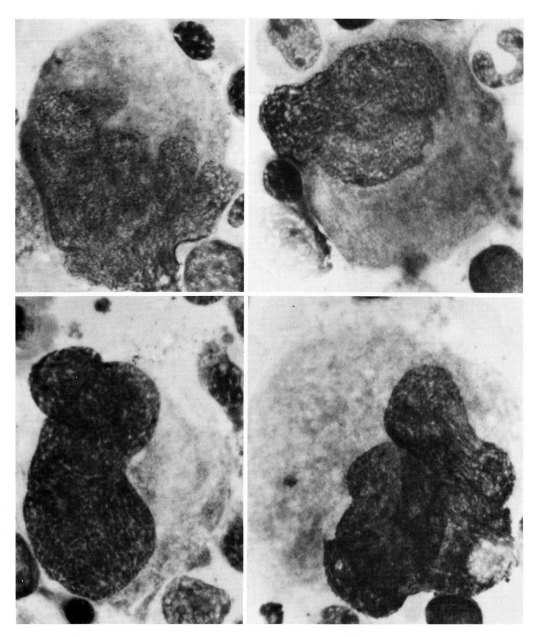

Figure 7–13   *Megakaryocytes with reticular-appearing lobulated nuclei.*

Megakaryocytes With Reticular-Appearing Nuclei. In one type of megakaryocyte, nuclear chromatin has a coarse, spongy, or reticular appearance with either no lobulations or a single lobulation (Fig. 7–13). Some of these cells may have as many as three or four lobulations. Megakaryocytes of this type occur in immune thrombocytopenic purpura and in thrombotic thrombocytopenic purpura.

Megakaryocytes With Coarsely Fenestrated Nuclear Chromatin. Megakarycytes may show chromatin strands that appear wide in caliber and are separated widely from adjacent chromatin strands, imparting a spongy appearance to the nuclear chromatin (Fig. 7–14). Chromatin aggregates are small and few, and cytoplasm is usually pale gray with few granules. Megakaryocytes like these are found in patients with myeloproliferative disorders and in immune thrombocytopenic purpura. Nuclei of these cells show few or no lobulations.

Megakaryocytes With Multiple Large, Dense Aggregates of Chromatin. Megakaryocytes found in marrows of patients with myeloproliferative disorders and immune thrombocytopenic purpura have a single unlobulated nucleus, or occasionally the nucleus shows one or two lobulations. Nuclear chromatin appears coarse, with numerous large aggregates of chromatin dispersed throughout the nucleus (Fig. 7–15). Cytoplasm is usually pale and hypogranular, and there may be cytoplasmic excrescences that represent platelet formation at the cell periphery.

Megakaryocytes With Dense Nuclear Chromatin and a Single Unlobulated Nucleus. Cells that have dense nuclear chromatin showing little or no detail of chromatin strands and few or no lobulations of the nucleus are found in patients with immune thrombocytopenic purpura and in thrombotic thrombocytopenic purpura (Fig. 7–16). In many of these megakaryocytes, cytoplasmic excrescences resembling large hypergranular platelets can be found along cytoplasmic margins. Cytoplasm of these megakaryocytes is usually deeply basophilic but sometimes shows occasional sparse granularity.

(Text continued on page 321)

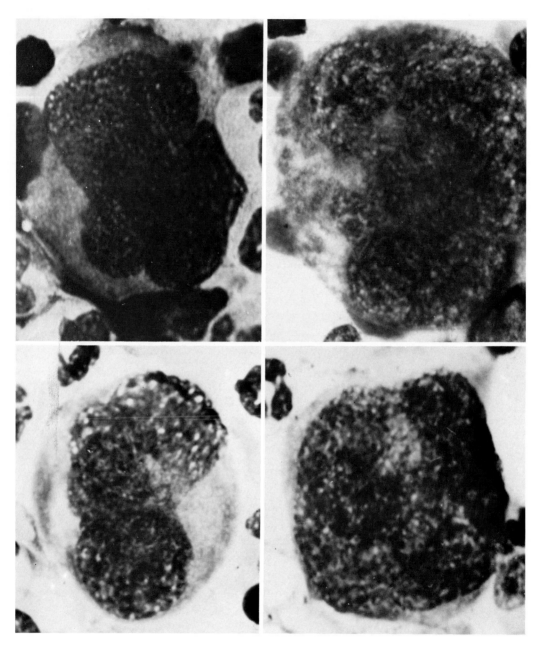

Figure 7–14   *Megakaryocytes with coarsely reticular-appearing strands of nuclear chromatin.*

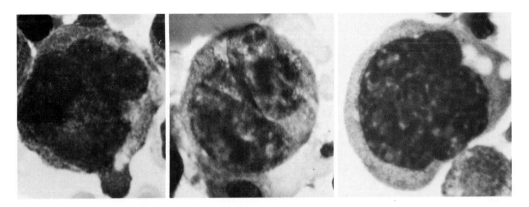

Figure 7–15   *Megakaryocytes with prominent dense aggregates of nuclear chromatin.*

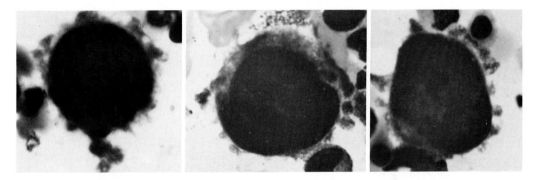

Figure 7–16   *Megakaryocytes with unlobulated nucleus, dense nuclear chromatin, and platelet excrescences at cytoplasmic borders.*

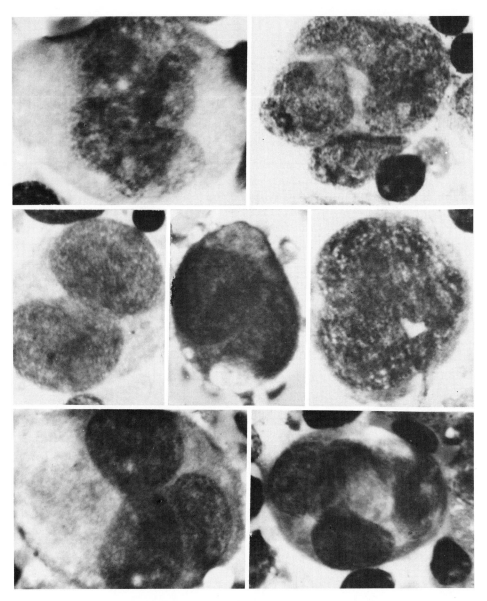

Figure 7–17   *Megakaryocytes, immune thrombocytopenic purpura, demonstrating basophilic, hypogranular cytoplasm. Abnormalities of nuclear size and configuration are also shown.*

Cytoplasmic Abnormalities

Hypogranularity of the Cytoplasm. The cytoplasm usually appears clear and basophilic in most areas (Fig. 7–17). Granularity as seen in normal megakaryocytes is either absent or sparse. Megakaryocytes with basophilic cytoplasm of this type are found in immune thrombocytopenic purpura and in thrombotic thrombocytopenic purpura.

Multiple Cytoplasmic Vacuoles. Some megakaryocytes from patients with immune thrombocytopenic purpura contain numerous cytoplasmic vacuoles (Fig. 7–18 and Plate 2A). In some of these cells, vacuoles are arranged around the periphery of the cell, as though platelet production at the periphery were impeded as the result of vacuole formation at the cellular margins.

In some patients with immune thrombocytopenic purpura, small or intermediate-sized lymphocytes may seem to appear within the cytoplasm of megakaryocytes. These cells are believed to exercise immune functions within the cytoplasm of the megakaryocytes.

Erythrocytophagy by Megakaryocytes. In megakaryocytes from patients with thrombotic thrombocytopenic purpura and monocytic leukemia, erythrocytes appear to lie within cytoplasmic vacuoles (Fig. 7–19). These may represent phagocytic vacuoles.

Figure 7–18 *Megakaryocyte, immune thrombocytopenic purpura, showing numerous cytoplasmic vacuoles.*

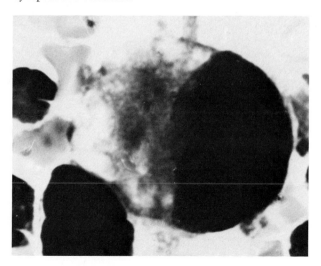

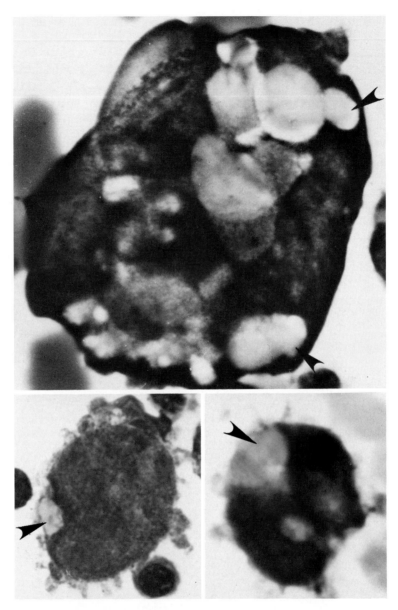

Figure 7–19   *Erythrocytophagy* (arrows) *by megakaryocytes in thrombotic thrombocytopenic purpura* (bottom insets) *and in monocytic leukemia (unusually large megakaryocyte at top).*

Immune Thrombocytopenia

In immune thrombocytopenic purpura, some megakaryocytes appear normal. However, many of them demonstrate abnormalities of the nucleus and cytoplasm. Although suggestive of immune thrombocytopenic purpura, these abnormalities are probably not diagnostic of this condition. Megakaryocytes are often increased in number (Fig. 7–20 but may be normal or decreased. In immune thrombocytopenic purpura, numerous small and large megakaryocytes are observed and show dense nuclear chromatin and multiple cytoplasmic vacuoles (Fig. 7–20 through 7–22 and Plate 2*A*). In some megakaryocytes, vacuoles are predominant within the cytoplasm of the cell (Fig. 7–21), whereas in others, vacuoles are predominant along the cell borders (Fig. 7–22). The cytoplasm is often basophilic and hypogranular.

Figure 7–20 *Increased numbers of immature-appearing megakaryocytes, immune thrombocytopenic purpura.*

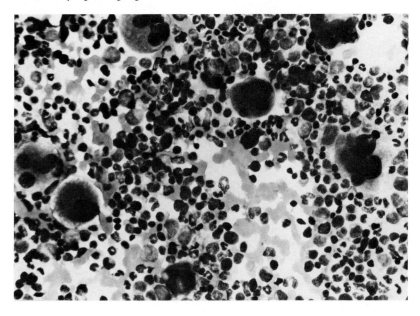

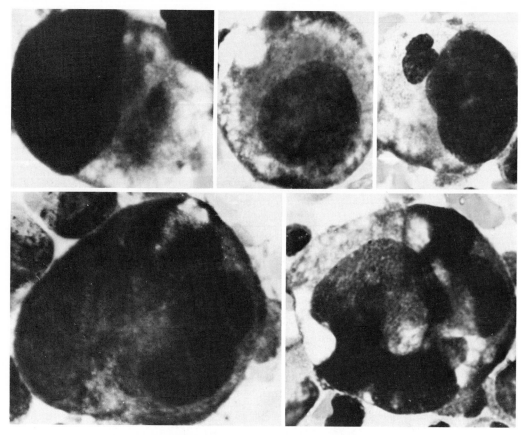

Figure 7–21 *Aberrant-appearing megakaryocytes, immune thrombocytopenic purpura, illustrating numerous cytoplasmic vacuoles and hypogranular cytoplasm.*

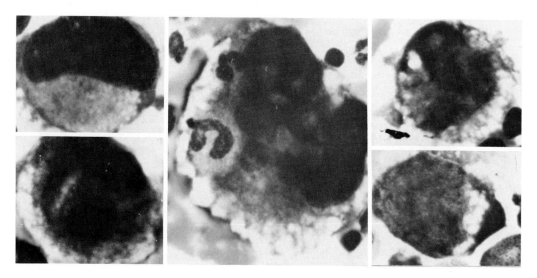

Figure 7–22 *Megakaryocytes with numerous vacuoles, principally around the cytoplasmic borders, immune thrombocytopenic purpura.*

324

Thrombotic Thrombocytopenic Purpura (TTP)

In TTP, a fulminating disorder characterized by thrombocytopenia, Coombs-negative hemolytic anemia, shifting neurologic signs, and hyaline thrombotic lesions of capillaries. Increased numbers of megakaryocytes are found in the bone marrow. Along with megakaryocytosis, markedly increased numbers of megaloblastoid intermediate macronormoblasts are found (Fig. 7–23), as well as increased numbers of hemohistiocytes, reticulum cells, and large erythroid "islands" containing a central reticulum cell or macrophage surrounded by developing erythroblasts (Fig. 7–24). Increased numbers of proerythroblasts may also occur. Megakaryocytic abnormalities can be distinctive and along with typical capillary lesions constitute the marrow manifestations of this disorder.

Figure 7–23   *Increased numbers of megaloblastoid intermediate macronormoblasts, thrombotic thrombocytopenic purpura.*

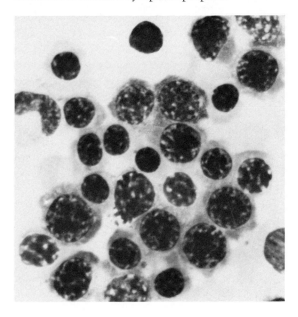

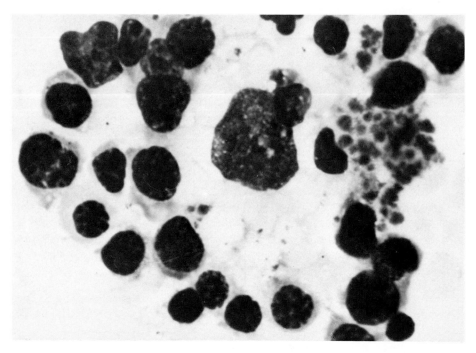

Figure 7–24   *Erythroid island, thrombotic thrombocytopenic purpura.*

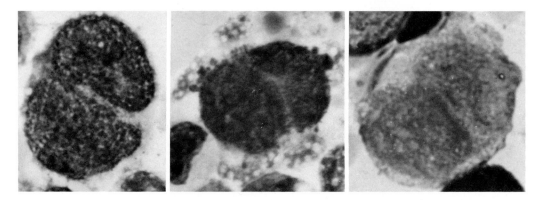

Figure 7–25   *Small binuclear megakaryocytes with finely reticular nuclear chromatin and scant hypogranular cytoplasm, thrombotic thrombocytopenic purpura.*

Megakaryocytes With Finely Reticular Nuclear Chromatin. Megakaryocytes with finely reticular nuclear chromatin are unusually small and contain hypogranular cytoplasm (Fig. 7–25). Several cytoplasmic excrescences, often containing hypergranular material, may be found. Some of these megakaryocytes are binuclear. Others have one nuclear lobulation or are unlobulated. Individual nonspecific abnormalities of megakaryocytes often include large megakaryocytes with single unlobulated nuclei containing coarsely fenestrated chromatin and hypogranular cytoplasm, megakaryocytes with multiple separate nuclei and relatively agranular cytoplasm, and large megakaryocytes with nuclear and cytoplasmic features resembling those found in megakaryoblasts.

Reticular Nucleus With Nuclear "Hole." Megakaryocytes may demonstrate a large multilobular nucleus with coarse-appearing chromatin strands and often a prominent "hole" in the nucleus (Fig. 7–26). Dense aggregates of chromatin can occur, and partially disconnected nuclear lobulations can be seen.

Figure 7–26 *Megakaryocytes, thrombotic thrombocytopenic purpura, demonstrating nuclear "hole."*

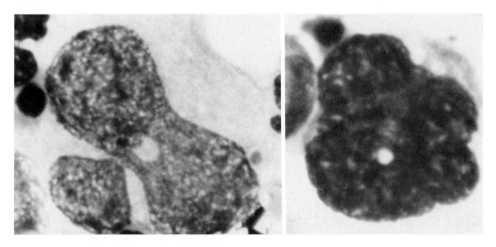

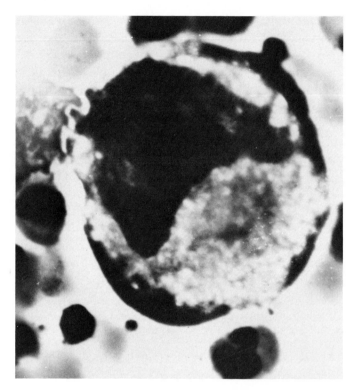

Figure 7–27   *Megakaryocyte, thrombotic thrombocytopenic purpura. Cytoplasm contains numerous small vacuoles, some of which appear confluent.*

Megakaryocytes With Vacuolated Cytoplasm. Cells with basophilic vacuolated cytoplasm appear similar to those in immune thrombocytopenic purpura (Fig. 7–27). In some instances, vacuoles are large and confluent and seem to fill the cell cytoplasm.

Megakaryocytes With Vacuolated Cytoplasmic Borders. As in immune thrombocytopenic purpura, megakaryocytes with vacuolated cytoplasmic borders may represent cytologic manifestations of toxic and/or immunologic damage to the megakaryocyte membrane and cytoplasm and perhaps contribute to thrombocytopenia (Fig. 7–28). Some of these megakaryocytes have pseudopodia containing numerous cytoplasmic vacuoles.

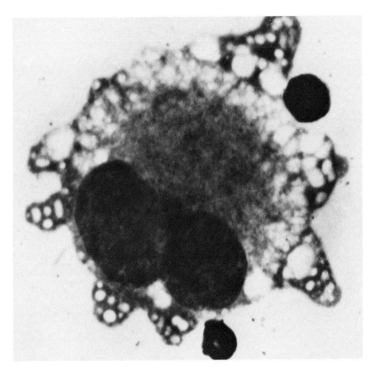

Figure 7–28   *Megakaryocyte, thrombotic thrombocytopenic purpura. Cytoplasmic borders show numerous vacuoles of various sizes.*

Megakaryocytes Demonstrating Erythrocytophagy. In cells showing erythrocytophagy, mature erythrocytes occur within what appears to be phagocytic vacuoles (Fig. 7–29). Several erythrocytes can be found within one megakaryocyte. Phagocytosis of erythrocytes by megakaryocytes can also be found in marrows of patients with monocytic leukemia, particularly those in which increased numbers of reticulum cells and hemohistioblasts are found. In some patients with thrombotic thrombocytopenic purpura, polymorphonuclear leukocytes seem to lie within phagocytic vacuoles (Fig. 7–30), suggesting that leukocytes are also phagocytized by megakaryocytes in this disorder.

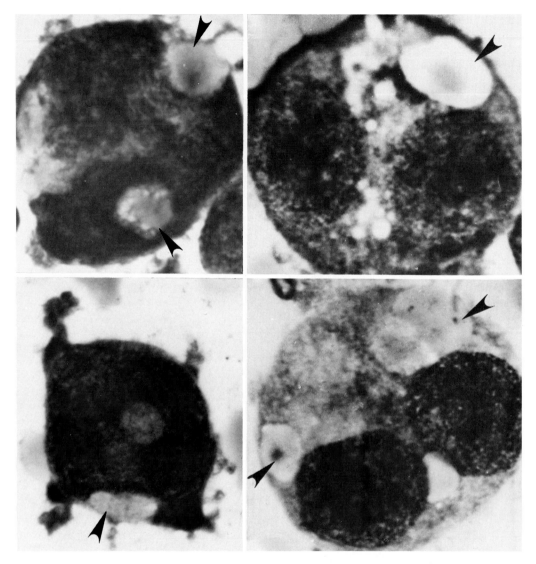

Figure 7–29   *Megakaryocytes, thrombotic thrombocytopenic purpura, showing erythrocytophagy* (arrows) *by megakaryocytes.*

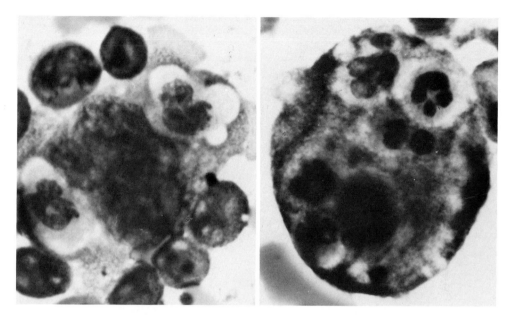

Figure 7–30   *Megakaryocytes, thrombotic thrombocytopenic purpura, illustrating phagocytosis of leukocytes by megakaryocytes.*

Giant Platelet Disorders

Giant platelet disorders are characterized by mild hemorrhagic diathesis, thrombocytopenia, and large platelets in the peripheral blood. Most frequently encountered entities include the May-Hegglin anomaly and the Bernard-Soulier syndrome. In both instances, increased numbers of megakaryocytes may occur in the marrow. Some of the megakaryocytes appear normal, and others demonstrate what may be distinctive abnormalities.

May-Hegglin Anomaly

This heredofamilial disorder is characterized by Döhle bodies in leukocytes and by large platelets and thrombocytopenia.

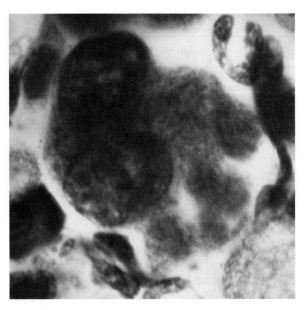

Figure 7–31　　*Megakaryocyte, May-Hegglin anomaly, demonstrating large sequestrations of hypergranular material in the cytoplasm. These sequestrations probably represent large platelets.*

Hypergranular Cytoplasm Containing Large Platelets. Cytoplasm of megakaryocytes contains prominent sequestrations of granules that appear as large confluent platelets (Fig. 7–31). Some megakaryocytes have voluminous cytoplasm that contains many platelet sequestrations. Other megakaryocytes have prominent, darkly staining nuclei with only a few platelets adherent to them and virtually no cytoplasm. Appearance of these types of megakaryocytes suggests a progressive disruption of the cytoplasm, leading to the elaboration of large platelets (Fig. 7–32). Nuclei of these megakaryocytes are usually dense and homogenous. In other instances, they may show a coarsely reticular pattern.

Megakaryocytes With Finely Reticular Nuclear Chromatin. Nuclear chromatin is finely attenuated with numerous large chromatin aggregates connected to each other by thick and thin strands of chromatin (Fig. 7–33). Cytoplasm is clear and hypogranular.

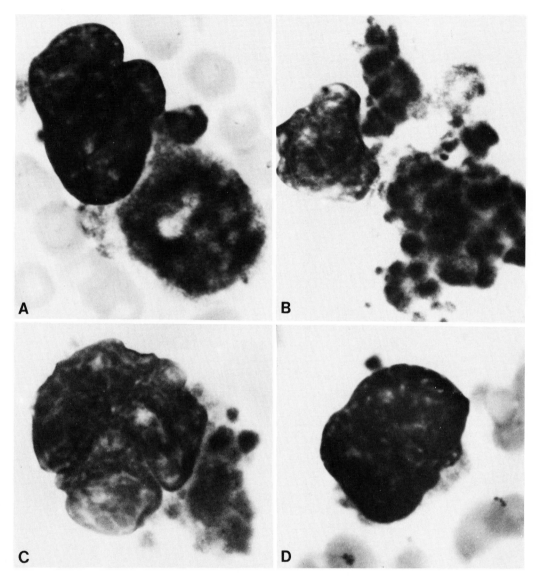

Figure 7–32 *Megakaryocytes, May-Hegglin anomaly. A through D depict possible sequence of dissolution of megakaryocytes. Cytoplasm contains large sequestrations of granular material. These sequestrations are probably precursors of platelets.*

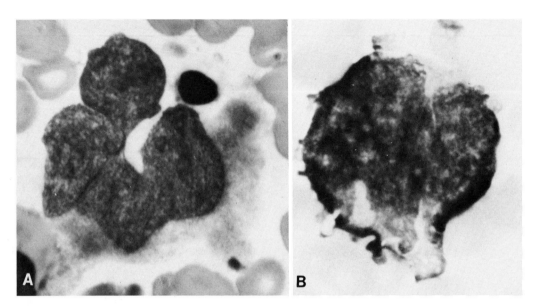

Figure 7–33   *Megakaryocytes, May-Hegglin anomaly. (A) Megakaryocyte with finely reticular nuclear chromatin. (B) Megakaryocyte with numerous aggregates of chromatin and clear granular cytoplasm.*

Bernard-Soulier Syndrome

In this hereditary disorder, giant platelets, abnormal platelet function tests, and a mild to moderate hemorrhagic diathesis occur.

Convoluted Nucleus. A seemingly distinctive nuclear abnormality in megakaryocytes of the Bernard-Soulier syndrome is a nucleus showing multiple convolutions and infoldings (Fig. 7–34). Nuclear chromatin shows numerous large aggregates. Cytoplasm may be hypogranular.

Multiple Nuclear Lobulations. The nucleus of the megakaryocyte shows multiple nuclear lobulations. Some demonstrate a coarsely reticular chromatin pattern with few small aggregates of chromatin. Cytoplasm of these megakaryocytes is often hypogranular.

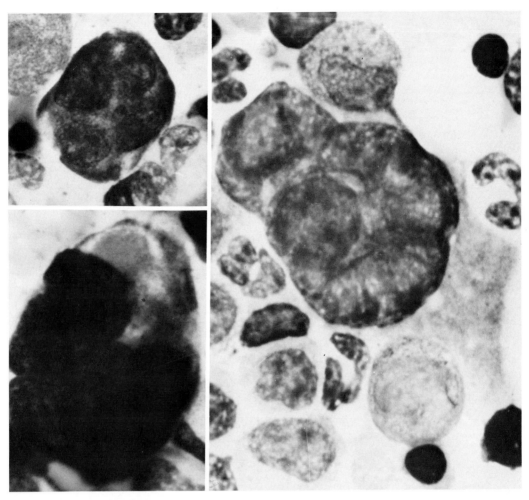

Figure 7–34   *Megakaryocytes from a patient with Bernard-Soulier syndrome. Nuclei of these cells show numerous convolutions, and chromatin appears dense with numerous aggregates.*

Thrombocytosis

In patients who have rheumatoid arthritis, thalassemia, or iron deficiency anemia and increased numbers of platelets, megakaryocytes in the marrow appear morphologically normal. In other disorders characterized by thrombocytosis, such as myeloproliferative disorders, megakaryocytes often demonstrate morphologic abnormalities.

Essential Thrombocythemia. In essential thrombocythemia, a myeloproliferative disorder, marrows are hypercellular and show increased numbers of granulocytic precursors, particularly promyelocytes. Increased numbers of basophils and eosinophils are also found. Megakaryocytes are increased in number (Fig. 7–35) and in typical cases can be gigantic (Fig. 7–36 and Plate 2*C*). These cells have multiple nuclear lobulations and voluminous hypergranular cytoplasm.

Figure 7–35   *Marrow, essential thrombocythemia, illustrating markedly increased numbers of large megakaryocytes having multiple nuclear lobulations.*

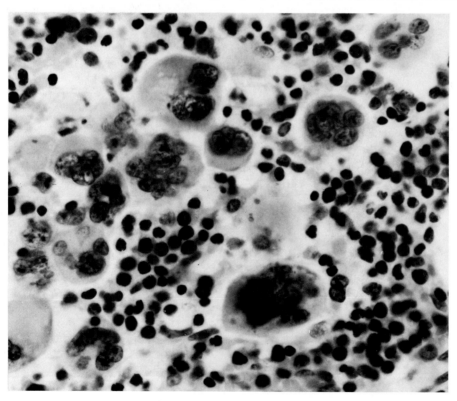

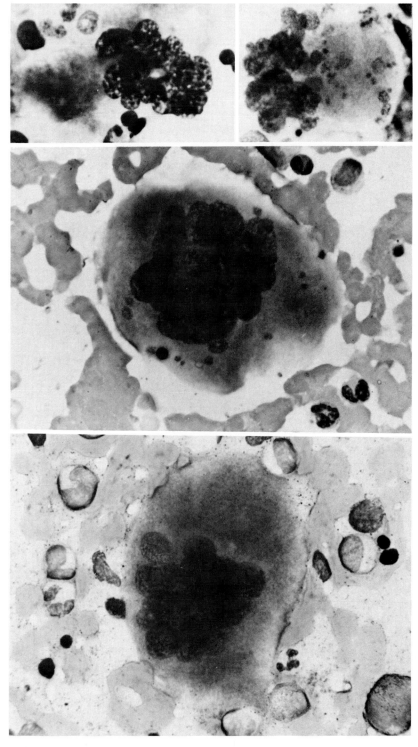

Figure 7–36   *Essential thrombocythemia, demonstrating giant megakaryocytes with voluminous cytoplasm and multilobular nuclei.*

In essential thrombocythemia, it is believed that the normal negative feedback mechanism of peripheral platelets upon size and replication of megakaryocytes in the marrow is lacking. Accordingly, the megakaryocytes function autonomously, leading to their unusually large size. Megakaryocytes in this disorder often occur in clusters of four to eight large cells. Sheets of platelets may surround them.

Agnogenic Myeloid Metaphasia. As noted earlier (Chap. 5), megakaryocytosis of the marrow is a prominent feature of agnogenic myeloid metaplasia. In the cellular phases of this disease, increased numbers of granulocytic precursors, particularly promyelocytes and myelocytes, may occur along with increased numbers of megakaryocytes. Some of these megakaryocytes appear normal. Other cells can be small micromegakaryocytes with few or no nuclear lobulations, coarsely reticular chromatin, and richly granular cytoplasm (Fig. 7–37). Megakaryocytes resembling those in agnogenic myeloid metaplasia also occur in marrows from patients with chronic granulocytic leukemia.

On H and E section of marrow biopsy, megakaryocytes often occur in clusters and are associated with collagen strands and increased numbers of fibroblasts having oval or elongated nuclei. In conjunction with increased numbers of collagen strands, fibroblasts, and megakaryocytes, deposition of reticulin fibers can be demonstrated.

Acute Megakaryocytic Myelosis. A rare disorder, acute megakaryocytic myelosis may represent an accelerated phase of agnogenic myeloid metaplasia. In some instances, megakaryocytic hyperplasia is associated with large numbers of hypogranular giant platelets and dwarf megakaryocytes in the bloodstream. Hematologic abnormalities of this type have been noted as a terminal or blast phase of chronic granulocytic leukemia.

Identification of primitive-appearing cells in the blood as megakaryocytes or megakaryocytic precursors in the blast phase of chronic granulocytic leukemia has been facilitated with the use of a specific platelet peroxidase reaction, detectable with both light microscopic and ultrastructural techniques.

On marrow aspiration, increased numbers of large and small megakaryocytes having few or no nuclear lobulations can be seen. Nuclei have delicate-appearing nuclear chromatin strands, and cytoplasm stains pale gray with indistinct granularity. In severe cases, marrow is virtually replaced by megakaryocytes. "Dwarf" megakaryocytes are seen frequently (Fig. 7–38).

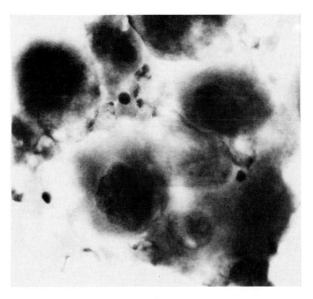

Figure 7–37   *Micromegakaryocytes in marrow of patient with agnogenic myeloid metaplasia.*

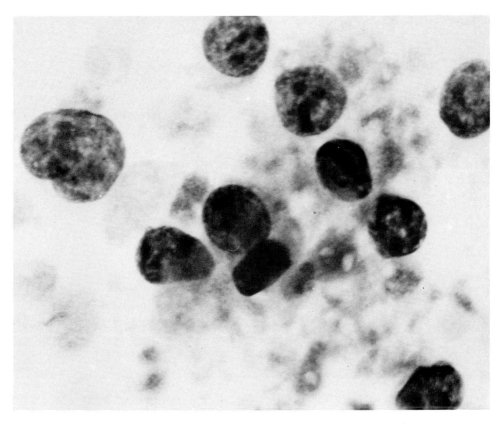

Figure 7–38   *Dwarf megakaryocytes in marrow of patient with acute megakaryocytic myelosis.*

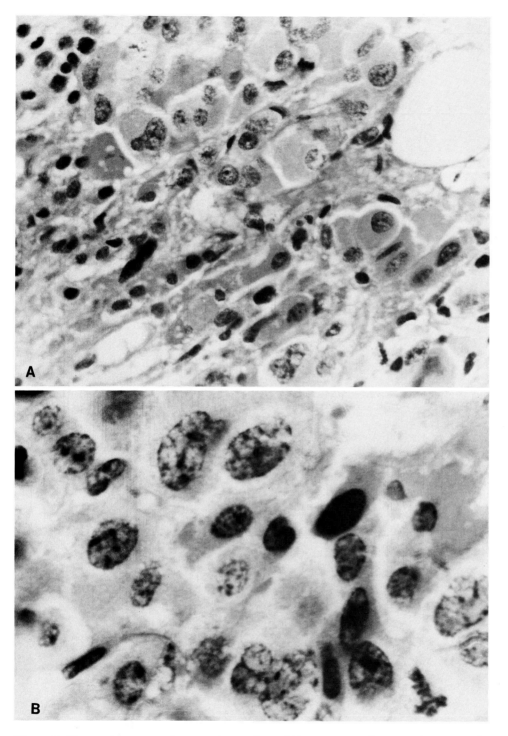

Figure 7–39   *Acute megakaryocytic myelosis. (A) Low magnification of marrow showing numerous immature megakaryocytes. (B) Higher-power view of immature megakaryocytes with small oval to round nuclei and intensely staining cytoplasm.*

On H and E section, primitive-appearing cells representing megakaryocytes are observed (Fig. 7–39 and Plate 2D). These cells have eosinophilic-staining cytoplasm and indistinct cellular borders and vary considerbly in size and shape, indicating considerable pleomorphism of megakaryocytes.

Cytochemistry of Megakaryocytes

Using routine panoptic stains, typical megakaryocytes are identified easily on the basis of their large size and darkly staining nucleus and cytoplasm. In both normal and pathologic marrows, small megakaryocytes, including micromegakaryocytes and megakaryoblasts, may be difficult to identify and to distinguish from atypical promyelocytes or large reticulum cells. Identification of megakaryoblasts in the terminal megakaryocytic leukemia phase of chronic granulocytic leukemia or in acute megakaryocytic myelosis may also be difficult using morphologic criteria alone.

For these reasons, a number of cytochemical and immunologic techniques have been developed for identification of megakaryocytes and their precursors. Using conventional cytochemical stains, megakaryocytes show intense activity of fluoride-resistant nonspecific esterase. They also exhibit intense unipolar or focal activity of acid phosphatase. With the PAS stain, megakaryocytes stain intensely and diffusely and may contain numerous chunklike aggregates of glycogen. With the methyl green-pyronine stain, megakaryocytes stain intensely with pyronine, indicating their high content of RNA.

More recently, megakaryocytes in normal and pathologic bone marrow specimens have been identified on the basis of a unique staining reaction with the oxazine dye rhodanile blue. Synthesized by a reaction between rhodamine blue and Nile blue to form an amide, rhodanile blue has been recognized as a metachromatic dye, but up to now has been used rarely in hematopathology. Used in an aqueous solution as a single-agent direct stain on ribonuclease-treated slides, rhodanile blue stains megakaryocytes metachromatically and intensely. Megakaryocytes stain bright pink, a color not found in other types of bone marrow or blood cells (Plate 4F). On the basis of enzymatic digestion studies, the metachromasia was due in part to a high content of acid mucopolysaccharide in the cytoplasm of megakaryocytes. Similarly, megakaryocytes can be identified on the basis of a metachromatic staining reaction of the cytoplasm using the basic cationic textile dye Lycramine brilliant blue JL.

Immunologically based techniques for identification of megakaryocytes have also been reported. These methods include immunoperoxidase and 5-nucleotidase in megakaryocytes, identification of
platelet factor 4, detection of 5-hydroxytryptamine organelles in
megakaryocytes, identification of β thromboglobulin, detection of
anti–factor VIII antigen, and demonstration of antiplatelet antibodies
in megakaryocytes. Currently, the immunoperoxidase techniques for
identification of megakaryoblasts are among the most sensitive of
those available and are particularly useful in identification of
megakaryoblasts in the megakaryoblastic phase of chronic granulocytic leukemia.

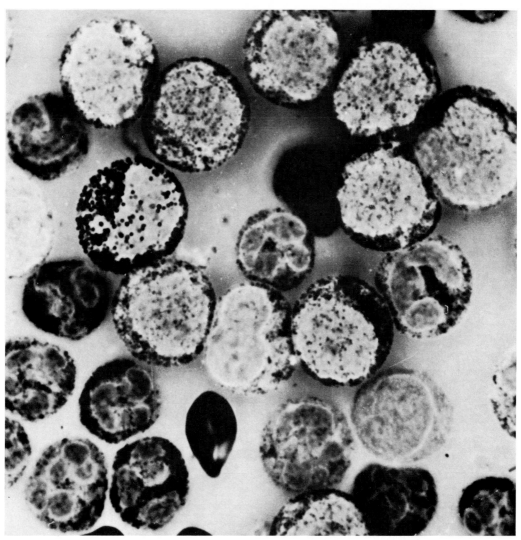

Granules in leukemic blasts from a patient with acute myelomonocytic leukemia (M4), as demonstrated by merocyanine 540 stain.

8 Cytochemistry of Marrow Cells

For more than a century, synthetic organic dyestuffs have been used to impart a color or colors to blood cells, either alive, as in a supravital stain, or fixed in the traditional way. Based on the perception of differences in these colors by the naked eye through the microscope and in recent years by instruments using image analysis, blood and bone marrow cells in health and disease have been distinguished from one another and classified.[16]

Cytochemistry of blood and bone marrow cells began with Ehrlich in 1879, since the colors imparted to blood cells by his triacid stain (acid orange, basic fuchsin, and methyl green) represented interactions between a dyestuff and cellular constituents to produce colored reaction products. Ehrlich's triacid stain was soon supplanted by the now-familiar Romanowsky stain and its variants, most of which contain eosin, methylene blue, and one or more of the azures in varying combinations and chemical modifications. In the case of both the triacid stain and the Romanowsky-type mixtures, characterization of the reaction products between individual dyestuffs and cellular constituents has not as yet been achieved.

Although pragmatically useful and forming the cornerstone of morphologic hematology as we know it today, the panoptic stains of the Romanowsky type have limitations. Early in the history of morphologic hematology, it became apparent that using visual perceptive techniques based on the Romanowsky stain alone, one could not identify certain types of "primitive" cells in cases of acute leukemia. In an effort to distinguish cells by a distinctive property rather than by appearance alone, the peroxidase stain was applied to morphologic hematology nearly 80 years ago. Since it distinguishes cells of granulocytic origin from those of lymphoid origin on an "all-or-none" basis with respect to peroxidase content, it became rapidly integrated into the study of leukemic blood cells. To this day, and particularly with newer chromogens and immunologic applications, the peroxidase reaction remains one of the most valuable cytochemical stains in hematopathology.

With the use of inhibitors, as well as the application of other stains such as the periodic acid–Schiff reagent and the stain for non-specific esterase activity, it is now possible to confirm morphologic observations and to quantitate small numbers of cells of a particular type in a specimen of bone marrow. With continuing applications of dyestuffs to hematology, particularly in the area of flow cytometry, we can anticipate that our ability to identify cells and to make distinctions between normal and abnormal cells of the same cytologic type will improve in the near future.

Tests for Iron

In hemosiderin, iron exists as ferric hydroxide in the form of aggregates of ferritin. Various tests can be used to identify hemosiderin in cells and in tissues.

Prussian Blue

Prussian blue reagent is an acidified solution of sodium nitroprusside. When this reagent is used, iron is demonstrated as bright blue green granular deposits (Fig. 8–1). Most of these deposits are intracellular, but some may be extracellular. Prussian blue can be used to demonstrate the presence of pathologic "ringed" sideroblasts in certain refractory anemias characterized by increased iron stores

Figure 8–1 *Prussian blue stain, chronic erythremic myelosis. Aggregates of hemosiderin are depicted.*

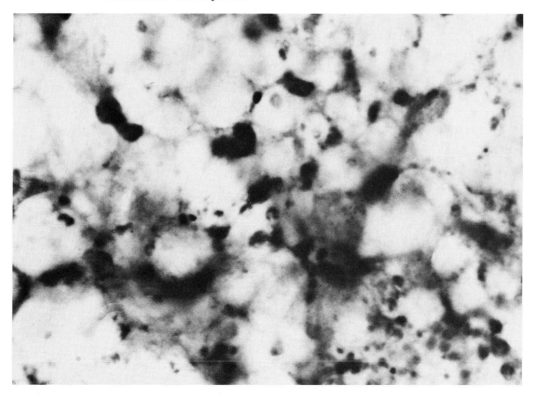

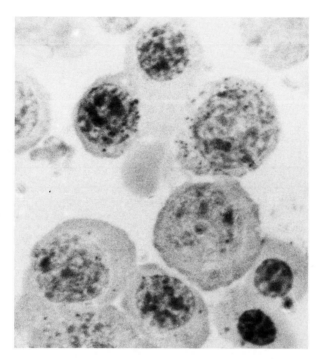

Figure 8–2   *Prussian blue stain, chronic erythremic myelosis, demonstrating siderotic granules in the cytoplasm. These represent iron in mitochondria.*

(Fig. 8–2) and to confirm the diagnosis of iron deficiency in cases in which the serum iron and total iron binding capacity do not provide a clear-cut answer. Patterns of iron deposits in the marrow have been thought to be of diagnostic usefulness. Large aggregates of hemosiderin occur in certain refractory anemias characterized by slow iron turnover. In hemolytic anemias, in which iron turnover is rapid, a "small particle" iron pattern is seen.

Fixative (formalin-methanol)

37% Formalin   10 ml

100% Methanol   90 ml

(store in refrigerator)

Solutions

A. 2% HCl

Concentrated HCl	2 ml
Distilled H_2O	100 ml

B. 2% Potassium ferrocyanide

Potassium ferrocyanide	2 g
Distilled H_2O	100 ml

(shelf life 6 weeks)

C. 0.1% Nuclear fast red

Nuclear fast red	0.1 g
Aluminum sulfate	5.0 g
Distilled H_2O	100 ml

Mix and filter through Whatman No. 1 paper.

Procedure

1. Fix coverslips in Coplin jar for 30 minutes.
2. Rinse in distilled H_2O.
3. Mix equal parts solution A and B.
4. Pour solution (step 3) into Coplin jar for 30 minutes.
5. Rinse in distilled H_2O.
6. Counterstain with 0.1% nuclear fast red for 1 minute.
7. Wash in distilled H_2O.
8. Air dry and mount with Permount.[1]

Alizarin Red S

Alizarin red S reacts with ferric iron, giving a bright purple salt composed of iron and alizarin. In a 15-minute test, this anthraquinone dye can be used to demonstrate iron in ringed sideroblasts. Iron in these cells appears as a purple perinuclear "halo" or as discrete blocks of purple-staining material (Fig. 8–3).[8]

Bromochlorophenol Blue

Bromochlorophenol blue forms a bright blue insoluble precipitate with ferric iron. The precipitate is composed of the dye and iron. In a 60-second test, bromochlorophenol blue can be used to rapidly demonstrate iron in ringed sideroblasts and in macrophages (Fig. 8–4). Iron appears as discrete dark blue particles.[12]

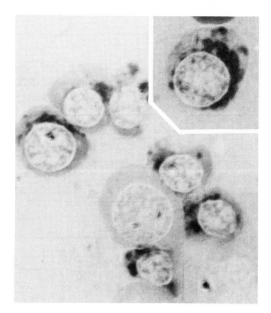

Figure 8–3   *Alizarin red S stain for sideroblasts, chronic erythremic myelosis. Iron in mitochondria appears as purple-staining coccoid structures and/or purple perinuclear halo.*

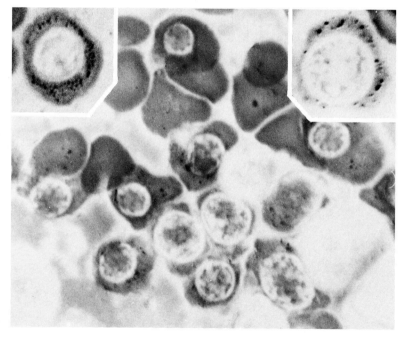

Figure 8–4   *Bromochlorophenol blue stain, demonstrating black punctate areas that represent iron in mitochondria of ringed sideroblasts from a patient with chronic erythremic myelosis.*

Tests That Demonstrate Abnormalities of the Glycogen Biosynthetic Pathway

Normally, glycogen is degraded in part as a result of the action of phosphorylase enzymes. However, it is believed that the reaction can be reversible and that phosphorylase may be involved in biosynthesis of glycogen in some types of abnormal cells.

Periodic Acid–Schiff (PAS) Test

First applied to blood cells by Astaldi and co-workers and subsequently by Quaglino and Hayhoe, the PAS test demonstrates glycogen within the cell. Normal polymorphonuclear leukocytes and megakaryocytes contain abundant glycogen. Normal lymphocytes may contain small amounts of glycogen. In normal erythroblasts, glycogen cannot be detected with the PAS stain. In hematopathology, the greatest usefulness of the PAS stain is its ability to demonstrate abnormally increased amounts of glycogen in pathological erythroid precursors, and in leukemic lymphoblasts. The appearance of the PAS-positive substance may be diffuse, granular, or a combination of the two.

Punctate-appearing aggregates of PAS-positive material can be seen in lymphoblasts from patients with acute lymphoblastic leukemia (Fig. 8–5 and Plate 4*B*) and in proerythroblasts from patients with chronic erythremic myelosis (Fig. 8–6, *inset*). In this disorder, diffuse PAS positivity is found in late intermediate macronormoblasts (Fig. 8–6). Large aggregates occur in erythroblasts from patients with Di Guglielmo syndrome, particularly acute erythremic myelosis and erythroleukemia (Fig. 8–7 and Plate 4*A*). PAS positivity is also found in erythroid precursors from patients with iron deficiency and thalassemia and in lymphocytoid plasma cells from patients with macroglobulinemia. Megaloblasts from patients with deficiency of vitamin B_{12} as in pernicious anemia contain PAS-positive material in a granular pattern in proerythroblasts and as a diffuse staining in intermediate megaloblasts (Fig. 8–8).[11]

As yet, mechanisms responsible for deposition of glycogen are unknown. Possibly increased activity of phosphorylase may facilitate glycogen synthesis and accumulation. Alternatively, increased deposits of glycogen may also occur as a result of decreased activity of enzymes involved in degradation of glycogen.

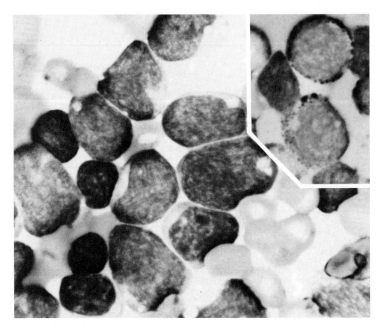

Figure 8–5   *Lymphoblasts, acute lymphoblastic leukemia. Inset shows prominent aggregates of PAS-positive material in cytoplasm of lymphoblasts.*

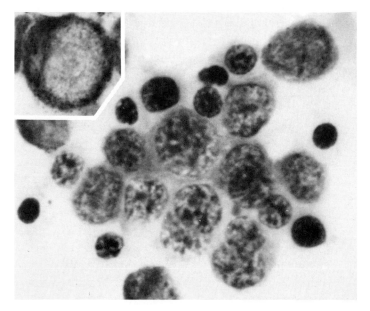

Figure 8–6   *PAS reaction, erythroblasts in chronic erythremic myelosis. In early erythroblasts and proerythroblasts, the reaction in punctate (inset), whereas in more mature erythroblasts, the reaction is usually diffuse.*

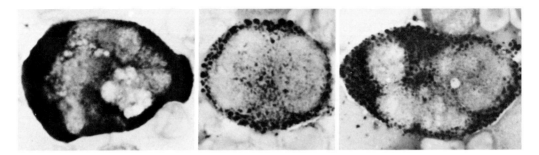

Figure 8–7 *PAS reaction, erythroleukemia erythroblasts, showing unusually intense blocklike aggregates of PAS-positive material.*

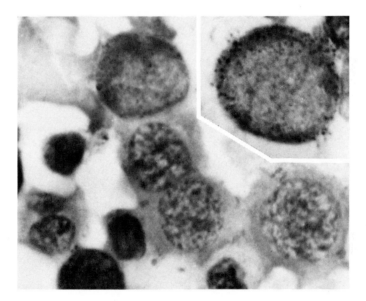

Figure 8–8 *PAS stain in megaloblasts, untreated pernicious anemia. In early megaloblasts and proerythroblasts, the PAS reaction is punctate (inset), whereas in more mature megaloblasts, the reaction is diffuse.*

Method. Periodic acid oxidizes glycols and related compounds to aldehydes. The aldehydes then can react with the Schiff's reagent (leukofuchsin) to release fuchsin and stain the cellular components containing the oxidizable compounds. A variety of intracellular compounds react with the PAS reagents. In blood and bone marrow cells glycogen appears to be the compound primarily responsible because the staining can be blocked by digestion with amylase.

Solutions

1. Schiff's reagent

Basic fuchsin	1.0 g
Sodium metabisulfite	2.0 g
IN HCl	10.0 ml
Distilled H_2O	200.0 ml
Activated charcoal	1.0 g

Bring H_2O to boiling, remove from heat, and very slowly add basic fuchsin. When fuchsin is dissolved, cool and filter. Add sodium metabisulfite and IN HCl. Let solution bleach for 24 hours. Add charcoal and shake for 1 minute. Filter through Whatman No. 1 filter paper. Solution should appear colorless. Store in refrigerator. Discard when reagent becomes light pink.

2. 1% Periodic acid

Periodic acid	1 g
Distilled H_2O	100 ml

Procedure

1. In staining jar, fix blood films or marrows in esterase fixative (*vide infra*) for 15 minutes.
2. Wash well in distilled H_2O.
3. Place in periodic acid for 10 minutes.
4. Wash in distilled H_2O for 5 minutes.
5. Place in Schiff's reagent for 30 minutes.
6. Wash in distilled H_2O for 5 minutes.
7. Counterstain with Mayer's hematoxylin for 8 minutes.
8. Wash in distilled H_2O.
9. "Blue" in NH_4OH water (six drops of 28% NH_4OH per 500 ml H_2O; six quick dips).
10. Wash in distilled H_2O.
11. Air dry and mount with Permount.[1, 2]

Diastase may be used to confirm that the staining reaction was due to glycogen.

Phosphorylase Activity

As noted above, phosphorylase is usually regarded as an enzyme involved in the catabolism of glycogen. In cells that show PAS positivity, activity of phosphorylase is also strong and usually parallels the type of diffuse or granular pattern found in the PAS-positive cells from the same individual (Fig. 8–9). These findings suggest that in abnormal and perhaps neoplastic cells such as those found in acute lymphoblastic leukemia or Di Guglielmo syndrome, phosphorylase

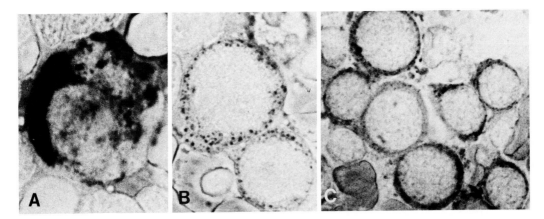

Figure 8–9   *Phosphorylase activity. (A) Erythroleukemia erythroblast. (B) Pernicious anemia megaloblast. (C) Megaloblastoid intermediate macronormoblasts in chronic erythremic myelosis.*

acts to facilitate the biosynthesis and consequent deposition of glycogen, visible as PAS-positive material. As another possible pathogenetic mechanism, increased glycogen may induce increased activity of phosphorylase to facilitate glycogen breakdown.[13]

Tests That Demonstrate Abnormalities of Nucleic Acids and Nucleoproteins

Feulgen Stain

Feulgen stain demonstrates DNA and at present may not have immediate clinical application in routine hematopathology.

Pyronine Stain

Combined with methyl green as a nuclear counterstain, pyronine demonstrates RNA in the cytoplasm of cells. Intense pyroninophilia is seen in pernicious anemia megaloblasts (Fig. 8–10), in some leukemic blasts, and in myeloma cells. In normal bone marrows, proerythroblasts, early intermediate normoblasts, megakaryocytes, and plasma cells demonstrate increased RNA. Pyroninophilia is also characteristic of immunoblasts in angioimmunoblastic lymphadenopathy and is typical of Burkitt's lymphoma cells (Fig. 8–11).

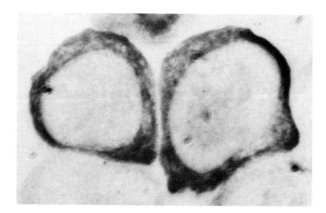

Figure 8–10   *Methyl green-pyronine stain, megaloblasts in pernicious anemia, demonstrating intense cytoplasmic pyroninophilia due to increased RNA.*

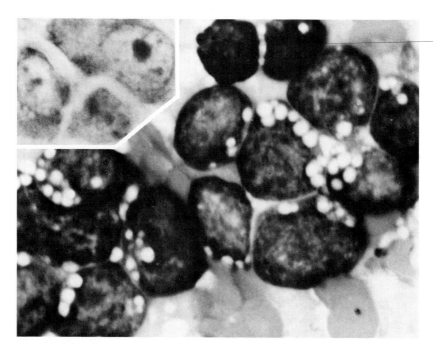

Figure 8–11   *Vacuolated neoplastic lymphoid cells, Burkitt's lymphoma. Inset shows intense pyroninophilia in these cells using the methyl green-pyronine reaction.*

Method. Although not specific for RNA, pyronine Y stains RNA intensely red in cells. Methyl green stains DNA green and is used as the counterstain.

FAA Fixative

95% Ethanol	90 ml
Glacial acetic acid	5 ml
37% Formalin	5 ml

(store in refrigerator)

Staining Solution

Methyl green	0.5 g
Pyronine Y	0.2 g
Dissolve in 100 ml	0.10 M sodium acetate (1.36 g sodium acetate per 100 ml distilled H_2O)

Adjust to *p*H 4.4 with glacial acetic acid.

Procedure

1. Fix in cold FAA fixative for 1 hour.
2. Rinse in distilled H_2O.
3. Stain in methyl green-pyronine for 30 minutes.
4. Wash in distilled H_2O, air dry, and mount with Permount.

Ammoniacal Silver Stain

The ammoniacal silver stain distinguishes between lysine-rich and arginine-rich histones (basic nucleoproteins). Lysine-rich histones stain yellow to orange, whereas arginine-rich histones stain brown or black. A unique abnormality found in erythroid precursors of Di Guglielmo syndrome (acute and chronic erythremic myelosis and erythroleukemia) is the black-speckled appearance of the nucleus when this stain is used (Fig. 8–12). Similar findings are observed in erythroid precursors of thrombotic thrombocytopenic purpura (TTP). One interpretation of the speckled pattern is that arginine-rich histones are present in increased amounts and localized in areas of heterochromatin (metabolically repressed DNA) in nuclei of erythroblasts from patients with these disorders.[3, 4]

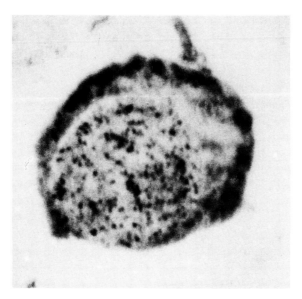

Figure 8–12   *Ammoniacal silver stain, proerythroblast, erythroleukemia, showing black punctate areas of arginine-rich histone in the nucleus. (Kass L: Preleukemic Disorders. Springfield, IL, Charles C Thomas, 1979).*

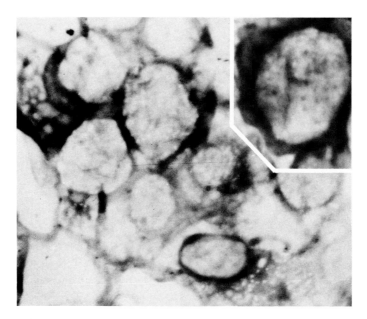

Figure 8–13   *Azure A stain, chronic erythremic myelosis, demonstrating pink metachromatic material in the nucleus (light gray filamentous-appearing material in nucleus).*

Azure A

After removal of nucleic acids with TCA (trichloroacetic acid) and subsequent staining with the blue thiazine dye azure A, nuclei of erythroid precursors from patients with Di Guglielmo syndrome show a unique pink metachromasia (Fig. 8–13). This metachromasia is not found in erythroid precursors in other disorders. Using biochemical, chromatographic, and electrophoretic techniques, the pink metachromasia was found to be due to methylated arginines present in the nuclei of erythroblasts in Di Guglielmo syndrome. It has been suggested that this nuclear metachromasia may be a useful diagnostic test for the Di Guglielmo syndrome group of disorders.[5]

Tests That Demonstrate Abnormalities of Cytoplasmic Components

Leukocyte Alkaline Phosphatase (LAP)

Alkaline phosphatase is found in secondary or specific granules. Normally, cells of the neutrophilic granulocytic series and particularly neutrophils show substantial activity of alkaline phosphatase. Using a conventional test for demonstration of this enzyme, a "score" can be enumerated, based on the intensity of the reaction product and the number of reaction products representing enzyme activity in specific granules.

A normal alkaline phosphatase score is 50 to 200 units. In typical chronic granulocytic leukemia and paroxysmal nocturnal hemoglobinuria (PNH), the alkaline phosphatase score is usually low (Fig. 8–14). When combined with other criteria, it may be of diagnostic usefulness, particularly in distinguishing chronic granulocytic leukemia from leukemoid reactions (in which the leukocyte alkaline phosphatase is normal or high) and from atypical cases of agnogenic myeloid metaplasia.

Method. Naphthol AS-MX phosphoric acid as the substrate is hydrolyzed to phosphate and an aryl naphtholamide by alkaline phosphatase. Aryl naphtholamide is coupled to the diazonium salt fast blue RR, forming an insoluble reaction product. This pigment is visible at sites of alkaline phosphatase activity.

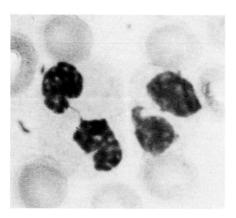

Figure 8–14
Alkaline phosphatase stain in neutrophils from a patient with chronic granulocytic leukemia. Little if any enzymatic activity can be detected.

Chemicals and Solutions

1. Fast blue RR salt capsule
2. Naphthol AS-MX phosphate alkaline solution (obtained commercially)
3. Mayer's hematoxylin solution.

Procedure

Fixing

1. After making films, allow them to air dry.
2. Using a Coplin jar, fix blood films in cold 10% formalin 90% methanol for 30 seconds.
3. Rinse thoroughly, but gently, with tap water.
4. Air dry.
5. Store in freezer.

Staining

1. Pipette 2 ml of naphthol AS-MX phosphate alkaline solution into an Erlenmeyer flask.
2. Add 48 ml of distilled water.
3. Add the contents of a fast blue RR salt capsule and mix thoroughly by shaking 15 to 30 seconds.
4. Filter through Whatman No. 2 filter paper onto blood films in a Coplin jar.
5. Incubate for 30 minutes at room temperature and away from direct light.
6. Wash gently with tap water.
7. Counterstain with Mayer's hematoxylin solution for 3 minutes.
8. Wash with tap water for 20 seconds, dry, and mount with immersion oil on labeled glass slide.

Table 8–1   *Precipitated Azo Dye in Cytoplasm*

Cell Ratings	Size of Granule	Intensity of Stain
0	No precipitated dye in cytoplasm	
1+	Small	Faint to moderate
2+	Small to medium	Moderate to strong
3+	Medium to large	Strong
4+	Medium and large	Brilliant

Multiply the number of cells counted in each rating by that rating. Add the totals together to give the total number of units. Normal is 11 to 95 units.

Most peripheral blood films and marrows from patients with untreated chronic granulocytic leukemia have a score between 0 and 11. Patients with polycythemia vera or with myeloid metaplasia or a leukemoid reaction as seen in severe infections usually have a LAP score ranging from the high end of the normal range to substantially above 95. Patients with paroxysmal nocturnal hemoglobinuria or congenital hypophosphatasia generally have a low LAP score.[2]

Alizarin Red S in Pernicious Anemia

Alizarin red S stains the cytoplasm of megaloblasts from patients with untreated pernicious anemia (or vitamin B_{12} deficiency due to other causes) a bright pink color (Fig. 8–15). After specific treatment with vitamin B_{12}, the color becomes yellow. On the basis of test

Figure 8–15   *Pink staining of cytoplasm of pernicious anemia megaloblasts with alizarin red S.*

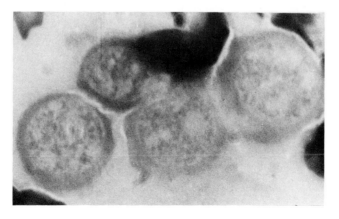

tube experiments, the pink color is believed to be due in large part to excessive amounts of methylmalonyl CoA found in deficiency of vitamin B_{12}. Because excess methylmalonyl CoA results from decreased activity of the coenzyme B_{12}-dependent methylmalonyl CoA mutase enzyme, the "pink" megaloblasts may constitute cytochemical evidence for the known metabolic block in deficiency of vitamin B_{12}.[6]

Lysozyme

The sulfonated dis-azo dye Biebrich scarlet is used. If cells containing lysozyme are preincubated with *N*-acetylglucosamine oligosaccharides prior to Biebrich scarlet, subsequent staining with this dye is greatly diminished, presumably because the oligosaccharides compete with Biebrich scarlet for the active site of the lysozyme molecule (Fig. 8–16). This test may be of diagnostic usefulness in the cytochemical categorization of various types of acute leukemia, since blasts from patients with monocytic leukemia contain abundant lysozyme, whereas myeloblasts and lymphoblasts do not. These cytochemical reactions are paralleled by serum and urinary lysozyme levels in the same patients.[19]

Figure 8–16   *Strong reaction for lysozyme in cytoplasm of neoplastic monocytes (dark gray cytoplasmic rim). Inset shows lack of stainability of cytoplasm with Biebrich scarlet after preincubation with oligosaccharides.*

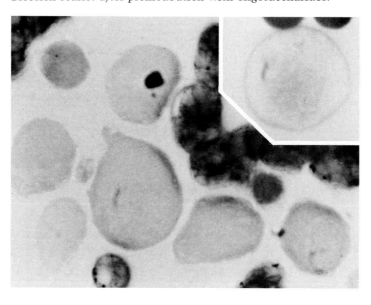

Acid Phosphatase

Using naphthol AS-TR phosphate as the substrate at an acid *p*H, activity of acid phosphatase can be demonstrated. Hairy cells from patients with hairy cell leukemia show acid phosphatase activity that is resistant to inhibition by L-tartrate (Fig. 8–17*A* and *B*). Leukemic lymphoblasts of the T-cell convoluted type often contain unipolar localization of acid phosphatase activity (Fig. 8–17*C*). Monocytes are rich in acid phosphatase. In proerythroblasts and intermediate normoblasts, acid phosphatase activity is frequently localized in a unipolar area (Figure 8–17*D*). In normal plasma cells, acid phosphatase activity appears as a chunklike reaction product. In megakaryocytes, acid phosphatase activity is intense and often concentrated in one area of the cell.

Method. Acid phosphatase hydrolyzes naphthol AS-TR phosphate. Released alpha naphthol combines with hexazotized pararosaniline to form a colored insoluble reaction product at the site(s) of enzymatic activity.

Fixative (buffered formalin-acetone)

Na_2HPO_4	20 mg
KH_2PO_4	100 mg
H_2O	30 ml
Acetone	45 ml
37% Formalin *p*H 6.6	25 ml

Store in refrigerator at 4°C.

Solutions

A. Acetate buffer (0.1M *p*H5)

a. Sodium acetate	2.0 gm
Distilled H_2O	250 ml

Store in refrigerator at 4°C.

b. 0.1N HCl

Concentrated HCl	0.835 ml
Distilled H_2O	91.7 ml

c. Distilled H_2O	75 ml

To 20 ml solution a add 5 ml solution b.
Then add 75 ml solution c. Check *p*H
and adjust to *p*H 5.0.

(Text continued on page 364)

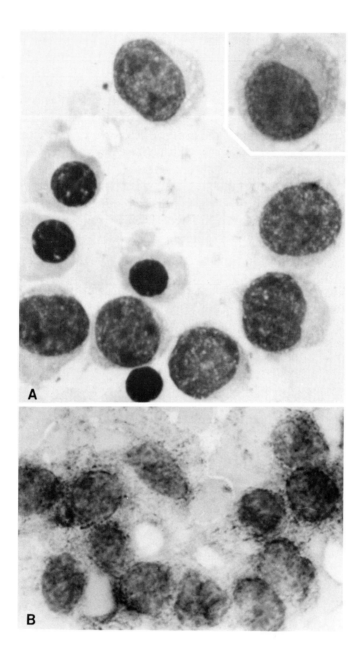

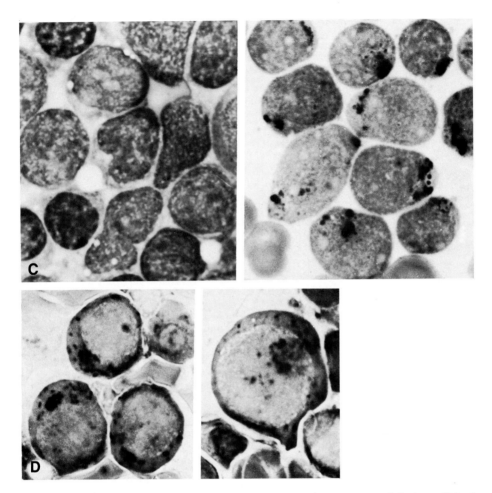

Figure 8–17
(opposite
and above)

(A) *Hairy cells from bone marrow of a patient with hairy cell leukemia.* (B) *Strong tartrate-resistant acid phosphatase activity in hairy cells.* (C) *T-cell convoluted leukemic lymphoblasts* (left) *and unipolar acid phosphatase activity in these cells* (right). (D) *Proerythroblasts from the bone marrow of a patient with paroxysmal nocturnal hemoglobinuria. Intense focal activity of acid phosphatase is seen. Similar focal localization although less activity of acid phosphatase is found in normal proerythroblasts and normoblasts.*

B. Pararosaniline

     Pararosaniline hydrochloride   1 gm
     Distilled H_2O 20 ml
     Concentrated HCl   5 ml

Store in dark at room temperature.

C. 4% Sodium nitrite

     Sodium nitrite   0.2 g
     Distilled H_2O 5 ml

Make freshly each time.

D. Naphthol AS-BI phosphoric acid   40 mg
E. N,N-dimethylformamide   4 ml
F. L(+) tartaric acid   300 mg
G. 1% Aqueous methyl green buffered with 0.1N sodium acetate to pH 4.2. Extract with chloroform until solvent is clear.

Procedure:

1. Fix bone marrow films for 30 seconds and wash in distilled H_2O.
2. Mix 71.2 ml acetate buffer (pH 5.0) with 40 mg naphthol AS-BI phosphoric acid dissolved in 4 ml N,N-dimethylformamide.
3. Mix 2.4 ml pararosaniline with 2.4 ml sodium nitrite for 1 minute. Add this solution to the solution in step 2 to make a total volume of 80 ml.
4. For the tartrate-resistant acid phosphatase reaction add 300 mg L(+) tartaric acid to 40 ml of the mixture in step 3.
5. Adjust the pH of both mixtures to 5.1 with a saturated solution of sodium hydroxide.
6. Filter solution and pour into a Coplin jar.
7. Incubate slides in solution at 37°C for 1 hour.
8. Wash slides with distilled H_2O.
9. Counterstain with 1% aqueous methyl green for 2 minutes.
10. Rinse in distilled H_2O, air dry, and mount on a cleaned labeled slide.[21]

Sudan Black B

A dis-azo dye (C.I. solvent black 3), Sudan black B is used to identify immature cells of granulocytic origin, such as leukemic myeloblasts (Fig. 8–18). As yet, substances that have affinity for Sudan black B have not been identified or characterized but are believed to be lipids and sterols. Generally, immature cells like myeloblasts and pro-

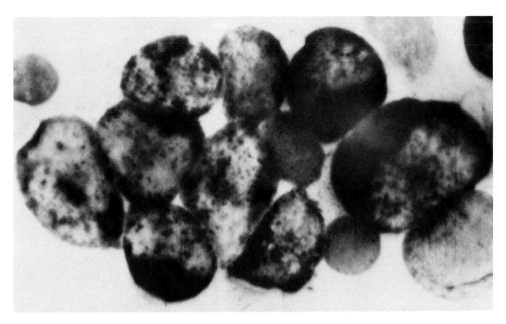

Figure 8–18   *Sudan black B stain, leukemic myeloblasts.*

myelocytes stain weakly with Sudan black B, and more mature cells like bands and neutrophils stain strongly; occasionally, some leukemic myeloblasts may show stainability by Sudan black B and no activity of myeloperoxidase.

Solutions

1. Formalin 37% aqueous solution
2. Sudan black B stock solution, made by dissolving 0.3 g Sudan black B powder in 100 ml absolute ethanol. The dye is poorly soluble in ethanol and may take up to several days to dissolve.
3. Buffer solution, made by combining 16 g phenol with 30 ml absolute ethanol and adding this mixture to a solution of 0.3 g $Na_2PO_4 \cdot 12\ H_2O$ in 100 ml distilled water
4. Staining solution, made by mixing 60 ml Sudan black B stock solution with 40 ml buffer. Filter by suction, and store at room temperature for no longer than several weeks before making a new solution.
5. Mayer's or Harris's hematoxylin can be used as a counterstain.

Procedure

1. Fix air-dried films of bone marrow or blood in formalin vapor for 10 minutes.

2. Immerse fixed film in Sudan black B staining solution in a Coplin jar for 60 minutes.
3. Wash in 70% ethanol for 2 or 3 minutes to remove excess stain.
4. Wash in tap water and counterstain for 10 minutes in hematoxylin solution.
5. Wash in tap water for 5 minutes, air dry, and mount face down with immersion oil or aqueous mounting medium for conventional light microscopy.[2]

Myeloperoxidase

Myeloperoxidase is a lysosomal enzyme found in cells of granulocytic origin, including monocytes (Fig. 8–19). Immature neutrophilic granulocytes like promyelocytes contain abundant peroxidase activity. This is due in large part to the high content of lysosomes (primary granules) in these immature cells. In bands and neutrophils, myeloperoxidase activity is less than in promyelocytes or myelocytes. Myeloblasts in myeloblastic leukemia contain myeloperoxidase activity (Fig. 8–20). Myeloperoxidase activity can also be detected in the cytoplasm of abnormal erythroblasts in erythroleukemia (Fig. 8–21) and suggests that these erythroblasts may contain granulocytic properties. A variety of chromogens, including 3-amino-9-ethylcarbazole, benzidine,[18] and O-tolidine, can be used to indicate the reaction. Because of its reputed carcinogenicity, benzidine is used infrequently at the present time.

Figure 8–19   *Normal monocyte (A) and polymorphonuclear leukocyte (B) demonstrating peroxidase activity. Benzidine stain.*

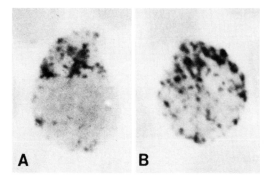

A   B

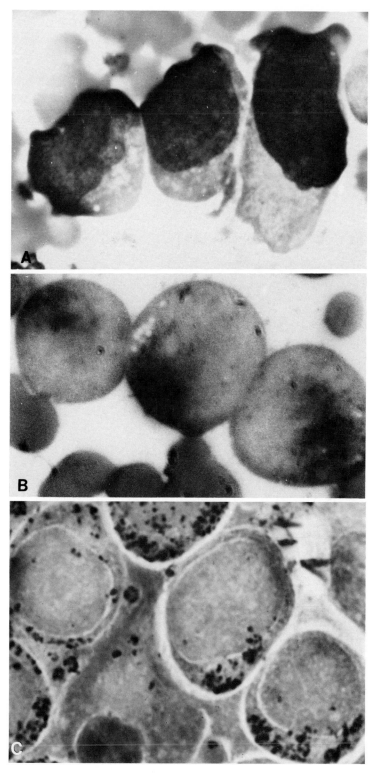

Figure 8–20   (A) *Myeloblasts from a patient with myeloblastic leukemia. (B) Strong peroxidase activity (black) in myeloblasts, using O-tolidine. (C) Strong peroxidase activity (black) in leukemic myeloblasts, using benzidine.*

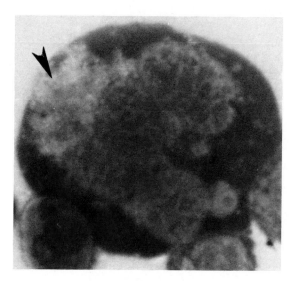

Figure 8–21   *Peroxidase activity* (arrow) *in cytoplasm of erythroblast, erythroleukemia, using O-tolidine.*

Method. Hydrogen peroxide and the catalytic action of peroxidase reduce 3-amino-9-ethylcarbazole to a colored compound. Myeloperoxidase activity is represented by red orange granular-appearing deposits.

Fixative   **(Buffered formalin acetone, pH 6.6)**

Na_2HPO_4	100 mg
KH_2PO_4	500 mg
Distilled H_2O	150 ml
Acetone	225 ml
37% Formalin	125 ml

Solutions

1. Stain at pH 5.5

3-amino-9-ethylcarbazole	30 mg
Dimethylsulfoxide	6 ml
0.3% Fresh hydrogen peroxide	0.4 ml
0.2M Acetate buffer pH 5.0	50 ml

    A. 0.6 ml acetic acid in 500 ml distilled H_2O

acetic acid

O
‖
HOCCH₃

O
‖
O-C-CH₃

esterase
H₂O

acetate

CH₃

N=N—

CH₃

⊕
N≡N

Fast Garnet GBC Salt

OH

α-naphthol

O
‖
O-C-CH₂CH₂CH₃

esterase
H₂O

butyrate

O
‖
HOCCH₂CH₂CH₃

n-butyric acid

OH

azo dye –
colored reaction
product

N=N

CH₃

N=N

CH₃

Chemical reactions involved in demonstration of nonspecific esterase activity. Alpha naphthol is liberated from synthetic substrates by the action of nonspecific esterase. Alpha naphthol forms a colored insoluble reaction products with an azo dye, such as fast blue BBN or fast garnet GBC.

Specific Esterase. Specific esterase is an enzyme that is believed to be characteristic of cells of granulocytic origin. Specific esterase activity can be demonstrated with the use of naphthol ASD-chloroacetate as the substrate (Fig. 8–23). Specific esterase activity occurs in both primary and secondary granules of granulocytes (Fig. 8–24) and is also found in blasts from patients with acute myeloblastic (Fig. 8–25) and myelomonocytic leukemia (Fig. 8–26) and in erythroblasts from patients with acute erythremic myelosis and erythroleukemia (Fig. 8–27).[9, 10]

(Text continued on page 374)

B. 1.15 g sodium acetate in 500 ml dis

Add 10 ml A to 40 ml B to make 0
In a 100-ml beaker, dissolve the 3-
the dimethylsulfoxide. Add acetate
beaker, and add 0.3% hydrogen pei
as described below.

2. Mayer's hematoxylin

α -naphthyl

Procedure

1. Fix smears in buffered formalin acetoɪ
2. Incubate smears in filtered stain for 2
3. Wash gently in running water.
4. Counterstain in Mayer's hematoxylir
5. Wash, air dry, and mount in aqueous

As alternatives to the peroxidase re
1),[14] as shown in Plate 4*E*, and Niagara
described as single-agent stains that are
of both primary and secondary granule

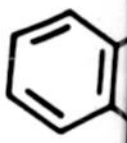

α - naphthyl

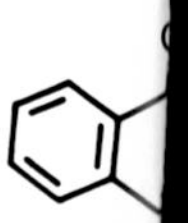

Esterases

Esterases are ubiquitous enzymes tha
matic ester bonds. Over the past deca
tests have been developed to detect t
in cells. In these tests, synthetic subs
reaction and dye couplers are used to
plexes with the product(s) of the enz
ing site(s) of enzymatic activity.

Figure 8–22

Chemically, enzymatic catalysis
of alpha naphthol from the syntheti
substance reacts with a diazo salt, s
garnet GBC, to form a colored insol
lar localization of esterase activity.

Diazo salts vary in their sensiti
GBC may be a more sensitive couɪ
ase reaction than fast blue BBN.

B. 1.15 g sodium acetate in 500 ml distilled H$_2$O.

Add 10 ml A to 40 ml B to make 0.2M acetate buffer *p*H 5.0. In a 100-ml beaker, dissolve the 3-amino-9-ethylcarbazole with the dimethylsulfoxide. Add acetate buffer, filter into another beaker, and add 0.3% hydrogen peroxide. Stain is ready for use as described below.

2. Mayer's hematoxylin

Procedure

1. Fix smears in buffered formalin acetone for 15 seconds.
2. Incubate smears in filtered stain for 2½ minutes.
3. Wash gently in running water.
4. Counterstain in Mayer's hematoxylin for 3 minutes.
5. Wash, air dry, and mount in aqueous mounting medium.

As alternatives to the peroxidase reaction, Saturn blue (acid blue 1),[14] as shown in Plate 4*E*, and Niagara sky blue 6 B[15] have been described as single-agent stains that are useful for the demonstration of both primary and secondary granules in granulocytic cells.

Esterases

Esterases are ubiquitous enzymes that hydrolyze aliphatic and aromatic ester bonds. Over the past decade, a variety of cytochemical tests have been developed to detect the presence of esterase activity in cells. In these tests, synthetic substrates are used for the esterase reaction and dye couplers are used to form colored insoluble complexes with the product(s) of the enzymatic reaction, thereby localizing site(s) of enzymatic activity.

Chemically, enzymatic catalysis by esterases leads to liberation of alpha naphthol from the synthetic substrates (Fig. 8–22). This substance reacts with a diazo salt, such as fast blue BBN or fast garnet GBC, to form a colored insoluble salt that indicates the cellular localization of esterase activity.

Diazo salts vary in their sensitivity. For example, fast garnet GBC may be a more sensitive coupling reagent for the specific esterase reaction than fast blue BBN.

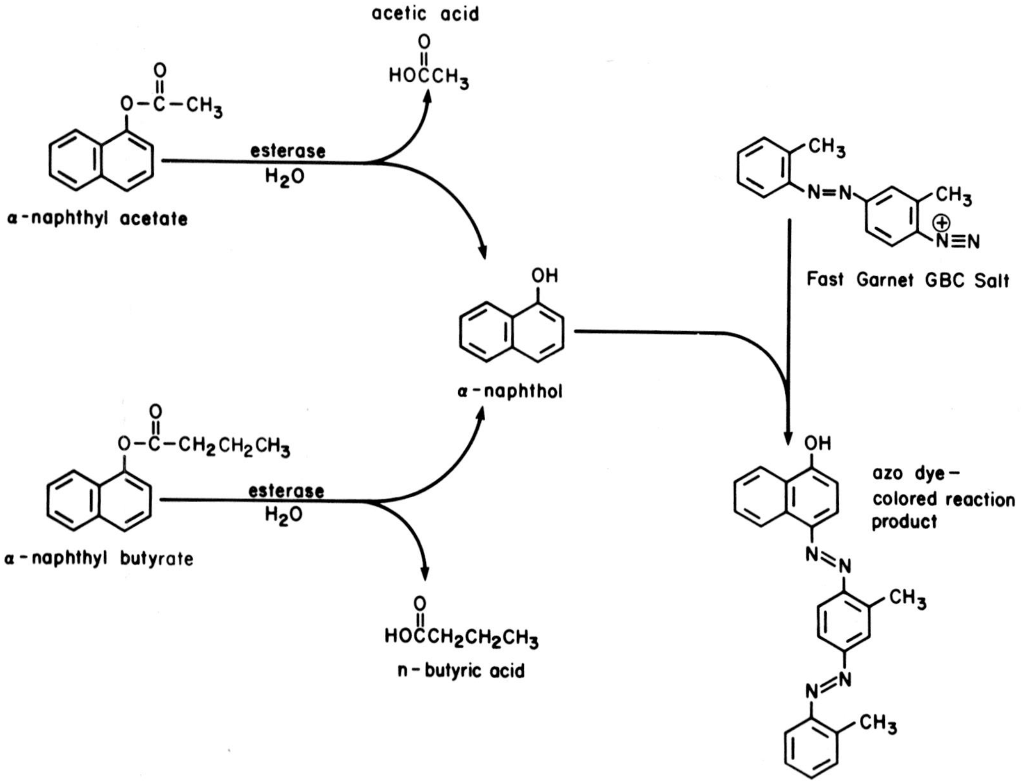

Figure 8–22   *Chemical reactions involved in demonstration of nonspecific esterase activity. Alpha naphthol is liberated from synthetic substrates by the action of nonspecific esterase. Alpha naphthol forms a colored insoluble reaction products with an azo dye, such as fast blue BBN or fast garnet GBC.*

Specific Esterase. Specific esterase is an enzyme that is believed to be characteristic of cells of granulocytic origin. Specific esterase activity can be demonstrated with the use of naphthol ASD-chloroacetate as the substrate (Fig. 8–23). Specific esterase activity occurs in both primary and secondary granules of granulocytes (Fig. 8–24) and is also found in blasts from patients with acute myeloblastic (Fig. 8–25) and myelomonocytic leukemia (Fig. 8–26) and in erythroblasts from patients with acute erythremic myelosis and erythroleukemia (Fig. 8–27).[9, 10]

(Text continued on page 374)

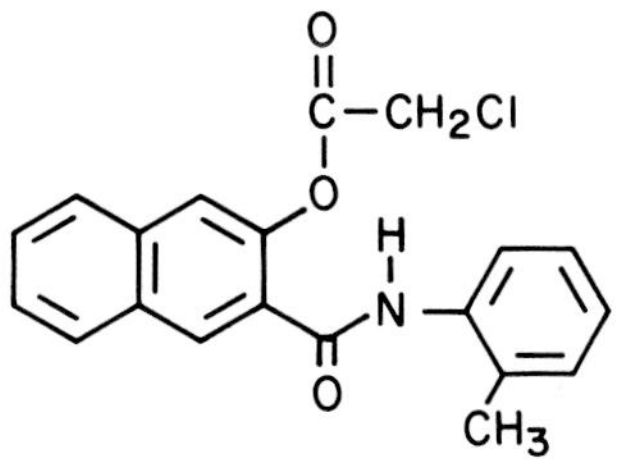

Figure 8–23   *Naphthol ASD-chloroacetate.*

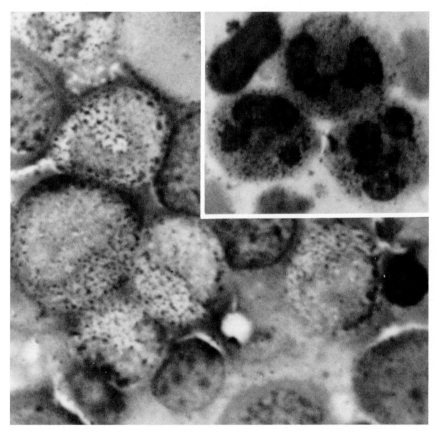

Figure 8–24   *Specific esterase activity in immature granulocytes (punctate black) and in mature polymorphonuclear leukocytes (inset).*

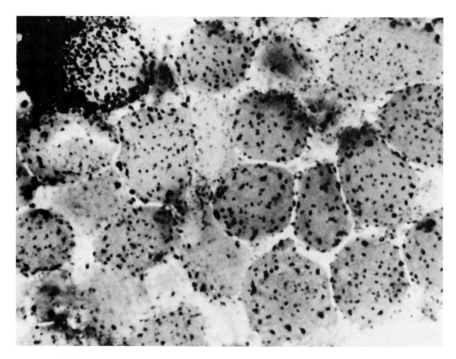

Figure 8–25   *Myeloblasts, myeloblastic leukemia, showing specific esterase activity (punctate black).*

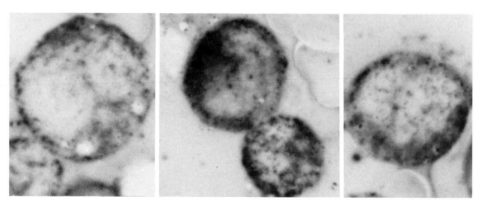

Figure 8–26   *Neoplastic monocytes, acute myelomonocytic leukemia, demonstrating nonspecific esterase activity (diffuse gray) and specific esterase (punctate black). (Kass L: Preleukemic Disorders. Springfield, IL., Charles C Thomas, 1979)*

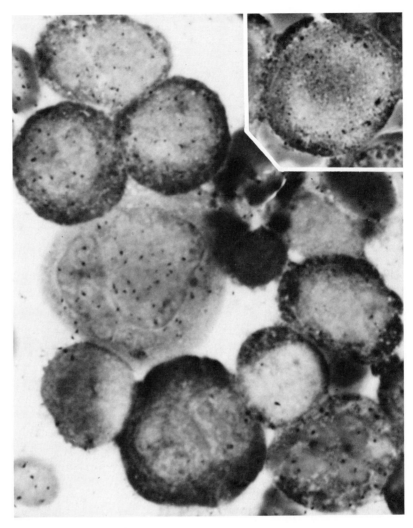

Figure 8–27   *Neoplastic erythroblasts, erythroleukemia, showing strong activity of nonspecific esterase (diffuse gray) and specific esterase (punctate black).*

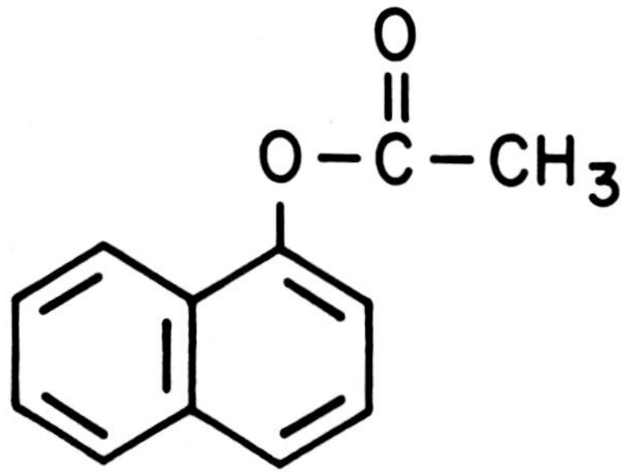

Figure 8–28   *Alpha naphthyl acetate.*

Nonspecific Esterase. Cytochemical tests for identifying nonspecific esterases have been developed using various synthetic substrates such as alpha naphthyl acetate and alpha naphthyl butyrate.[16, 20] Sensitivity or lack of sensitivity to organophosphate inhibitors or to sodium fluoride is a valuable addition to the nonspecific esterase reaction, since different types of nonspecific esterases have differing sensitivities to fluoride inhibition. Using alpha naphthyl acetate as the substrate (Fig. 8–28), nonspecific esterase activity that can be inhibited by fluoride is found in normal monocytes and macrophages, pernicious anemia megaloblasts, leukemic blasts from patients with monocytic leukemia (Fig. 8–29), histiocytic lymphoma cells (Fig. 8–30), hairy cell leukemia, and erythroblasts from patients with Di Guglielmo syndrome.

Using alpha naphthyl butyrate as substrate (Fig. 8–31), nonspecific esterase activity is found in cells of monocytic or macrophage origin. Consequently, fluoride-sensitive nonspecific esterase using alpha naphthyl acetate and particularly alpha naphthyl butyrate is regarded by some as a specific marker for cells of monocytic or macrophage origin. Along these lines, nonspecific esterase activity can be demonstrated with the use of alpha naphthyl butyrate in hairy cell from patients with hairy cell leukemia (Fig. 8–32). Fluoride-resistant nonspecific esterase demonstrable with these substrates is found in cells of granulocytic or megakaryocytic origin.[20]

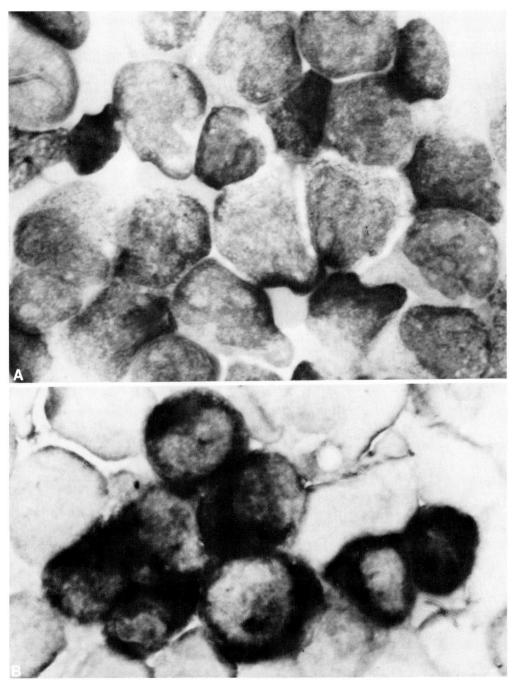

Figure 8–29 (A) *Neoplastic monocytes, monocytic leukemia* (B) *Strong activity of nonspecific esterase in neoplastic monocytes.*

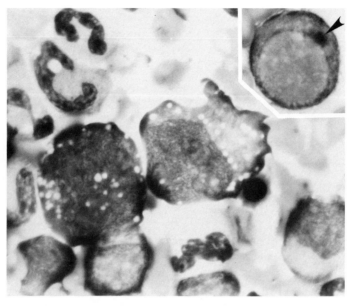

Figure 8–30   *Neoplastic cells from a patient with histiocytic lymphoma involving bone marrow. Inset shows unipolar nonspecific esterase activity (arrow) in histiocytic lymphoma cell.*

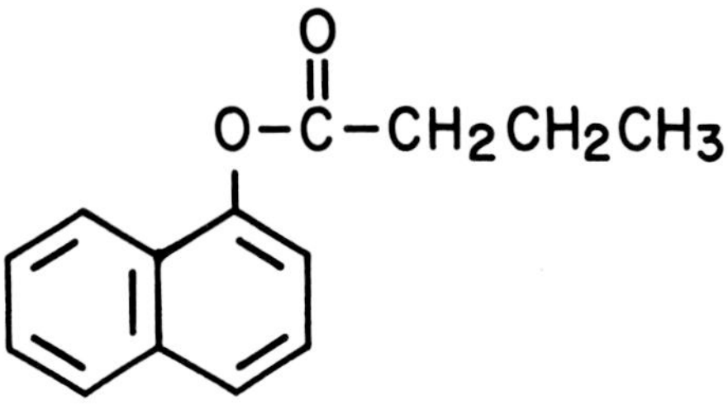

Figure 8–31   *Alpha naphthyl butyrate.*

Combined Esterases. In certain pathologic cells, activities of both specific esterase and nonspecific esterase are demonstrable. In these cells, as found in acute erythremic myelosis (De Guglielmo syndrome), erythroleukemia, and monocytic leukemia, the presence of specific esterase activity constitutes evidence for granulocytic differentiation in a cell that is morphologically erythroid or monocytic, as the case may be (Fig. 8–33).

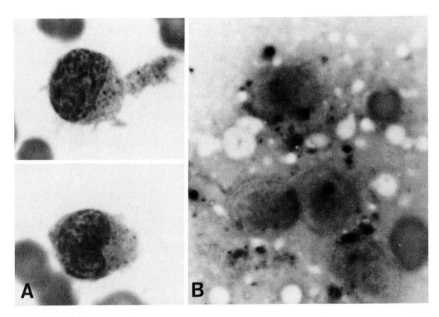

Figure 8–32   (A) *Nonspecific esterase activity in hairy cells, alpha naphthyl butyrate.* (B) *Nonspecific esterase in hairy cells from spleen of a patient with hairy cell leukemia, alpha naphthyl butyrate.*

In some instances (e.g., monocytic leukemia), the cells may demonstrate morphologic properties of the two cell lines. In acute erythremic myelosis and erythroleukemia, the presence of specific esterase activity in erythroblasts reflects a common myeloblastic stem cell for the abnormal erythroblasts and perhaps their propensity to precede the development of myeloblastic or monocytic leukemia.

In monocytic leukemia, the presence of specific esterase activity is consistent with the belief that monocytic leukemia is a morphologic variant of myeloblastic leukemia. Additionally, using fast garnet GBC as the dye indicator rather than fast blue BBN to demonstrate specific esterase activity, the enzyme is detectable in monocytes from patients with so-called histiomonocytic leukemia diagnosed on the basis of currently accepted morphologic criteria.

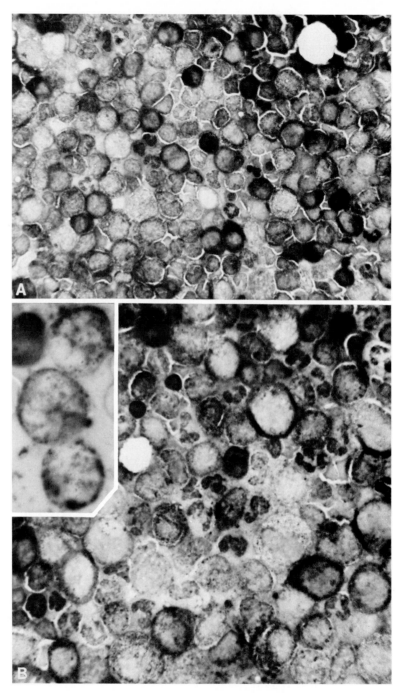

Figure 8–33 (A and B) Low-power and higher-power views of marrow from a patient with acute myelomonocytic leukemia, showing reactions for specific and nonspecific esterase. Diffuse gray and black areas represent nonspecific esterase activity, whereas punctate black areas represent specific esterase activity. Inset shows leukemic monocytes containing specific and nonspecific esterase activities.

These findings raise questions about the distinction of histiomono-cytic leukemia as an entity separate and distinct from monocytic leukemia. Perhaps histiomonocytic and myelomonocytic leukemias are part of a broad spectrum of monocytic leukemias and vary from one another in part of the basis of qualitative differences in specific and nonspecific esterase activities.

Method. Esterases liberate alpha naphthol from synthetic substrates. Alpha naphthol couples with sensitized pararosaniline or with a diazo salt, such as fast blue BBN, to form a colored, insoluble precipitate at the site(s) of enzymatic activity. In the nonspecific esterase stain, the reaction product is orange to orange brown. In the specific esterase stain, the reaction product is dark blue.

Chemicals

1. Naphthol AS-D chloroacetate	1 mg
2. Alpha naphthyl acetate	10 mg
3. Fast blue BBN	4 mg

Solutions

1. Buffered formalin acetone (esterase fixative)

Na_2HPO_4	20 mg
KH_2PO_4	100 mg
Distilled H_2O	30 ml
Acetone	45 ml
37% Formalin	25 ml

Adjust to pH 6.6

2. Phosphate buffer (0.15; pH 7.6)
   a. Na H_2PO_4 (monobasic)
      per 1000 ml distilled H_2O 20.7 g
   b. Na_2HPO_4 (dibasic)
      per 1000 ml distilled H_2O 21.3 g
   c. Mix 130 ml of a and 870 ml of b, and adjust to pH 7.6

3. 4% Sodium nitrite—must be made freshly before use with fresh sodium nitrite.

Sodium nitrate	0.2 g
Distilled H_2O	5 ml

4. 1% Methyl green

Sodium acetate	1.4 g
Methyl green	1.0 g

Mix with 100 ml distilled H_2O, and adjust to pH 4.2 with acetic acid.

5. Pararosaniline

Pararosaline hydrochloride	1 mg
Distilled H_2O	20 ml
Concentrated HCl	2 ml

Heat solution to dissolve dye, cool, and filter. Store in refrigerator no longer than 2 months.

6. New fuchsin

New fuchsin	1 g
Distilled H_2O	20 ml
Concentrated HCl	2 ml

Heat solution to dissolve dye, cool, and filter. Store in refrigerator. Either pararosailine (step 5) or new fuchsin (step 6) can be used.

Procedure for Specific Esterase

1. Fix films in esterase fixative for 30 to 45 seconds.
2. Add a few drops dimethylformamide to 1 mg naphthol AS-D chloroacetate. Use a 15-ml beaker.
3. Add 9.5 ml phosphate buffer.
4. Add 5 mg fast blue BBN.
5. Mix well and filter directly onto films.
6. Incubate at room temperature for 40 minutes.
7. Wash with distilled H_2O.
8. Counterstain with 1% methyl green for 2 minutes.
9. Wash in distilled H_2O, air dry, and mount with Permount on cleaned glass slides.

Procedure for Nonspecific Esterase

1. In staining jars, fix blood and bone marrow films in esterase fixative for 30 to 45 seconds.
2. Wash thoroughly in distilled water.
3. Make fresh 4% sodium nitrite solution.
4. Mix 0.5 ml of pararosaniline or new fuchsin and 0.5 ml sodium nitrite. Let react for 1 minute only to effect hexazotization.
5. Add a few drops of acetone to 10 mg alpha naphthyl acetate. Use a 15-ml beaker.
6. Add 0.6 ml of step 4 solution to step 5.
7. Add 8.9 ml phosphate buffer to step 6. Using concentrated HCl or NaOH, adjust to *p*H 6.1. Filter and pour into a Coplin jar, containing bone marrow films.
8. Incubate for 1½ hours at room temperature. For fluoride inhibition, dissolve 75 mg sodium fluoride in 50 ml filtered incubation mixture and incubate coverslips for 90 minutes at room temperature in a small Coplin jar.

9. Wash coverslips in distilled H_2O.
10. Counterstain in 1% methyl green for 2 minutes.
11. Wash in distilled H_2O.
12. Air dry and mount with Permount.[20]

Although it is best to store the films in the freezer, films may be kept at room temperature for at least 2 weeks without appreciable change in enzyme activity. Also, if fast garnet GBC is used to demonstrate either specific or nonspecific esterase activity, mounting media containing organic solvent (*e.g.*, Permount) cannot be used, since the red reaction product that forms is soluble in these substances. Furthermore, fast garnet GBC cannot be used in the combined esterase solution, since these reactions depend on color differences in each of the dye couplers (pararosaniline and fast blue BBN) to distinguish between the two types of esterases.[7, 9, 10, 20]

Rhodanile Blue

Rhodanile blue is a basic cationic oxazine dyestuff formed by condensation of rhodamine B with Nile blue to form the amide. Used as an aqueous solution applied to blood and bone marrow cells fixed in methanol, rhodanile blue stains the cytoplasm of mature and immature megakaryocytes a bright pink color as seen in Figure 8–34 and Plate 4F. This bright pink metachromasia is not abolished by pretreatment of the fixed cells with either diastase or ribonuclease, and the staining contrast may actually be enhanced after ribonuclease treatment. After pretreatment of fixed cells with hyaluronidase, subsequent staining with rhodanile blue does not produce pink staining of megakaryocyte cytoplasm, indicating that the metachromatic staining reaction was due largely to the high content of acid mucopolysaccharides in the cytoplasm of megakaryocytes.[17]

Method. As an aqueous stain applied to methanol-fixed cells, rhodanile blue stains the cytoplasm of normal and abnormal megakaryocytes a bright pink color. On the basis of enzyme digestion techniques, this pink metachromasia may be due in large part to detection of increased amounts of acid mucopolysaccharide in megakaryocytes by rhodanile blue.

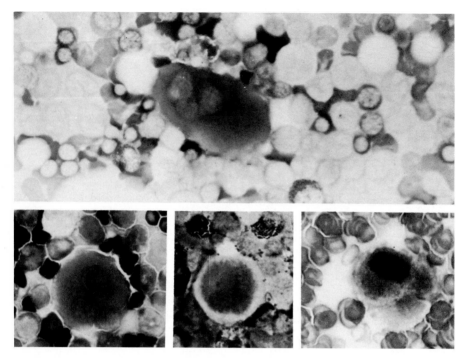

Figure 8–34   (Top) *Normal megakaryocyte.* (Bottom, left to right) *Megakaryocyte in chronic erythremic myelosis, micromegakaryocyte in chronic granulocytic leukemia, micromegakaryocyte in preleukemia. Rhodanile blue stain after ribonuclease digestion.*

Fixative

1. Absolute methanol

Ribonuclease solution

A. Sodium acetate, 1.4 g in 10 ml distilled water.
B. Magnesium sulfate, 2.46 g in 10 ml distilled water
C. Combine A and B and add 80 ml distilled water.
D. Dissolve 4 mg ribonuclease-A in 50 ml of C for working solution.

Make freshly each time before use.

Procedure

1. In a small Coplin jar, fix coverslips containing blood or bone marrow cells for 5 minutes in absolute methanol.
2. Wash coverslips in distilled water.

3. Treat surface of coverslip containing cells with ribonuclease solution for 60 minutes at 37°C.
4. Wash with distilled water, then flood the surface of the coverslips with a 1% aqueous solution of rhodanile blue.
5. Stain 10 minutes, wash coverslips with running distilled water for 3 minutes, air dry, and mount with Permount on clean labeled slide.

Rhodanile blue is a metachromatic dye that produces bright pink metachromatic staining of the cytoplasm of megakaryocytes. This pink metachromasia is more intense in mature megakaryocytes than in immature megakaryocytes like micromegakaryocytes. Compared to more tedious immunologic or ultrastructural techniques (Chap. 7), rhodanile blue is a simple direct stain that facilitates identification of megakaryocytes in normal and pathologic marrow specimens as well as dwarf megakaryocytes in peripheral blood samples. Detection of what may be acid mucopolysaccahride in the cytoplasm of megakaryocytes suggests that rhodanile blue may represent a useful addition to those immunologic techniques already available for megakaryocyte identification. Further experience with the dye applied to identification of megakaryoblasts in the megakaryoblastic phase of chronic granulocytic leukemia will help to determine the ability of the dyestuff to identify these primitive cells.

Cytochemical Tests in Acute Leukemias

A useful "battery" of tests for the acute leukemias would include the following:

1. PAS
2. Myeloperoxidase
3. Nonspecific esterase with and without fluoride inhibition
4. Acid phosphatase

On the basis of these three tests, and combined with cell-specific monoclonal antibodies when appropriate, one should be able to distinguish between the various typical forms of acute leukemias.[16] Lymphoblasts show punctate PAS-positive material and weak or negative reaction for nonspecific esterase and absent activity of myeloperoxidase. Blasts in monocytic leukemia demonstrate weak PAS positivity, strong fluoride-sensitive nonspecific esterase activity, and weak myeloperoxidase activity. Myeloblasts demonstrate weak PAS positivity, weak nonspecific esterase activity, and punctate myeloperoxidase activity. In some patients who have atypical morphologic forms of acute leukemia, blasts may demonstrate confusing cytochemical reactions. For example, these leukemic blasts contain large aggregates of PAS-positive material and strong activity of specific esterase, suggesting that they possess properties of lymphoblasts and myeloblasts. Measurement of activity of terminal deoxynucleotidyl transferase may facilitate identification of these cells as lymphoblasts, if activity is elevated substantially.

Cytochemical Tests in Refractory Anemias

A useful "battery" of tests for refractory anemias would include the following:

1. Prussian blue
2. PAS
3. Ammoniacal silver
4. Azure A

References

1. Dacie JV, Lewis SM: Practical Haematology, 4th ed. New York, Grune & Stratton, 1968
2. Hayhoe FGJ, Quaglino D, Doll R: Haematological Cytochemistry. Edinburg, Churchill Livingstone, 1982
3. Kass L: Demonstration of histones in proerythroblasts in pernicious anemia and the Di Guglielmo syndrome. J Histochem Cytochem 20:817, 1972
4. Kass L: Nuclear "speckling" in pernicious anemia proerythroblasts and megaloblasts. Blood 41:549, 1973
5. Kass L: Metachromatic staining of basic nucleoproteins in chronic erythremic myelosis. Am J Clin Pathol 62:21, 1974
6. Kass L: Pink staining of pernicious anemia megaloblasts by alizarin red S. Am J Clin Pathol 62:511, 1974
7. Kass L: Cytochemical abnormalities of atypical erythroblasts in acute erythremic myelosis. Acta Haematol 54:321, 1975
8. Kass L: Rapid detection of ringed sideroblasts in erythremic myelosis. Arch Pathol 99:225, 1975
9. Kass L: Esterase activities in acute myelomonocytic leukemia. Am J Clin Pathol 67:485, 1977
10. Kass L: Esterase activities in erythroleukemia. Am J Clin Pathol 67:368, 1977
11. Kass L: Periodic acid–Schiff-positive megaloblasts in pernicious anemia. Am J Clin Pathol 67:368, 1977

12. Kass L, Eickholt M: Rapid demonstration of ringed sideroblasts with bromochlorophenol blue. Am J Clin Pathol 70:738, 1978
13. Kass L, Hadi MZ: Phosphorylase activity in chronic erythremic myelosis. Am J Clin Pathol 64:503, 1975
14. Kass L: Saturn blue: A new stain for granulocytic cells. Arch Pathol Lab Med *104:*551, 1980
15. Kass L: Niagara sky blue 6B—A new stain for granulocytic cells. Am J Clin Pathol 74:801, 1980
16. Kass L: Advances in the cytochemistry of blood cells. Clin Lab Annu 3:101, 1984
17. Kass L: Identification of human megakaryocytes with rhodanile blue. Arch Pathol Lab Med 109:320, 1985
18. Sato A, Yoshimatsu SH: The peroxidase reaction in epidemic encephalitis. Am J Dis Child 29:301, 1925
19. Scholnik A, Kass L: A direct and cytochemical method for the identification of lysozyme in various tissues. J Histochem Cytochem 21:65, 1973
20. Yam LT, Li CY, Crosby WH: Cytochemical identification of monocytes and granulcoytes. Am J Clin Pathol 55:283, 1971
21. Yam LT, Li CY, Lam KW: Tartrate-resistant acid phosphatase in the reticulum cells of leukemic reticuloendotheliosis. N Engl J Med 284:357, 1971

Differential Cell Count in Normal Bone Marrow Aspirate

Reticulum cell	up to 2%
Hemohistioblast	up to 1%
Hemohistiocyte	up to 1%
Proerythroblast	up to 5%
Early normoblast ⎫	up to 20%
Intermediate normoblast ⎭	
Late normoblast	up to 15%
Myeloblast	up to 3%
Promyelocyte	up to 5%
Myelocyte	10%–20%
Metamyelocyte ⎫	8%–35%
Band ⎭	
Polymorphonuclear leukocyte	10%–20%
Eosinophil myelocyte	up to 4%
Mature eosinophil	up to 4%
Basophil myelocyte	up to 1%
Mature basophil	up to 1%
Lymphocyte	up to 25%
Plasma cell	up to 5%
Monocyte	up to 1%
Megakaryocyte	up to 1%

Appendix

Procedures for Performing Aspiration and Biopsy of Bone Marrow

Introduction

Biopsies of marrow are composed of a generous sample of marrow and bone. Because they involve a large sample quantity, biopsies provide a more representative assessment of marrow and bone pathology than marrow aspirates. In evaluating possible marrow involvement by lymphomas and carcinomas and in cases of "dry taps," marrow biopsies are indispensable. They are also necessary to evaluate disorders such as agnogenic myeloid metaplasia, in which determination of the architecture of the marrow is essential. Detection of subtle morphologic changes in nuclear chromatin and cytoplasm is made better on aspirates of bone marrow than on biopsies, since cellular structures are altered more drastically by conventional formalin and/or mercuric chloride fixation than by methanol fixation, which is used in most panoptic stains.

Clinical indications for performing an aspiration and/or biopsy of the bone marrow include the following:

1. Unexplained anemia
2. Unexplained leukopenia
3. Unexplained thrombocytopenia
4. Unexplained polymorphonuclear leukocytosis
5. Unexplained monocytosis
6. Unexplained lymphocytosis
7. Unexplained eosinophilia
8. Unexplained thrombocytosis
9. Presence of immature erythroid cells (normoblasts) and/or immature granulocytic cells (myeloblasts, promyelocytes, myelocytes) in the blood
10. Pancytopenia
11. Suspected carcinomatosis
12. Hodgkin's disease and non-Hodgkin's lymphomas (lymphocytic lymphoma and histiocytic lymphoma), to ascertain extent of disease
13. Lysosomal storage disease such as Gaucher's disease or Niemann-Pick disease
14. Unexplained splenomegaly
15. Dysproteinemias
16. Unexplained hypercalcemia
17. Fever of unknown origin

In many disorders, examination of an aspirate and biopsy of bone marrow can provide important information regarding the pathophysiology of an underlying disorder(s). However, in relatively few instances, marrow samples are actually diagnostic of a primary disorder. These include the following:

1. Megaloblastic anemia resulting from deficiency of vitamin B_{12}, folate, or both
2. Acute leukemias
3. Preleukemic disorders characterized by myeloblastosis
4. Sideroblastic anemias
5. Hereditary erythroblastic multinuclearity
6. Iron deficiency anemia
7. Chronic granulocytic leukemia, although it may be difficult to distinguish this disorder from a leukemoid reaction on the basis of a marrow sample alone
8. Chronic lymphocytic leukemia
9. Hairy cell leukemia

10. Osteopetrosis
11. Paget's disease
12. Agnogenic myeloid metaplasia
13. Carcinomatosis of the marrow
14. Lysosomal storage diseases
15. Essential thrombocythemia
16. Granulomatous diseases
17. Hodgkin's disease and non-Hodgkin's lymphoma
18. Angioimmunoblastic lymphadenopathy
19. Thrombotic thrombocytopenic purpura
20. Dysproteinemias, such as multiple myeloma and Waldenström's macroglobulinemia
21. Hypoplastic anemia
22. Chédiak-Higashi syndrome

Bone Marrow Aspiration and Biopsy

Aside from surgical specimens of bone and bone marrow that are obtained at operation, most aspirations and biopsies of bone marrow are obtained from the anterior iliac crest or posterior iliac crest. Aspirations may be obtained conveniently from the sternum, but because of the thinness of the sternal bone, biopsies are not usually obtained from it. In some instances, marrow can be obtained from spinous processes of vertebrae.

In performing an aspiration of marrow from the sternum, an Illinois needle may be used. Using a skin cleansing technique of iodine followed by isopropyl alcohol, the area immediately under the sternal angle (angle of Louis) in the fourth intercostal space is located. With 2% xylocaine local anesthetic, the skin overlying the marrow site is infiltrated, and anesthetic is injected carefully into the subcutaneous tissue and periosteum. With a surgical blade, a small incision is made in the skin. After the needle guard has been moved upward, the needle is introduced into the sternum with a gentle back and forth screwing motion. Entry into the marrow cavity is signified by a "give" feeling.

A 12.0-ml plastic syringe containing 0.2 ml aqueous heparin (1000 units/ml) is attached to the top of the marrow needle after the obturator is removed. With an abrupt pull on the barrel of the syringe, approximately 1.0 to 2.0 ml of marrow particles and sinusoidal blood are aspirated into it. Using sterile technique, the marrow needle is withdrawn carefully and a pressure dressing is placed over the aspiration site. After 24 hours, the dressing can be removed. In patients who have thrombocytopenia, additional pressure should be applied to the aspiration site after removal of the needle to prevent undue bleeding.

In performing an aspiration and biopsy of marrow from the anterior iliac crest, an Illinois needle can be used for the aspiration and a Jamshidi needle for the biopsy. Alternatively, a Jamshidi needle can be used for both the aspiration and biopsy. After localization of the rolled-under edge of the iliac crest and the anterior iliac spine, skin is cleansed and anesthetized and the aspiration needle is introduced at an angle parallel to the table or bed on which the patient is lying. Marrow is aspirated as described above.

In performing aspirations on children, anesthetic can be given with a needle "gun" and the aspiration needle introduced from above between the two plates of the iliac crest and aimed toward the pubic symphysis. In situations in which the posterior iliac crest has received therapeutic amounts of radiation, it may be necessary to perform a biopsy from the anterior iliac crest. A Jamshidi biopsy needle is introduced from above between the two plates of the iliac crest as described, and marrow is aspirated into a heparinized syringe. Following this maneuver, the needle is advanced several more centimeters without the obturator and a biopsy is taken.

In performing a biopsy from the posterior iliac crest, the posterior iliac spine is located. In most persons, this landmark is prominent and is located lateral to the sacral prominences. In obese persons, the posterior iliac spine is more difficult to locate. After cleansing the skin and infiltrating with local anesthetic, an incision is made over the posterior iliac spine and the Jamshidi needle is introduced directly into the posterior iliac spine with a firm screwing motion. After entry into the marrow cavity, signified by a "give" feeling and a firm fixation of the needle shaft in the bone, marrow is aspirated quickly into a heparinized syringe. After this has been accomplished, the needle is advanced another 1 to 2 cm without the obturator, rotated several times, and withdrawn carefully. With a metal wire, the biopsy specimen is removed from the shaft of the needle and placed in appropriate fixative.

If a person is allergic to xylocaine, subcutaneous and periosteal anesthesia can be attempted with diphenhydramine. Although once thought to interfere with staining reactions, heparin can be used to anticoagulate marrow samples without difficulty, provided that films of the marrow aspirate are stained with Wright's stain within 4 hours after making them and washed well after staining.

Failure to obtain an aspirate of marrow may be due to improper placement of the needle or to blockage of the shaft of the needle by bone or connective tissue. Rotation of the needle accompanied by slight advancement may correct this problem. Alternatively, failure to obtain an aspirate of marrow may be due to intramedullary pathology, such as carcinomatosis of the marrow, osteopetrosis, agnogenic myeloid metaplasia, acute leukemia, megaloblastic anemia, and hairy cell leukemia. In these instances, a "dry tap" can result from a routine marrow aspiration, necessitating a biopsy to establish the diagnosis. If only a biopsy core can be obtained, imprints of the marrow biopsy should be made by grasping the biopsy with a clean forceps and gently touching the biopsy to the surfaces of cleaned glass coverslips.

Coverslip Films of Marrow Aspirates

After obtaining the aspirate of marrow in a heparinized syringe, marrow is expressed from the syringe onto a clean glass slide (Fig. A-1).

The slide is tilted gently onto a piece of filter paper, allowing excess blood to absorb onto the filter paper and leaving marrow particles behind on the glass slide (Fig. A-2). In most instances, marrow particles appear white or pink and appear deep pink or red in disorders of erythropoiesis in which there is erythroblastic hyperplasia of the bone marrow.

Using a Pasteur pipette to which a rubber nipple has been attached, gentle pressure is applied to the rubber nipple, and particles of marrow along with small amounts of sinusoidal blood are aspirated into the pipette (Fig. A-3). Care should be taken to avoid aspiration of marrow particles into the barrel of the pipette, since it is difficult to express them onto coverslips if they are located too high in the pipette.

A particle of marrow with a small amount of sinusoidal blood is expressed from the pipette onto the center of a clean glass coverslip (Fig. A-4). Excess sinusoidal blood is aspirated from the coverslip with a Pasteur pipette.

(Text continued on page 395)

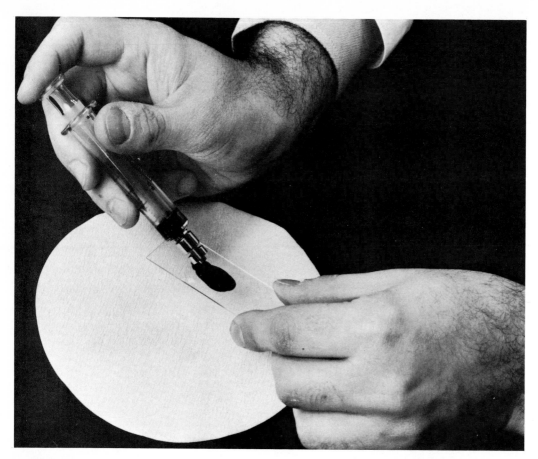

Figure A–1   Express marrow particles and sinusoidal blood onto a clean glass slide.

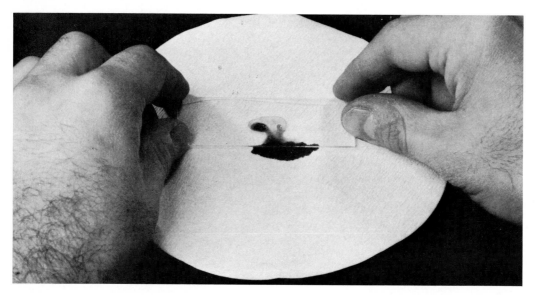

Figure A–2   Tilt the glass slide onto a piece of filter paper, allowing sinusoidal blood to be absorbed by the filter paper and leaving marrow particles on the glass slide.

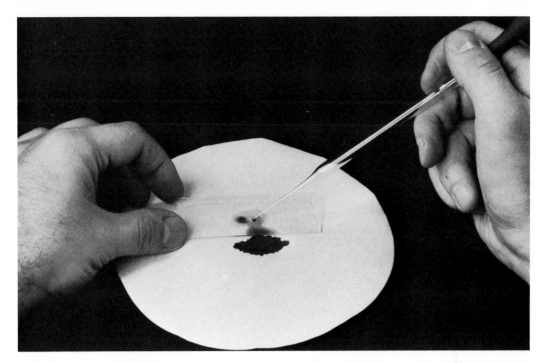

Figure A–3   *Pick up particles of marrow with a Pasteur pipette.*

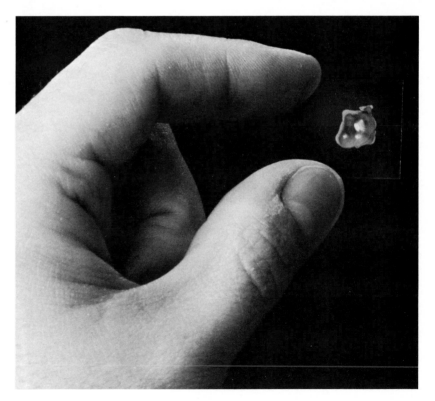

Figure A–4   *Deposit marrow particles onto a glass coverslip.*

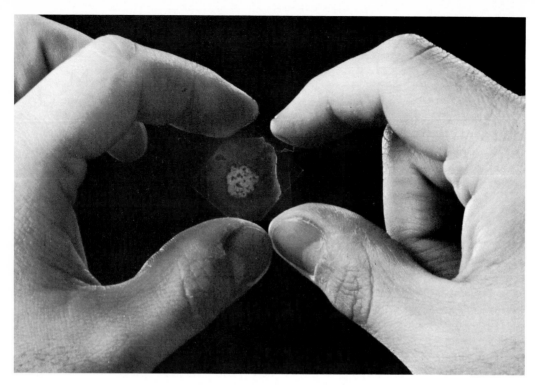

Figure A–5   *Place another coverslip diagonally across the coverslip containing marrow particles. Press coverslips together gently, allowing marrow particles to spread evenly between the two coverslips.*

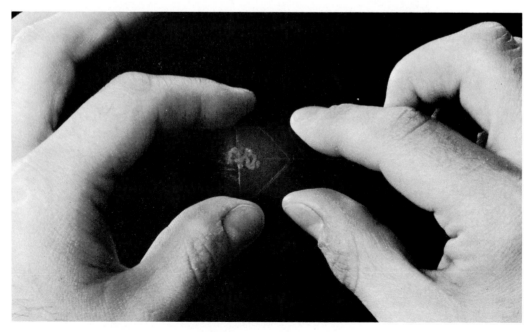

Figure A–6   *Drag the top coverslip gently over the bottom coverslip to spread marrow particles evenly.*

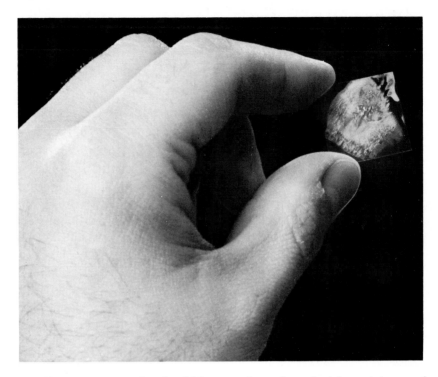

Figure A–7   *Ideally marrow particles should be spread evenly and with a minimum of cellular distortion or disruption.*

A second glass coverslip is placed diagonally across the coverslip containing the marrow particle(s) (Fig A-5).

The top coverslip is gently dragged across the bottom coverslip to make the marrow spread preparation (Fig. A-6). It may be necessary to press the coverslips together gently prior to pulling the film. Vigorous pressure on the two coverslips may squash and distort cells, making interpretation of cellular morphology difficult and in some instances impossible.

A well-spread film is depicted in Figure A-7. After staining with Wright's stain or Wright's-Giemsa stain, cellular morphology and much of the architecture of the marrow are preserved. In general, morphologic features of marrow cells are preserved better in coverslip-film preparations of marrow particles than in smears of marrow flecks made between glass slides.

Fixation and Staining of Marrow Biopsies

After the core of marrow has been obtained, it should be placed into fixative prior to embedding and sectioning. Although various types of fixatives have been employed, those that incorporate mercury salts in them, such as Zenker's fixative, seem to provide the best preservation of nuclear and cytoplasmic details and the least amount of shrinkage. When using solutions containing mercury, proper precautions for environmental safety should be used.

Accordingly, marrow biopsy cores are placed in a solution of 1 ml 40% formaldehyde and 9 ml B5 fixative (made by mixing 900 ml distilled water, 60 g mercuric chloride, and 15 g sodium acetate at a final pH of 5.8). Formaldehyde and fixative are mixed immediately prior to use. Biopsies are allowed to fix for at least 2 hours, and the formalin fixative is decanted. To the biopsy is added 5% nitric acid to decalcify the specimen, and the biopsy is exposed to nitric acid for 2 hours. With care, nitric acid is removed and 70% ethanol is added to the container. The specimen can be processed in the conventional manner and stained with H and E, Giemsa, or other types of panoptic stains such as Maximow's stain (hematoxylin and eosin-azure II). Alternatively, biopsy cores can be fixed and embedded in glycol methacrylate. One-micron thick sections can be cut and sections stained with a Romanowsky-type stain, or for a variety of enzymes as described by Beckstead and Bainton.

If sections of marrow particles are desired, these particles should be removed from the glass slide after aspiration and a number of them placed into the fixative in a manner identical to the marrow biopsy core. However, after fixation for 2 hours, the fixative is decanted and 70% ethanol is added. After addition of the alcohol, marrow particles are processed in the conventional manner.

At the time of aspiration, at least ten extra coverslip preparations of marrow and/or biopsy imprints are made for cytochemical studies. For long-term preservation, these coverslips should be stored at $-30°C$. Some cytochemical tests, such as Prussian blue stain, specific esterase reaction, and PAS stain, can be performed on formalin-fixed tissues. Other stains, such as peroxidase, must be performed on either unfixed tissue or tissue fixed in a special manner.

Bibliography

Bone Marrow Structure

Doan CA: Bone marrow: Normal and pathologic physiology with special reference to diseases involving the cells of the blood. In Downey H (ed): Handbook of Hematology, vol 3, p 1839, New York, Paul B Hoeber, 1938

Tavassoli M, Yoffey JM: Bone Marrow Structure and Function. New York, Alan Liss, 1983

Autoimmune Hemolytic Anemia

Cazzola M, Barosi G et al: Cold haemagglutinin disease with severe anaemia, reticulocytopenia and erythroid bone marrow. Scand J Haematol 30:25, 1983

Issitt PD: Autoimmune hemolytic anemia and cold hemagglutinin disease: Clinical disease and laboratory findings. Prog Clin Pathol 7:137, 1978

Petz LD: Drug-induced immune haemolytic anaemia. Clin Haematol 9:455, 1980

Petz LD: Autoimmune hemolytic anemia. Hum Pathol 14:251, 1983

Stefanelli M, Barosi G et al: Quantitative assessment of erythropoiesis in haemolytic disease. Br J Haematol 45:297, 1980

Acute Erythremic Myelosis

Di Guglielmo G: Eritremie acute. Boll Soc Med Chir Ser Pavia 1:665, 1916

Di Guglielmo G: Le Malattie Eritremiche ed Eritroleucemiche. Rome, II Pensiero Scientifico Editore, 1962

Refractory Anemia

Astaldi G, Rondanelli EG et al: An abnormal substance present in the erythroblasts of thalassaemia major: Cytochemical investigations. Acta Haematol 12:145, 1954

Bjorkman SE: Chronic refractory anemia with sideroblastic bone marrow: A study of four cases. Blood 11:250, 1956

Bowman WD Jr: Abnormal ("ringed") sideroblasts in various hematologic and non-hematologic disorders. Blood 18:662, 1961

Brain MC, Herdan A: Tissue iron stores in sideroblastic anaemia. Br J Haematol 11:107, 1965

Catovsky D, Shaw MT et al: Sideroblastic anaemia and its association with leukaemia and myelomatosis: A report of five cases. Br J Haematol 20:385, 1971

Dacie JV, Smith MD et al: Refractory normoblastic anaemia: A clinical and haematological study of seven cases. Br J Haematol 5:56, 1959

Dameshek W, Baldini M: Editorial: The Di Guglielmo syndrome. Blood 13:192, 1958

Di Guglielmo G, Quattrin DN: Mielosi eritremica cronica. Haematologica 24:1, 1942

Downey H: Monocytic leucemia and leucemic reticulo-endotheliosis. In Downey H (ed): Handbook of Hematology, vol 2, p 1273. New York, Paul B Hoeber, 1938

Eastman P, Wallerstein RO et al: Conversion of polycythemia vera to chronic Di Guglielmo's syndrome. JAMA 204:1141, 1968

Eastman PM, Schwartz R et al: Distinctions between idiopathic ineffective erythropoiesis and Di Guglielmo's disease: Clinical and biochemical differences. Blood 40:487, 1972

Hayhoe FGJ, Quaglino D: Refractory sideroblastic anaemia and erythraemic myelosis: Possible relationship and cytochemical observations. Br J Haematol 6:381, 1960

Johnstone JM: The appearance and significance of tissue mast cells in human bone marrow. J Clin Pathol 7:275, 1954

Kass L: Metachromatic staining of basic nucleoproteins in chronic erythremic myelosis. Am J Clin Pathol 62:21, 1974

Kass L: Annotation: Biochemical abnormalities in chronic erythraemic myelosis. Br J Haematol 35:169, 1977

Kass L, Peters CL: Nonspecific esterase activity in pernicious anemia and chronic erythremic myelosis: A cytochemical and electrophoretic study. Am J Clin Pathol 68:273, 1977

Kass L, Schnitzer B: Refractory Anemia. Springfield, IL, Charles C Thomas, 1975

Khaleeli M, Keane WM et al: Sideroblastic anemia in multiple myeloma: A preleukemic change. Blood 41:17, 1973

Kushner JP, Lee GR et al: Idiopathic refractory sideroblastic anemia: Clinical and laboratory investigation of 17 patients and review of the literature. Medicine 50:139, 1971

Peterson HR Jr, Bowlds CF et al: Familial Di Guglielmo syndrome. Cancer 54:932, 1984.

Petz LD, Goodman JR et al: Refractory normoblastic ("sideroblastic") anemia: Clinical and electron microscopic observations. Am J Clin Pathol 45:581, 1966

Quaglino D, Hayhoe FGJ: Periodic-acid-Schiff positivity in erythroblasts with special reference to Di Guglielmo's disease. Br J Haematol 6:26, 1960

Rosenthal DS, Moloney WC: Refractory dysmyelopoietic anemia and acute leukemia. Blood 63:314, 1984

Schnitzer B, Kass L: Refractory sideroblastic anemia (chronic erythremic myelosis). Am J Clin Pathol 60:343, 1973

Schwartz SO, Critchlow J: Erythremic myelosis (Di Guglielmo's disease): Critical review with report of four cases, and comments on erythroleukemia. Blood 7:765, 1952

Schwarz E: Cellular gigantism and pluripolar mitosis in human hematopoiesis. Am J Anat 79:75, 1946

Sondergaard-Petersen H: Erythrophagocytosis by pathological erythroblasts in the Di Guglielmo syndrome: A study of 18 cases. Scand J Haematol 13:260, 1974

Sullivan AL, Weintraub LR: Sideroblastic anemias: An approach to diagnosis and management. Med Clin North Am 57:335, 1973

Refractory Anemia with Excess Blasts

Armitage JO, Dick FR et al: Effect of chemotherapy for the dysmyelopoietic syndrome. Cancer Treat Rep 65:601, 1981

Dreyfus B, Rochant H, Sultan C et al: Les anémies refractaires avec excess de myeloblastes dans la moelle. Presse Medicale 78:359, 1970

Greenberg PL: The smoldering myeloid leukemic states: Clinical and biologic features. Blood 61:1035, 1983

Knospe WH, Gregory SA: Smoldering acute leukemia: Clinical and cytogenetic studies in six patients. Arch Intern Med 127:910, 1971

Najean Y Pecking A, Broquet M: Anémies refractaires avec myeloblastose partielle. Analyse d'un protocole, groupant 79 cas. Nouv Rev Fr Hematol 16:67, 1976

Rheingold JJ, Kaufman R et al: Smoldering acute leukemia. N Engl J Med 268:812, 1963

Van Slyck EJ, Rebuck JW et al: Smoldering acute granulocytic leukemia: Observations on its natural history and morphologic characteristics. Arch Intern Med 143:37, 1983

Weisdorf DJ, Oken MM et al: Auer rod positive dysmyelopoietic syndrome. Am J Hematol 11:397, 1981

Erythroleukemia

Al-Hilali MM, Edgcumbe JO et al: Chronic lymphatic leukaemia terminating as erythroleukaemia. Postgrad Med J 57:585, 1981

Andersson LC, Gahmberg CG et al: Glycophorin A as a cell surface marker of early erythroid differentiation in acute leukemia. Int J Cancer 24:717, 1979

Bank A, Larsen PR et al: Di Guglielmo's syndrome after polycythemia. N Engl J Med 275:489, 1966

Beaven GH, Coleman PN et al: Occurrence of haemoglobin H in leukaemia: A further case of erythroleukaemia. Acta Haematol 59:37, 1978

Cowall DE, Pasquale DN et al: Paroxysmal nocturnal hemoglobinuria terminating as erythroleukemia. Cancer 43:1914, 1979

Di Guglielmo G: Richerche di hematologia: I. Un caso di eritroleucemia. Folia Med 3:386, 1917

Di Guglielmo G: Eritroleucemia e piastrinemia. Folia Med 6:1, 1920

Ekblom M, Borgstrom G et al: Erythroid blast crisis in chronic myelogenous leukemia. Blood 62:591, 1983

Ellerton JA, deVeber GA et al: Erythroleukemia in a renal transplant recipient. Cancer 43:1924, 1979

Ellims PH, Van der Weyden MB et al: Erythroleukemia following drug induced hypoplastic anemia. Cancer 44:2140, 1979

Gabuzda TG, Shute HE et al: Regulation of erythropoiesis in erythroleukemia. Arch Intern Med 123:60, 1969

Goldhirsch A, Pirovino M et al: Acute erythroleukemia following chemotherapy for Hodgkin's disease. Am J Med Sci 280:53, 1980

Greaves MF, Sieff C et al: Monoclonal antiglycophorin as a probe for erythroleukemias. Blood 61:645, 1983

Kass L: Esterase activity in erythroleukemia. Am J Clin Pathol 67:368, 1977

Kass L: Enzymatic abnormalities in erythroleukemia. Acta Haematol 59:302, 1978

Marks PA, Rifkind RA: Erythroleukemic differentiation. Annu Rev Biochem 47:419, 1978

McClure PD, Thaler MM et al: Chronic erythroleukemia with chromosome mosaicism: Report of a case in a 5-year-old boy. Arch Intern Med 115:697, 1965

Miura AB: Multiple vacuole formation in erythroblasts in an erythroleukaemic patient. Scand J Haematol 16:183, 1976

Newcomb MM, Balducci L et al: Erythroleukemia: In vitro studies of erythropoiesis. Am J Hematol 5:291, 1978

Phillips BA, Yarbro JW et al: Acquired Pelger-Huet anomaly in erythroleukemia. J Surg Oncol 2:407, 1970

Pinkus GS, Said JW: Intracellular hemoglobin—a specific marker for erythroid cells in paraffin sections: An immunoperoxidase study of normal, megaloblastic, and dysplastic erythropoiesis, including erythroleukemia and other myeloproliferative disorders. Am J Pathol 102:308, 1981

Prindull G, Jentsch E et al: Fanconi's anaemia developing erythroleukaemia. Scand J Haematol 23:59, 1979

Roggli VL, Saleem A: Erythroleukemia: A study of 15 cases and literature review. Cancer 49:101, 1982

Rosenthal S, Canellos GP et al: Erythroblastic transformation of chronic granulocytic leukemia. Am J Med 63:116, 1977

Rotzak R, Kaplinsky N et al: Giant marker chromosome in Fanconi's anemia transforming into erythroleukemia in an adult. Acta Haematol 67:214, 1982

Scott RB, Ellison RR et al: A clinical study of twenty cases of erythroleukemia (di Guglielmo's syndrome). Am J Med 37:162, 1964

Skinnider LF, Ghadially FN: Glycogen in erythroid cells. Arch Pathol 95:139, 1973

Stavem P, Hjort PF et al: Ring-shaped nuclei of granulocytes in a patient with acute erythroleukaemia. Scand J Haematol 6:31, 1969

Steel NR, Carr D et al: Erythroleukaemia following treatment of Hodgkin's disease. Clin Lab Haematol 4:417, 1982

Tada T, Nitta M et al: Acute myelofibrosis terminating in erythroleukemic state. Am J Clin Pathol 78:102, 1982

Taher A, Gilbert E et al: Erythroblastic islands in erythroleukemia. Am J Pediatr Hematol Oncol 3:121, 1981

Megaloblastic Anemia

Amess JA, Burman JF et al: Severe megaloblastic bone marrow change associated with unsuspected mild vitamin B_{12} deficiency. Clin Lab Haematol 3:231, 1981

Bessis MC: Living Blood Cells and Their Ultrastructure. New York, Springer-Verlag, 1973

Cabot RC: Ring bodies (nuclear remnants?) in anemic blood. J Med Res 9:15, 1903

Chanarin I: The Megaloblastic Anaemias, 2nd ed. Oxford, Blackwell Scientific Publications, 1979

Downey H: The megaloblast-normoblast problem: A cytologic study. J Lab Clin Med 39:837, 1952

Fudenberg H, Estren S: Non-Addisonian megaloblastic anemia: The intermediate megaloblast in the differential diagnosis of pernicious and related anemias. Am J Med 25:198, 1958

Isaacs R: The leucocytes in pernicious anemia—physiology, pathology and clinical significance. J Clin Invest 6:28, 1928

Jones OP: Cytological studies of biopsied pernicious anemia bone marrow during relapse. Proc Soc Exp Biol Med 34:694, 1936

Jones OP: Morphologic, physiologic, chemical and biologic distinction of megaloblasts. Arch Pathol 35:752, 1943

Kass L: A clockface chromatin pattern in the intermediate megaloblast of vitamin B_{12} or folate deficiency. Blood 32:711, 1968

Kass L: Demonstration of histones in proerythroblasts in pernicious anemia and the Di Guglielmo syndrome. J Histochem Cytochem 20:817, 1972

Kass L: Pink staining of pernicious anemia megaloblasts by alizarin red S. Am J Clin Pathol 62:511, 1974

Kass L: Origin and composition of Cabot rings in pernicious anemia. Am J Clin Pathol 64:53, 1975

Kass L: Detection of methionine in pernicious anemia megaloblasts and other types of erythroid precursors. Am J Clin Pathol 65:504, 1976

Kass L: Unusual morphologic abnormalities of megaloblasts in pernicious anemia and folate deficiency. Am J Clin Pathol 65:195, 1976

Kass L: Cytochemical detection of homocysteine in pernicious anemia and in chronic erythremic myelosis. Am J Clin Pathol 67:53, 1977

Kass L: Periodic acid-Schiff-positive megaloblasts in pernicious anemia. Am J Clin Pathol 67:371, 1977

Kass L, Hadi MZ: Phosphorylase activity in chronic erythremic myelosis. Am J Clin Pathol 64:503, 1975

Kiossoglou KA, Mitus WJ et al: Chromosomal aberrations in pernicious anemia: Study of three cases before and after therapy. Blood 25:662, 1965

Peabody FW: The pathology of the bone marrow in pernicious anemia. Am J Pathol 3:179, 1927

Peabody FW, Broun GO: Phagocytosis of erythrocytes in the bone marrow, with special reference to pernicious anemia. Am J Pathol 1:169, 1925

Rozenszajn L, Leibovich M et al: The esterase activity in megaloblasts, leukaemic and normal haemopoietic cells. Br J Haematol 14:605, 1968

Schleicher EM: Giant orthochromatic erythroblasts: Their importance for the promegaloblast and pronormoblast problem. J Lab Clin Med 29:127, 1944

Stuart J, Skowron PN: A cytochemical study of marrow enzymes in megaloblastic anaemia. Br J Haematol 15:443, 1968

Tudhope GR, Wilson GM: Anaemia in hypothyroidism: Incidence, pathogenesis, and response to treatment. Q J Med 29:513, 1960

Wallerstein RO, Pollycove M: Bone marrow hemosiderin and ferrokinetics patterns in anemia: I. Pernicious anemia. Arch Intern Med 101:418, 1958

Wickramasinghe SN, Cooper EH et al: A study of erythropoiesis by combined morphologic, quantitative cytochemical and autoradiographic methods: Normal human bone marrow, vitamin B_{12} deficiency and iron deficiency anemia. Blood 31:304, 1968

Wickramasinghe SN, Pratt JR: Myelocyte proliferation in pernicious anaemia. Acta Haematol 44:37, 1970

Lymphocyte Identification

Bevan A, Burns GF et al: Cytochemistry of human T-cell subpopulations. Scand J Immunol 11:223, 1980

Davey FR, Dock NL et al: Cytochemical reactions in resting and activated T-lymphocytes. Am J Clin Pathol 74:174, 1980

Ellner JJ: Suppressor cells of man. Clin Immunol Rev 1:119, 1981

Heumann D, Colombatti M et al: Human large granular lymphocytes contain an esterase activity usually considered as specific for the myeloid series. Eur J Immunol 13:254, 1983

Landay A, Clement LT, Gross CE: Phenotypically and functionally distinct subpopulations of human lymphocytes with T cell markers also exhibit different cytochemical patterns of staining for lysosomal enzymes. Blood 63:1067, 1984

Pangalis GA, Waldman SR et al: Cytochemical findings in human nonneoplastic blood and tonsillar B and T lymphocytes. Am J Clin Pathol 69:314, 1978

Pinkus GS, Hargreaves HK et al: Alpha-naphthyl acetate esterase activity—a cytochemical marker for T lymphocytes: Correlation with immunologic studies of normal tissues, lymphocytic leukemias, non-Hodgkin's lymphomas, Hodgkin's disease, and other lymphoproliferative disorders. Am J Pathol 97:17, 1979

Quesada JR, Murphy SG: Histochemical patterns of human T lymphocyte subpopulations with nonspecific esterase staining. Int Arch Allergy Appl Immunol 68:138, 1982

Yourno J, Burkart P et al: Nonspecific esterase of B lymphocytes from a case of chronic lymphocytic leukemia and of normal T lymphocytes: Similar constellations of isoenzymes. Blood 60:24, 1982

Infectious Mononucleosis

Krause JR, Kaplan SS: Bone marrow findings in infectious mononucleosis and mononucleosis-like diseases in the older adult. Scand J Haematol 28:15, 1982

McKenna RW, Parkin J et al: Ultrastructural, cytochemical, and membrane surface marker characteristics of the atypical lymphocytes in infectious mononucleosis. Blood 50:505, 1977

Thomas WJ, Yasaka K et al: Hand-mirror lymphocytes in infectious mononucleosis. Blood 55:925, 1980

Chronic Lymphocytic Leukemia and Lymphocytic Lymphoma

Aisenberg AC, Wilkes B: Lymphosarcoma cell leukemia: The contribution of cell surface study to diagnosis. Blood 48:707, 1976

Aisenberg AC, Wilkes BM et al: T-cell chronic lymphocytic leukemia. Report of a case studied with monoclonal antibody. Am J Med 72:695, 1982

Andres TL, Kadin ME: Immunologic markers in the differential diagnosis of small round cell tumors from lymphocytic lymphoma and leukemia. Am J Clin Pathol 79:546, 1983

Baccarani M, Cavo M et al: Staging of chronic lymphocytic leukemia. Blood 59:1191, 1982

Bakri K, Ezdinli EZ et al: T-suppressor cell chronic lymphocytic leukemia: Phenotypic characterization by monoclonal antibodies. Cancer 54:284, 1984

Bartl R, Frisch B et al: Assessment of marrow trephine in relation to staging in chronic lymphocytic leukaemia. Br J Haematol 51:1, 1982

Boldt DH, Nelson MO: Lymphocyte subpopulations in chronic lymphocytic leukemia detected by lectin binding and flow cytometry. Cancer 51:2083, 1983

Brunning RD, McKenna RW: Bone marrow manifestations of malignant lymphoma and lymphoma-like conditions. Pathol Annu 14(pt. 1):1, 1979

Catovsky D, Galton DAG: Myelomonocytic leukaemia supervening on chronic lymphocytic leukaemia. Lancet 1:478, 1971

Catovsky D, Galetto J et al: Cytochemical profile of B and T leukaemic lymphocytes with special reference to acute lymphoblastic leukaemia. J Clin Pathol 27:767, 1974

Catovsky D, Costello C: Cytochemistry of normal and leukaemic lymphocytes: A review. Basic Appl Histochem 23:255, 1979

Cohen HJ: B-cell lymphosarcoma cell leukemia: Dynamics of surface-membrane immunoglobulin: Value for differentiation from chronic lymphocytic leukemia. Ann Intern Med 88:317, 1978

Come SE, Jaffe ES et al: Non-Hodgkin's lymphomas in leukemia phase: Clinicopathologic correlations. Am J Med 69:667, 1980

Costello C, Catovsky D et al: Chronic T-cell leukemias: I. Morphology, cytochemistry and ultrastructure. Leuk Res 4:463, 1980

Dick F, Bloomfield CD et al: Incidence, cytology, and histopathology of non-Hodgkin's lymphomas in the bone marrow. Cancer 33:1382, 1974

Economopoulos T, Fotopoulos S et al: "Prolymphocytoid" cells in chronic lymphocytic leukaemia and their prognostic significance. Scand J Haematol 28:238, 1982

Ferraini M, Romagnani S et al: A lymphoproliferative disorder of the large granular lymphocytes with natural killer activity. J Clin Immunol 3:30, 1983

Foa R, Catovsky D et al: Clinical staging and immunological findings in chronic lymphocytic leukemia. Cancer 44:483, 1979

Foucar K, McKenna RW et al: Incidence and patterns of bone marrow and blood involvement by lymphoma in relationship to the Lukes-Collins classification. Blood 54:1417, 1979

Foucar K, Rydell RE: Richter's syndrome: A blastic transformation of chronic lymphocytic leukemia. Minn Med 64:613, 1981

Garrett JV, Scarffe JH et al: Abnormal peripheral blood lymphocytes and bone marrow infiltration in non-Hodgkin's lymphoma. Br J Haematol 42:41, 1979

Gastl G, Niederwieser D et al: Human large granular lymphocytes and their relationship to natural killer cell activity in various disease states. Blood 64:288, 1984

Gray JL, Jacobs A et al: Bone marrow and peripheral blood lymphocytosis in the prognosis of chronic lymphocytic leukemia. Cancer 33:1169, 1974

Han T, Barcos M et al: Bone marrow infiltration patterns and their prognostic significance in chronic lymphocytic leukemia: Correlations with clinical, immunologic phenotypic, and cytogenetic data. J Clin Oncol 2:562, 1984

Isaacs R: Lymphosarcoma cell leukemia. Ann Intern Med 11:657, 1937

Itoh K, Tsuchikawa K et al: A case of chronic lymphocytic leukemia with properties characteristic of natural killer cells. Blood 61:940, 1983

Kay NE, Zarling JM: Impaired natural killer activity in patients with chronic lymphocytic leukemia is associated with a deficiency of azurophilic cytoplasmic granules in putative NK cells. Blood 63:305, 1984

Kim H, Heller P et al: Monoclonal gammopathies associated with lymphoproliferative disorders: A morphologic study. Am J Clin Pathol 59:282, 1973

Koziner B, Filippa DA et al: Characterization of malignant lymphomas in leukemic phase by multiple differentiation markers of mononuclear cells: Correlation with clinical features and conventional morphology. Am J Med 63:556, 1977

Koziner B, Kempin S et al: Characterization of B-cell leukemias: A tentative immunomorphological scheme. Blood 56:815, 1980

Kulenkampff J, Janossy G et al: Acid esterase in human lymphoid cells and leukaemic blasts: A marker for T lymphocytes. Br J Haematol 36:231, 1977

Lipshutz MD, Mir R et al: Bone marrow biopsy and clinical staging in chronic lymphocytic leukemia. Cancer 46:1422, 1980

Manoharan A, Catovsky D et al: Simultaneous or spontaneous occurrence of lympho- and myeloproliferative disorders: A report of four cases. Br J Haematol 48:111, 1981

McKenna RW, Bloomfield CD et al: Nodular lymphoma: Bone marrow and blood manifestations. Cancer 36:428, 1975

Mills KH, Cawley JC: Suppressor T cells in B-cell chronic lymphocytic leukaemia: Relationship to clinical stage. Leuk Res 6:653, 1982

Mintzer DM, Hauptman SP: Lymphosarcoma cell leukemia and other non-Hodgkin's lymphomas in leukemic phase. Am J Med 75:110, 1983

Miyamoto Y, Yamaguchi K, Nishimura H et al: Familial adult T-cell leukemia. Cancer 55:181, 1985

Palutke M, Eisenberg L et al: Natural killer and suppressor T-cell chronic lymphocytic leukemia. Blood 62:627, 1983

Pandolfi F, Strong DM et al: Characterization of a suppressor T-cell chronic lymphocytic leukemia with ADCC but not NK activity. Blood 56:653, 1980

Pangalis GA, Nathwani BN et al: Malignant lymphoma, well differentiated lymphocytic: Its relationship with chronic lymphocytic leukemia and macroglobulinemia of Waldenström. Cancer 39:999, 1977

Peterson LC, Bloomfield CD et al: Morphology of chronic lymphocytic leukemia and its relationship to survival. Am J Med 59:316, 1975

Peterson LC, Bloomfield CD et al: Relationship of clinical staging and lymphocyte morphology to survival in chronic lymphocytic leukaemia. Br J Haematol 44:563, 1980

Phyliky RL, Li CY et al: T-cell chronic lymphocytic leukemia with morphologic and immunologic characteristics of cytotoxic/suppressor phenotype. Mayo Clin Proc 58:709, 1983

Plesner T, Wilken M et al: The contribution of immunologic methods to the classification of leukemias and malignant lymphomas. Clin Lab Med 2:579, 1982

Reinherz EL, Nadler LM et al: T-cell-subset characterization of human T-CLL. Blood 53:1066, 1979

Rozman C, Hernandez-Nieto L et al: Prognostic significance of bone marrow patterns in chronic lymphocytic leukaemia. Br J Haematol 47:529, 1981

Rozman C, Montserrat E et al: Bone marrow histologic pattern—the best single prognostic parameter in chronic lymphocytic leukemia: A multivariate survival analysis of 329 cases. Blood 64:642, 1984.

Said JW, Pinkus GS: Immunologic characterization and ultrastructural correlations for 125 cases of B- and T-cell leukemias: Studies of chronic and acute lymphocytic, prolymphocytic, lymphosarcoma cell and hairy cell leukemia: Sezary's syndrome and other lymphoid leukemias. Cancer 48:2630, 1981

Simpkins H, Kiprov DD, Davis JL III: T cell chronic lymphocytic leukemia with lymphocytes of unusual immunologic phenotype and function. Blood 65:127, 1985

Skinnider LF, Tan L et al: Chronic lymphocytic leukemia: A review of 745 cases and assessment of clinical staging. Cancer 50:2951, 1982

Sugai S, Hirose Y et al: Leukemic lymphosarcoma (LLS) with monoclonal IgM: Idiotypic specificity on the cell surface and in the cytoplasm of lymphosarcoma cells. Blood 52:922, 1978

Uchiyama T, Yodoi J et al: Adult T-cell leukemia: Clinical and hematologic features of 16 cases. Blood 50:481, 1977

Volk JR, Kjeldsberg CR et al: T-cell prolymphocytic leukemia: Clinical and immunologic characterization. Cancer 52:2049, 1983

Yamaguchi K, Nishimura H et al: A proposal for smoldering adult T-cell leukemia: A clinicopathologic study of five cases. Blood 62:758, 1983

Yoo D, Lessin LS et al: Bone-marrow mast cells in lymphoproliferative disorders. Ann Intern Med 88:753, 1978

Prolymphocytic Leukemia

Bearman RM, Pangalis GA et al: Prolymphocytic leukemia: Clinical, histopathological, and cytochemical observations. Cancer 42:2360, 1978

Costello C, Catovsky D et al: Prolymphocytic leukaemia: An ultrastructural study of 22 cases. Br J Haematol 44:389, 1980

Diamond LW, Bearman RM et al: Prolymphocytic leukemia: Flow micro-fluorometric, immunologic, and cytogenetic observations. Am J Hematol 9:319, 1980

Enno A, Catovsky D et al: "Prolymphocytoid" transformation of chronic lymphocytic leukaemia. Br J Haematol 41:9, 1979

Galton DAG, Goldman JM et al: Prolymphocytic leukaemia. Br J Haematol 27:7, 1974

Katayama I, Aiba M et al: B-lineage prolymphocytic leukemia as a distinct clinicopathologic entity. Am J Pathol 99:399, 1980

Kjeldsberg CR, Bearman RM et al: Prolymphocytic leukemia: An ultrastructural study. Am J Clin Pathol 73:150, 1980

Kjeldsberg CR, Marty J: Prolymphocytic transformation of chronic lymphocytic leukemia. Cancer 48:2447, 1981

Lampert I, Catovsky D et al: The histopathology of prolymphocytic leukaemia with particular reference to the spleen: A comparison with chronic lymphocytic leukaemia. Histopathology 4:3, 1980

Acute Lymphoblastic Leukemia

Arkin CF, Kurtz SR et al: Acute B-cell leukemia occurring with Hodgkin's disease. Am J Clin Pathol 75:406, 1981

Bearman RM, Winberg CD et al: Terminal deoxynucleotidyl transferase activity in neoplastic and nonneoplastic hematopoietic cells. Am J Clin Pathol 75:794, 1981

Bennett JM, Catovsky D et al: Proposals for the classification of the acute leukaemias: French-American-British (FAB) co-operative group. Br J Haematol 33:451, 1976

Bloomfield CD: B & T markers in leukemia and lymphoma. Minn Med 62:499, 1979

Bloomfield CD: Classification and prognosis of acute lymphoblastic leukemia. Prog Clin Biol Res 58:167, 1981

Bollum FJ: Terminal deoxynucleotidyl transferase as a hematopoietic cell marker. Blood 54:1203, 1979

Brunning RD, McKenna RW et al: Bone marrow involvement in Burkitt's lymphoma. Cancer 40:1771, 1977

Burgio VL, Maccario R et al: Golgi-ANAE positivity in leukemic blast cells: A possible T-suppressor cell leukemia. Acta Haematol 66:122, 1981

Catovsky D, Galetto J et al: Cytochemical profile of T and B leukaemic lymphocytes with special reference to acute lymphoblastic leukaemias. J Clin Pathol 27:767, 1974

Clift RA, Wright DH et al: Leukemia in Burkitt's lymphoma. Blood 22:243, 1963

Colon-Otero G, Li C-Y et al: Erythrophagocytic acute lymphocytic leukemia with B-cell markers and with a 20 q − chromosome abnormality. Mayo Clin Proc 59: 678, 1984

Dick FR, Maca RD et al: Hodgkin's disease terminating in a T-cell immunoblastic leukemia. Cancer 42:1325, 1978

Dyment PG, Savage RA et al: Anomalous azurophilic granules in acute lymphoblastic leukemia. Am J Pediatr Hematol Oncol 4:207, 1982

Flandrin G, Brouet JC et al: Acute leukemia with Burkitt's tumor cells: A study of six cases with special reference to lymphocyte surface markers. Blood 45:183, 1975

Glassy EF, Sun NCJ et al: Hand-mirror cell leukemia: Report of nine cases and a review of the literature. Am J Clin Pathol 74:651, 1980

Gramatzki M, Strong DM, Duval-Arnould B, et al: Hand mirror variant of acute lymphoblastic leukemia. Evidence for early T-cell lineage in two cases by evaluation with monoclonal antibodies. Cancer 55:77, 1985

Grogan TM, Insalaco SJ et al: Acute lymphocytic leukemia with prominent azurophilic granulation and punctate acidic nonspecific esterase and phosphatase activity. Am J Clin Pathol 75:716, 1981

Hanaoka M, Shirakawa S et al: Adult T cell leukemia: Histological features of the lymphoid tissues. Adv Exp Med Biol 114:613, 1979

Hecht T, Forman SJ et al: Histochemical demonstration of terminal deoxynucleotidyl transferase in leukemia. Blood 58:856, 1981

Humphrey GB, Nesbit ME et al: Prognostic value of the periodic acid-Schiff (PAS) reaction in acute lymphoblastic leukemia. Am J Clin Pathol 61:393, 1974

Jansson S-E, Gripenberg J et al: Classification of acute leukaemia by light and electron microscope cytochemistry. Scand J Haematol 25:412, 1980

Komiyama A, Ogawa M et al: Unusual cytoplasmic inclusions in blast cells in acute leukemia. Arch Pathol Lab Med 100:590, 1976

Komiyama A, Yamada S et al: Childhood acute lymphoblastic leukemia with natural killer activity: Clinical and cellular features of three cases. Cancer 54:1547, 1984

Kueh YK: Acute lymphoblastic leukemia with brilliant cresyl blue erythrocytic inclusions—acquired hemoglobin H? N Engl J Med 307:193, 1982

McKenna RW, Brynes RK et al: Cytochemical profiles in acute lymphoblastic leukemia. Am J Pediatr Hematol Oncol 1:263, 1979

McKenna RW, Parkin J et al: Morphologic and ultrastructural characteristics of T-cell acute lymphoblastic leukemia. Cancer 44:1290, 1979

Minerbrook M, Schulman P et al: Burkitt's leukemia: A re-evaluation. Cancer 49:1444, 1982

Salsbury AJ: Nucleolar staining in the differentiation of acute leukaemias. Br J Haematol 13:768, 1967

Tricot G, Broeckaert-Van Orshoven A et al: Sudan black B positivity in acute lymphoblastic leukaemia. Br J Haematol 51:615, 1982

Watanabe S, Shimosato Y et al: Lymphoma and leukemia of T-lymphocytes. Pathol Annu 16 (pt. 2):155, 1981

Yanagihara ET, Naeim F et al: Acute lymphoblastic leukemia with giant intracytoplasmic inclusions. Am J Clin Pathol 74:345, 1980

Yourno J, Burkart P et al: Enzymologic classification of acute leukemias: Nonspecific esterase markers distinguish myeloid and lymphoid varieties. Blood 60:304, 1982

Hairy Cell Leukemia

Aiba M, Raffa PP et al: Significance of leukocyte alkaline phosphatase in hairy cell leukemia. Am J Clin Pathol 74:297, 1980

Bouroncle BA, Wiseman BK et al: Leukemic reticuloendotheliosis. Blood 13:609, 1958

Burke JS, Byrne GE Jr et al: Hairy cell leukemia (leukemic reticuloendotheliosis): I. A clinical pathologic study of 21 patients. Cancer 33:1399, 1974

Catovsky D: Hairy-cell leukaemia and prolymphocytic leukaemia. Clin Haematol 6:245, 1977

Golde DW, Saxon A et al: Macroglobulinemia and hairy-cell leukemia. N Engl J Med 296:92, 1977

Janckila AJ, Li CY et al: The cytochemistry of tartrate resistant acid phosphatase: Technical considerations. Am J Clin Pathol 70:45, 1978

Katayama I, Li CY et al: Ultrastructural cytochemical demonstration of tartrate-resistant acid phosphatase isoenzyme activity in "hairy cells" of leukemic reticuloendotheliosis. Am J Pathol 69:471, 1972

Krause JR: Aplastic anemia terminating in hairy cell leukemia: A report of two cases. Cancer 53:1533, 1984

Mitus WJ, Mednicoff IB et al: Neoplastic lymphoid reticulum cells in the peripheral blood: A histochemical study. Blood 17:206, 1961

Naeim F, Gatti RA et al: "Hairy cell" leukemia: A heterogeneous chronic lymphoproliferative disorder. Am J Med 65:479, 1978

Rubin AD, Douglas SD et al: Chronic reticulolymphocytic leukemia: Reclassification of "leukemic reticuloendotheliosis" through functional characterization of the circulating mononuclear cells. Am J Med 47:149, 1969

Schrek R, Donnelly WJ: "Hairy" cells in blood in lymphoreticular neoplastic disease and "flagellated" cells of normal lymph nodes. Blood 27:199, 1966

Yam LT, Li CY et al: Tartrate-resistant acid phosphatase isoenzyme in the reticulum cells of leukemic reticuloendotheliosis. N Engl J Med 284:357, 1971

Hodgkin's Disease

Cavalli P, Cazzola M et al: Reed-Sternberg cell leukaemia. Tumori 67:63, 1981

Han T, Stutzman L et al: Bone marrow biopsy in Hodgkin's disease and other neoplastic diseases. JAMA 217:1239, 1971

Kass L, Schnitzer B: Ammoniacal silver staining of Reed-Sternberg cell in Hodgkin's disease. Acta Haematol 48:288, 1972

O'Carroll DI, McKenna RW et al: Bone marrow manifestations of Hodgkin's disease. Cancer 38:1717, 1976

Strum SB, Park JK et al: Observation of cells resembling Sternberg-Reed cells in conditions other than Hodgkin's disease. Cancer 26:176, 1970

Weiss RB, Brunning RD et al: Hodgkin's disease in the bone marrow. Cancer 36:2077, 1975

Leukemic Phase of Histiocytic Lymphoma

Armitage JO, Dick FR et al: Diffuse histiocytic lymphoma complicating chronic lymphocytic leukemia. Cancer 41:422, 1978

Brynes RK, Golomb HM et al: The leukemic phase of histiocytic lymphoma: Histologic, cytologic, cytochemical, ultrastructural, immunologic and cytogenetic observations in a case. Am J Clin Pathol 69:550, 1978

Lowenbraun S, Sutherland JC et al: Transformation of reticulum cell sarcoma to acute leukemia. Cancer 27:579, 1971

Rehman KL, Rosner F et al: The leukemic phase of histiocytic lymphoma: Report of four cases. Am J Med Sci 268:353, 1974

Schnitzer B, Kass L: Leukemic phase of reticulum cell sarcoma (histiocytic lymphoma): A clinicopathologic and ultrastructural study. Cancer 31:547, 1973

Zeffren JL, Ultmann JE: Reticulum cell sarcoma terminating in acute leukemia. Blood 15:277, 1960

Angioimmunoblastic Lymphadenopathy

Brearley RL, Chapman J et al: Haematological features of angioimmunoblastic lymphadenopathy with dysproteinaemia. J Clin Pathol 32:356, 1979

Frizzera G, Moran EM et al: Angio-immunoblastic lymphadenopathy: Diagnosis and clinical course. Am J Med 59:803, 1975

Pangalis GA, Moran EM et al: Blood and bone marrow findings in angioimmunoblastic lymphadenopathy. Blood 51:71, 1978

Monocytic Leukemia

Altman AJ, Palmer CG et al: Juvenile "chronic granulocytic" leukemia: A panmyelopathy with prominent monocytic involvement and circulating monocyte colony-forming cells. Blood 43:341, 1974

Bearman RM, Kjeldsberg CR et al: Chronic monocytic leukemia in adults. Cancer 48:2239, 1981

Beattie JW, Seal RME et al: Chronic monocytic leukaemia. Q J Med 20:131, 1951

Broun GO Jr: Chronic erythromonocytic leukemia. Am J Med 47:785, 1969

Brynes RK, Golomb HM et al: Acute monocytic leukemia: Cytologic, histologic, cytochemical, ultrastructural, and cytogenetic observations. Am J Clin Pathol 65:471, 1976

Cawley JC, Burns GF et al: Morphological and immunological similarity of the monocytes from pure and mixed monocytic leukaemias. Scand J Haematol 21:233, 1978

Doan CA, Wiseman BK: The monocyte, monocytosis, and monocytic leukosis: A clinical and pathological study. Ann Intern Med 8:383, 1934

Downey H: Monocytic leucemia and leucemic reticulo-endotheliosis. In Downey H (ed): Handbook of Hematology, vol 2, p 1273. New York, Paul B Hoeber, 1938

Geary CG, Catovsky D et al: Chronic myelomonocytic leukaemia. Br J Haematol 30:289, 1975

Hurdle ADF, Garson OM et al: Clinical and cytogenetic studies in chronic myelomonocytic leukaemia. Br J Haematol 22:773, 1972

Jacobsen KM: Reticuloendotheliose-Monozytenleukose. Acta Med Scand 111:30, 1942

Kass L: Esterase reactions in acute myelomonocytic leukemia. Am J Clin Pathol 67:485, 1977

Kass L, Schnitzer B: Monocytes, Monocytosis, and Monocytic Leukemia. Springfield, IL, Charles C Thomas, 1973

Leder LD: The origin of blood monocytes and macrophages: A review. Blut 16:86, 1967

McKenna RW, Bloomfield CD et al: Acute monoblastic leukemia: Diagnosis and treatment of ten cases. Blood 46:481, 1975

Miescher PA, Farquet JJ: Chronic myelomonocytic leukemia in adults. Semin Hematol 11:129, 1974

Ryder RJ: Chronic monocytic leukaemia. Blut 14:47, 1966

Schmalzl F, Braunsteiner H: On the origin of monocytes. Acta Haematol 39:177, 1968

Scholnik AP, Kass L: A direct cytochemical method for the identification of lysozyme in various tissues. J Histochem Cytochem 21:65, 1973

Sexauer J, Kass L et al: Subacute myelomonocytic leukemia: Clinical, morphologic and ultrastructural studies of 10 cases. Am J Med 57:853, 1974

Shaw MT: Monocytic leukemias. Hum Pathol 11:215, 1980

Shaw MT, Bottomley SS et al: The relationship of erythromonocytic leukemia to other myeloproliferative disorders. Am J Med 55:542, 1973

Shaw MT, Nordquist RE: "Pure" monocytic or histiomonocytic leukemia: A revised concept. Cancer 35:208, 1975

Sinn CM, Dick FW: Monocytic leukemia. Am J Med 20:588, 1956

Tavassoli M, Shaklai M et al: Cytochemical diagnosis of acute myelomonocytic leukemia. Am J Clin Pathol 72:59, 1979

Tobelem G, Jacquillat C et al: Acute monoblastic leukemia: A clinical and biologic study of 74 cases. Blood 55:71, 1980

Yam LT, Li CY et al: Cytochemical identification of monocytes and granulocytes. Am J Clin Pathol 55:283, 1971

Zittoun R: Subacute and chronic myelomonocytic leukaemia: A distinct haematological entity (annotation). Br J Haematol 32:1, 1976

Histiocytoses

Cline MJ, Golde DW: A review and reevaluation of the histicytic disorders. Am J Med 55:49, 1973

Kim H, Pangalis GA et al: Ultrastructural identification of neoplastic histio-
    cytes—monocytes: An application of a newly developed cytochemical
    technique. Am J Pathol 106:204, 1982

Lee KS, Tobin MS et al: Acquired Gaucher's cells in Hodgkin's disease. Am
    J Med 73:290, 1982

Matsubara T, Yoshiya S et al: Histologic and histochemical investigation of
    Gaucher cells. Clin Orthop 166:233, 1982

Parkin JL, Brunning RD: Pathology of the Gaucher cell. Prog Clin Biol Res
    95:151, 1982

Peters SP, Lee RE et al: Gaucher's disease, a review. Medicine 56:425, 1977

Risdall RJ, Brunning RD et al: Malignant histiocytosis: A light- and elec-
    tron-microscopic and histochemical study. Am J Surg Pathol 4:439,
    1980

Scullin DC Jr, Shelburne JD et al: Pseudo-Gaucher cells in multiple mye-
    loma. Am J Med 67:347, 1979

Skoog DP, Feagler JR: T cell acute lymphocytic leukemia terminating as
    malignant histiocytosis. Am J Med 64:678, 1978

Tubbs RR, Sheibani K et al: Malignant histiocytosis: Ultrastructural and
    immunocytochemical characterization. Arch Pathol Lab Med 104:26,
    1980

Vardiman JW, Byrne GE Jr et al: Malignant histiocytosis with massive sple-
    nomegaly in asymptomatic patients: A possible chronic form of the dis-
    ease. Cancer 36:419, 1975

Varela-Duran J, Roholt PC et al: Sea-blue histiocyte syndrome: A secondary
    degenerative process of macrophages? Arch Pathol Lab Med 104:30,
    1980

Leukemoid Reaction

Anday EK, Harris MC: Leukemoid reaction associated with antenatal dexa-
    methasone administration. J Pediatr 101:614, 1982

Bordelon J, Stone MJ et al: Probable myeloblastic leukemoid reaction with
    disseminated sarcoidosis. South Med J 70:1378, 1977

Brodeur GM, Dahl GV et al: Transient leukemoid reaction and trisomy 21
    mosaicism in a phenotypically normal newborn. Blood 55:691, 1980

Eichenhorn MS, Van Slyck EJ: Marked mature neutrophilic leukocytosis: A
    leukemoid variant associated with malignancy. Am J Med Sci 284:32,
    1982

Narayana AS, Kelly DG et al: Leukaemoid reaction in a case of leiomyosar-
    coma of the bladder. Postgrad Med J 53:766, 1977

Okun DB, Tanaka KR: Profound leukemoid reaction in cytomegalovirus
    mononucleosis. JAMA 240:1888, 1978

Rosenfeld CS, Sloan B et al: Multiple hepatoma with leukemoid reaction.
    NY State J Med 82:359, 1982

Rubins J, Wakem CJ: Hypoglycemia and leukemoid reaction with hyperne-
    phroma. NY State J Med 77:406, 1977

Eosinophilia and Eosinophilic Leukemia

Brandt L, Mitelman R et al: Different composition of the eosinophilic bone marrow pool in reactive eosinophilia and eosinophilic leukaemia. Acta Med Scand 201:177, 1977

Chusid MJ, Dale DC et al: The hypereosinophilic syndrome: Analysis of fourteen cases with review of the literature. Medicine 54:1, 1975

Miller RR, Lewis JP et al: Acute eosinophilic leukemia associated with neutropenia. West J Med 123:399, 1975

Stavem P, Ly B et al: Light green crystals in May-Grunwald and Giemsa-stained bone marrow macrophages in patients with myeloid leukaemia. Scand J Haematol 18:67, 1977

Weinger RS, Andre-Schwartz J et al: Acute leukaemia with eosinophilia or acute eosinophilic leukaemia: A dilemma. Br J Haematol 30:65, 1975

Weller PF: Eosinophilia. J Allergy Clin Immunol 73:1, 1984

Weller PF, Goetzl EJ: The human eosinophil. Roles in host defense and tissue injury. Am J Pathol 100:793, 1980

Yam LT, Yam C-F et al: Eosinophilia in systemic mastocytosis. Am J Clin Pathol 73:48, 1980

Basophils

May ME, Waddell CC: Basophils in peripheral blood and bone marrow. A retrospective review. Am J Med 76:509, 1984

Mitchell EB, Askenase PW: Basophils in human disease. Clin Rev Allergy 1:427, 1983

Parkin JL, McKenna RW et al: Ultrastructural features of basophil and mast cell granulopoiesis in blastic phase Philadelphia chromosome-positive leukemia. J Natl Cancer Inst 65:535, 1980

Myeloperoxidase Deficiency

Catovsky D, Galton DA et al: Myeloperoxidase-deficient neutrophils in acute myeloid leukaemia. Scand J Haematol 9:142, 1972

Davis AT, Brunning RD et al: Polymorphonuclear leukocyte myeloperoxidase deficiency in a patient with myelomonocytic leukemia. N Engl J Med 285:789, 1971

Chronic Granulocytic Leukemia

Bainton DF: Neutrophil granules (annotation). Br J Haematol 29:17, 1975

Buyssens N, Bourgeois NH: Chronic myelocytic leukemia versus idiopathic myelofibrosis: A diagnostic problem in bone marrow biopsies. Cancer 40:1548, 1977

Gomez GA, Sokal JE et al: Prognostic features at diagnosis of chronic myelocytic leukemia. Cancer 47:2470, 1981

Kaplow LS: Cytochemistry of leukocyte alkaline phosphatase: Use of complex naphthol as phosphates in azo dye-coupling technics. Am J Clin Pathol 39:439, 1963

Karanas A, Silver RT: Characteristics of the terminal phase of chronic granulocytic leukemia. Blood 32:445, 1968

Koeffler HP, Golde DW: Chronic myelogenous leukemia—new concepts (pt. 1). N Engl J Med 304:1201, 1981

Korostoff NR, Sun NCJ et al: Atypical blast crisis in chronic myelogenous leukemia. JAMA 245:1245, 1981

Muehleck, SD, McKenna RW et al: Transformation of chronic myelogenous leukemia: Clinical, morphologic, and cytogenetic features. Am J Clin Pathol 82:1, 1984

O'Malley FM, Garson OM et al: Erythroblastic transformation of chronic granulocytic leukemia: A clinical and cytogenetic case study. Am J Hematol 14:371, 1983

Peterson LC, Bloomfield CD et al: Blast crisis as an initial or terminal manifestation of chronic myeloid leukemia: A study of 28 patients. Am J Med 60:209, 1976

Rosenthal S, Canellos GP et al: Characteristics of blast crisis in chronic granulocytic leukemia. Blood 49:705, 1977

Rosenthal S, Canellos GP et al: Erythroblastic transformation of chronic granulocytic leukemia. Am J Med 63:116, 1977

Shaw MT, Bottomley RH et al: Heterogeneity of morphological, cytochemical, and cytogenetic features in the blastic phase of chronic granulocytic leukemia. Cancer 35:199, 1975

Sjogren U: Morphologic studies of the erythropoietic part of bone marrow in myeloid leukaemias. Scand J Haematol 22:61, 1979

Spiers AS: The clinical features of chronic granulocytic leukaemia. Clin Haematol 6:77, 1977

Spiers ASD: Metamorphosis of chronic granulocytic leukaemia: Diagnosis, classification, and management. Br J Haematol 41:1, 1979

Theologides A: Unfavorable signs in patients with chronic myelocytic leukemia. Ann Intern Med 76:95, 1972

Velez-Garcia E, Santiago JV et al: Coexistence of chronic granulocytic leukemia and a lymphoproliferative disorder. Ann Intern Med 70:1219, 1969

Williams WC, Weiss GB: Megakaryoblastic transformation of chronic myelogenous leukemia. Cancer 49:921, 1982

Agnogenic Myeloid Metaplasia

Jackson H Jr, Parker F Jr et al: Agnogenic myeloid metaplasia of the spleen: A syndrome simulating other more definite hematologic disorders. N Engl J Med 222:985, 1940

Jennings WH, Li C-Y et al: Concomitant myelofibrosis with agnogenic myeloid metaplasia and malignant lymphoma. Mayo Clin Proc 58:617, 1983

Rappaport H: Tumors of the Hematopoietic System. Atlas of Tumor Pathology, sec. 3, fasc. 8. Washington, DC, Armed Forces Institute of Pathology, 1966

Ward HP, Block MH: The natural history of agnogenic myeloid metaplasia (AMM) and a critical evaluation of its relationship with the myeloproliferative syndrome. Medicine 50:357, 1971

Acute Myeloblastic Leukemia

Anner RM, Lennon JM et al: Prognostic significance of morphologic and cytochemical markers in adult acute leukemia. Am J Clin Pathol 69:494, 1978

Arthur DC, Bloomfield CD: Partial deletion of the long arm of chromosome 16 and bone marrow eosinophilia in acute nonlymphocytic leukemia: A new association. Blood 61:994, 1983

Bainton DF, Friedlander LM et al: Abnormalities in granule formation in acute myelogenous leukemia. Blood 49:693, 1977

Bessho F, Fujiu M et al: Acute nonlymphocytic leukemia showing abnormal nuclear lobulation. Am J Clin Pathol 75:684, 1981

Bloomfield CD, Brunning RD: Acute leukemia as a terminal event in non-leukemic hematopoietic disorders. Semin Oncol 3:297, 1976

Carey RW, Taft PD et al: Carcinocythemia (carcinoma cell leukemia): An acute leukemia-like picture due to metastatic carcinoma cells. Am J Med 60:273, 1976

Catovsky D, de Salvo Cardullo L et al: Cytochemical markers of differentiation in acute leukemia. Cancer Res 41:4824, 1981

Cuttner J, Seremetis S et al: Td-T-positive acute leukemia with monocytoid characteristics: Clinical, cytochemical, cytogenetic and immunologic findings. Blood 64:237, 1984

Diamond LW, Nathwani BN et al: Flow cytometry in the diagnosis and classification of malignant lymphoma and leukemia. Cancer 50:1122, 1982

Gallivan MVE, Lokich JJ: Carcinocythemia (carcinoma cell leukemia): Report of two cases with English literature review. Cancer 53:110, 1984

Glick AD, Paniker K et al: Acute leukemia of adults: Ultrastructural, cytochemical and histologic observations in 100 cases. Am J Clin Pathol 73:459, 1980

Gralnick HR, Galton DAG et al: Classification of acute leukemia. Ann Intern Med 87:740, 1977

Hayhoe FGJ, Quaglino D: Haematological Cytochemistry. Edinburgh, Churchill Livingstone, 1980

Hogge DE, Misawa S et al: Abnormalities of chromosome 16 in association with acute myelomonocytic leukemia and dysplastic bone marrow eosinophils. J Clin Oncol 2:550, 1984

Holden D, Lichtman H: Paroxysmal nocturnal hemoglobinuria with acute leukemia. Blood 33:283, 1969

Hull MT, Griep JA: Mixed leukemia, lymphatic and myelomonocytic. Am J Clin Pathol 74:473, 1980

Lanham GR, Bollum FJ et al: Simultaneous occurrence of terminal deoxynucleotidyl transferase and myeloperoxidase in individual leukemic blasts. Blood 64:318, 1984

LeBeau MM, Larson RA et al: Association of an inversion of chromosome 16 with abnormal marrow eosinophils in acute myelomonocytic leukemia. N Engl J Med 309:630, 1983

LeBien TW, McKenna RW et al: Use of monoclonal antibodies, morphology, and cytochemistry to probe the cellular heterogeneity of acute leukemia and lymphoma. Cancer Res 41:4776, 1981

Li CY: Immunocytochemical techniques for identifying leukemias. Mayo Clin Proc 59:185, 1984

Ligorsky RD, Axelrod AR et al: Acute myelomonocytic leukemia in a patient with macroglobulinemia and malignant lymphoma. Cancer 39:1156, 1977

Mertelsmann R, Tzvi Thaler H et al: Morphological classification, response to therapy, and survival in 263 adult patients with acute nonlympho-blastic leukemia. Blood 56:773, 1980

Morse H, Hays T et al: Acute nonlymphoblastic leukemia in childhood: High incidence of clonal abnormalities and nonrandom changes. Cancer 44:164, 1979

Neame PB, Soamboonsrup P, Browman G et al: Simultaneous or sequential expression of lymphoid and myeloid phenotypes in acute leukemia. Blood 65: 142, 1985

Needleman SW, Burns CP et al: Hypoplastic acute leukemia. Cancer 48:1410, 1981

Perentesis J, Ramsay NKC et al: Biphenotypic leukemia: Immunologic and morphologic evidence for a common lymphoid-myeloid progenitor in humans. J Pediatr 102:63, 1983

Schmalzl F, Huhn D et al: Cytochemistry and ultrastructure of pathologic granulation in myelogenous leukemia. Blut 27:243, 1973

Sjogren U: Erythroblastic islands and ineffective erythropoiesis in acute myeloid leukaemia. Acta Haematol 54:11, 1975

Sjogren U: Morphologic studies of the erythropoietic part of bone marrow in myeloid leukaemias. Scand J Haematol 22:61, 1979

Straus DJ, Andreeff M et al: The coexistence of acute myeloblastic leukemia and diffuse histiocytic lymphoma in the same patient as demonstrated by multiparameter analysis. Blood 54:1428, 1979

van Noorden CJ, Tas J et al: A new method for the enzyme cytochemical staining of individual cells with the use of a polyacrylamide carrier. His-tochemistry 74:171, 1982

Weiss RB, Brunning RD et al: Lymphosarcoma terminating in acute myelog-enous leukemia. Cancer 30:1275, 1972

Whiteside MG: Influence of classification systems on the treatment of leu-kemia. Pathology 14:295, 1982

Wolf DJ, Fialk MA et al: Unusual intracytoplasmic inclusions in acute myeloblastic leukemia. Am J Hematol 9:413, 1980

Youness E, Trujillo JM et al: Acute unclassified leukemia: A clinicopatho-logic study with diagnostic implications of electron microscopy. Am J Hematol 9:79, 1980

Zittoun R, Cadiou M et al: Prognostic value of cytologic parameters in acute myelogenous leukemia. Cancer 53:1526, 1984

Acute Promyelocytic Leukemia

Berger R, Bernheim A et al: Translocation t (15;17), leucemie aigue promye-locytaire et non promyelocytaire. Nouv Rev Fr Hematol 21:117, 1979

McKenna RW, Parkin J et al: Acute promyelocytic leukaemia: A study of 39 cases with identification of a hyperbasophilic microgranular variant. Br J Haematol 50:201, 1982

Paietta E, Dutcher JP, Wiernik P: Terminal transferase positive acute pro-myelocytic leukemia: in vitro differentiation of a T-lymphocytic/pro-myelocytic hybrid phenotype. Blood 65:107, 1985

Stavem P, Rørvik TO et al: Differing form of variant form of hypergranular promyelocytic leukaemia (M3), or transition between M3 and monocy-tic leukaemia? Scand J Haematol 26:149, 1981

Testa JR, Golomb HM et al: Hypergranular promyelocytic leukemia (APL): Cytogenetic and ultrastructural specificity. Blood 52:272,1978

Valdivieso M, Rodriquez V et al: Clinical and morphological correlations in acute promyelocytic leukemia. Med Pediatr Oncol 1:37, 1975

Acute Microgranular Promyelocytic Leukemia

Bennett JM, Catovsky D et al: A variant form of hypergranular promyelocy-tic leukemia (M3). Ann Intern Med 92:261, 1980

Edelman BB, Grossman NJ: Microgranular acute promyelocytic leukemia—a case with multiple Auer rods demonstrable only after staining for chlo-roacetate esterase. Am J Clin Pathol 79:621, 1983

Golomb HM, Rowley JD et al: "Microgranular" acute promyelocytic leuke-mia: A distinct clinical, ultrastructural, and cytogenetic entity. Blood 55:253, 1980

Savage RA, Hoffman GC et al: Morphology and cytochemistry of "micro-granular" acute promyelocytic leukemia (FAB M3m). Am J Clin Pathol 75:548, 1981

Treatment-Related Leukemia

Anderson RL, Bagby GC et al: Therapy-related preleukemic syndrome. Can-cer 47:1867, 1981

Cadman EC, Capizzi RL et al: Acute nonlymphocytic leukemia: A delayed complication of Hodgkin's disease therapy: Analysis of 109 cases. Can-cer 40:1280, 1977

Casciato DA, Scott JL: Acute leukemia following prolonged cytotoxic agent therapy. Medicine 58:32, 1979

Collins AJ, Bloomfield CD et al: Acute nonlymphocytic leukemia in patients with nodular lymphoma. Cancer 40:1748, 1977

Foucar K, McKenna RW et al: Therapy-related leukemia: A panmyelosis. Cancer 43:1285, 1979

Grunwald HW, Rosner F: Acute myeloid leukemia following treatment of Hodgkin's disease: A review. Cancer 50:676, 1982

Hoy WE, Packman CH et al: Evolution of acute leukemia in a renal transplant patient—? Relationship to azathioprine. Transplantation 33:331, 1982

Kjeldsberg CR, Nathwani BN et al: Acute myeloblastic leukemia developing in patients with mediastinal lymphoblastic lymphoma. Cancer 44:2316, 1979

McKenna RW, Parkin JL et al: Ultrastructural characteristics of therapy-related acute nonlymphocytic leukemia: Evidence for a panmyelosis. Cancer 48:725, 1981

Papa G, Alimena G et al: Acute nonlymphoid leukaemia following Hodgkin's disease: Clinical, biological and cytogenetic aspects of 3 cases. Scand J Haematol 23:339, 1979

Pedersen-Bjergaard J, Larsen SO: Incidence of acute nonlymphocytic leukemia, preleukemia, and acute myeloproliferative syndrome up to 10 years after treatment of Hodgkin's disease. N Engl J Med 307:965, 1982

Rosner F, Grunwald H: Hodgkin's disease and acute leukemia: Report of eight cases and review of the literature. Am J Med 58:339, 1975

Rosner F, Grunwald HW et al: Acute leukemia as a complication of cytotoxic chemotherapy. Int J Radiat Oncol Biol Phys 5:1705, 1979

Vardiman JW, Coelho A et al: Morphologic and cytochemical observations on the overt leukemic phase of therapy-related leukemia. Am J Clin Pathol 79:525, 1983

Vardiman JW, Golomb HM et al: Acute nonlymphocytic leukemia in malignant lymphoma: A morphologic study. Cancer 42:229, 1978

Weiss RB, Brunning RD et al: Lymphosarcoma terminating in acute myelogenous leukemia. Cancer 30:1275, 1972

Zarrabi MH, Rosner F et al: Non-Hodgkin's lymphoma and acute myeloblastic leukemia: A report of 12 cases and review of the literature. Cancer 44:1070, 1979

Preleukemia

Bennett JM, Catovsky D et al: Proposals for the classification of the myelodysplastic syndromes. Br J Haematol 51:189, 1982

Blair TR, Bayrd ED et al: Atypical leukemia. JAMA 198:139, 1966

Block M, Jacobson LO et al: Preleukemic acute human leukemia. JAMA 152:1018, 1953

Fisher WB, Armentrout SA et al: "Preleukemia": A myelodysplastic syndrome often terminating in acute leukemia. Arch Intern Med 132:226, 1973

Kass L: Preleukemic Disorders. Springfield, IL, Charles C Thomas, 1979

Linman JW: Myelomonocytic leukemia and its preleukemic phase. J Chronic Dis 22:713, 1970

Linman JW, Bagby C Jr: The preleukemic syndrome: Clinical and laboratory features, natural course, and management. Nouv Rev Fr Hematol 17:11, 1976

Linman JW, Saarni MI: The preleukemic syndrome. Semin Hematol 11:93, 1974

Meacham GC, Weisberger AS: Early atypical manifestations of leukemia. Ann Intern Med 41:780, 1954

Mitrou PS, Fischer M et al: Conversion of polycythemia vera to refractory anemia with hyperplastic bone marrow. Blut 36:41, 1978

Pierre RV: Preleukemic states. Semin Hematol 11:73, 1974

Saarni MI, Linman JW: Myelomonocytic leukemia: Disorderly proliferation of all marrow cells. Cancer 27:1221, 1971

Saarni MI, Linman JW: Preleukemia: The hematologic syndrome preceding acute leukemia. Am J Med 55:38, 1973

Vilter RW, Jarrold T et al: Refractory anemia with hyperplastic bone marrow. Blood 15:1, 1960

Wintrobe MM, Mitchell DM: Atypical manifestations of leukaemia. Q J Med 9:67, 1940

Zittoun R, Diebold J et al: Diagnostic des etats preleucemiques et des leucemies myelo-monocytaires et atypiques. Nouv Rev Fr Hematol 13:380, 1973

Multiple Myeloma

Bataille R, Durie BGM et al: Myeloma bone marrow acid phosphatase staining: A correlative study of 38 patients. Blood 55:802, 1980

Brunning RD, Parkin J: Intranuclear inclusions in plasma cells and lymphocytes from patients with monoclonal gammopathies. Am J Clin Pathol 66:10, 1976

Graham RC, Bernier GM: The bone marrow in multiple myeloma: Correlation of plasma cell ultrastructure and clinical state. Medicine 54:225, 1975

Reed M, McKenna RW et al: Morphologic manifestations of monoclonal gammopathies. Am J Clin Pathol 76:8, 1981

Rosner F, Grunwald H: Multiple myeloma terminating in acute leukemia: Report of 12 cases and review of the literature. Am J Med 57:927, 1974

Macroglobulinemia

Leonhard SA, Muhleman AF et al: Emergence of immunoblastic sarcoma in Waldenstrom's macroglobulinemia. Cancer 45:3102, 1980

Martelli MF, Falini B et al: Acute leukemia complicating Waldenstrom's macroglobulinemia. Haematologica 66:303, 1981

Ricci A Jr, Monahan RA et al: Unusual inclusions in plasmacytoid cells: Their occurrence in a patient with Waldenstrom's macroglobulinemia. Arch Pathol Lab Med 106:452, 1982

Megakaryocyte Identification

Breton-Gorius J, Guichard J: Ultrastructural localization of peroxidase activity in human platelets and megakaryocytes. Am J Pathol 66:277, 1972

Deng CT, Terasaki PI et al: A monoclonal antibody cross-reactive with human platelets, megakaryocytes and common acute lymphocytic leukemia cells. Blood 61:759, 1983

El-Mohandes E, Hayhoe FGJ: 5-Nucleotidase activity of megakaryoblasts in a case of acute megakaryoblastic leukaemia. Br J Haematol 53:523, 1983

Hourdille P, Fialon P et al: Mepacrine labelling test and uranaffin cytochemical reaction in human megakaryocytes. Thromb Haemost 47:232, 1982

Kanz L, Straub G et al: Identification of human megakaryocytes derived from pure megakaryocytic colonies (CFU-M), megakaryocytic erythroid colonies (CPU-GEMM) by antibodies against platelet associated antigens. Blut 45:267, 1982

Kass L: Megakaryocytes in the May-Heggelin anomaly. Arch Pathol 98:112, 1974

Kass L: Identification of human megakaryocytes with rhodanile blue. Arch Pathol Lab Med 109:320, 1985

Kass L: Lycramine brilliant blue JL: A new stain for megakaryocytes. Stain Technol 60:233, 1985

Kass L, Leichtman DA et al: Megakaryocytes in the giant platelet syndrome: A cytochemical and ultrastructural study. Thromb Haemost 38:652, 1977

Markovic OS, Shulman NR: Megakaryocyte maturation indurated by methanol inhibition of an acid phosphatase shared by megakaryocytes and platelets. Blood 50:905, 1977

Mazur EM, Hoffman R et al: Immunofluorescent identification of human megakaryocyte colonies using an antiplatelet glycoprotein antiserum. Blood 57:277, 1981

McLaren KM, Pepper DS: Immunological localisation of beta-thromboglobulin and platelet factor 4 in human megakaryocytes and platelets. J Clin Pathol 35:1227, 1982

Pizzolo G, Chilosi M et al: Detection of normal and malignant megakaryocytes by anti beta-thromboglobulin serum: An immunofluorescence study. Scand J Haematol 29:200, 1982

Ryo R, Proffitt RT et al: Platelet factor 4 antigen in megakaryocytes. Thromb Res 17:645, 1980

Schick PK, Weinstein MA: Marker for megakaryocytes: Serotonin accumulation in guinea pig megakaryocytes. J Lab Clin Med 98:607, 1981

Vainchenker W, Deschamps JF et al: Two monoclonal antiplatelet antibodies as markers of human megakaryocyte maturation: Immunofluorescent staining and platelet peroxidase detection in megakaryocyte colonies and in vitro cell from normal and leukemic patients. Blood 59:514, 1982

Micromegakaryocytes

Albrecht M, Fulle HH: Extremely small megakaryocytes in chronic myelocytic leukemia, acute leukemia and erythroleukemia. Klin Wochenschr 52:649, 1974

Rabellino EM, Levene RB et al: Human megakaryocytes: III. Characterization in myeloproliferative disorders. Blood 63:615, 1984

Smith WB, Ablin A et al: Atypical megakaryocytes in preleukemic phase of acute myeloid leukemia. Blood 42:535, 1973

Yamauchi K, Miyauchi J et al: Identification of circulating micromegakaryocytes in a case of erythroleukemia. Cancer 53:2668, 1984

Idiopathic Thrombocytopenic Purpura

Branehog I, Kutti J et al: The relation of thrombokinetics to bone marrow megakaryocytes in idiopathic thrombocytopenic purpura (ITP). Blood 45:551, 1975

Dameshek W, Miller EB: Megakaryocytes in idiopathic thrombocytopenic purpura, a form of hypersplenism. Blood 1:27, 1946

Diggs LW, Havlett JS: A study of the bone marrow from 36 patients with idiopathic (thrombocytopenic) purpura. Blood 3:1090, 1948

Pisciotta AV, Stefanini M et al: Studies on platelets: X. Morphologic characteristics of megakaryocytes by phase contrast microscopy and in patients with idiopathic thrombocytopenic purpura. Blood 8:703, 1953

Ridell B, Branehog I: The ultrastructure of the megakaryocytes in idiopathic thrombocytopenic purpura (ITP) in relation to thrombokinetics. Pathol Eur 11:179, 1976

Thrombotic Thrombocytopenic Purpura

Bukowski RM: Thrombotic thrombocytopenic purpura: A review. Prog Hemost Thromb 6:287, 1982

Kass L: Nuclear "speckling" in thrombotic thrombocytopenic purpura proerythroblasts. Am J Clin Pathol 59:869, 1973

Kass L, Schnitzer B: Extramedullary haematopoiesis in thrombotic thrombocytopenic purpura. Folia Haematol 106:32, 1979

Ridolfi RL, Bell WR: Thrombotic thrombocytopenic purpura: Report of 25 cases and review of the literature. Medicine 60:413, 1981

Essential Thrombocythemia

Gunz FW: Hemorrhagic thrombocythemia: A critical review. Blood 15:706, 1960

Kass L: Enzymatic abnormalities in megakaryocytes. Acta Haematol 49:133, 1973

Silverstein MN: Primary or hemorrhagic thrombocythemia. Arch Intern Med 122:18, 1968

Woodruff RK, Bell WR et al: Essential thrombocythaemia. Haemostasis 9:105, 1980

Megakaryocytic Leukemia

Allegra SR, Broderick PA: Acute aleukemic megakaryocytic leukemia: Report of a case. Am J Clin Pathol 55:197, 1971

Bain BJ, Catovsky D et al: Megakaryoblastic leukemia presenting as acute myelofibrosis: A study of four cases with the platelet-peroxidase reaction. Blood 58:206, 1981

Bearman RM, Pangalis GA et al: Acute ("malignant") myelosclerosis. Cancer 43:279, 1979

Breton-Gorius J, Reyes F et al: Megakaryoblastic acute leukemia: Identification by the ultrastructural demonstration of platelet peroxidase. Blood 51:45, 1978

Breton-Gorius J, Reyes F et al: The blast crisis of chronic granulocytic leukemia: Megakaryoblastic nature of cells as revealed by the presence of platelet peroxidase: A cytochemical study. Br J Haematol 39:295, 1978

Breton-Gorius J, Reyes F et al: Les leucemies aigues megacaryoblastiques (abstr). Nouv Rev Fr Hematol 23 (Suppl):14, 1981

Chan BWB, Flemans RJ et al: Acute leukemia with megakaryocytic predominance. Cancer 28:1343, 1971

Den Ottolander GJ, Te Velde J et al: Megakaryoblastic leukaemia (acute myelofibrosis): A report of three cases. Br J Haematol 42:9, 1979

Georgii A, Vykoupil KF et al: Chronic megakaryocytic granulocytic myelosis—CMGM: A subtype of chronic myeloid leukemia. Virchows Arch (Pathol Anat) 389:253, 1980

Habib A, Lee H et al: Acute myelogenous leukemia with megakaryocytic myelosis. Am J Clin Pathol 74:705, 1980

Huang M-J, Chin-Yang L et al: Acute leukemia with megakaryocytic differentiation: A study of 12 cases identified immunocytochemically. Blood 64:427, 1984

Innes DJ Jr, Mills SE et al: Megakaryocytic leukemia: Identification utilizing anti-factor VIII immunoperoxidase. Am J Clin Pathol 77:107, 1982

Jacobs P, le Roux I et al: Megakaryoblastic transformation in myeloproliferative disorders. Cancer 54:297, 1984

Koike T: Megakaryoblastic leukemia: The characterization and identification of megakaryoblasts. Blood 64:683, 1984

Mirchandani I, Palutke M: Acute megakaryocytic leukemia. Cancer 50:2866, 1983

Sultan C, Sigaux F et al: Acute myelodysplasia with myelofibrosis: A report of eight cases. Br J Haematol 49:11, 1981

Wang SE, Fligiel S et al: Acute megakaryocytic leukemia following chemotherapy for a malignant teratoma. Arch Pathol Lab Med 108:202, 1984

Cytochemistry of Blood Cells

Beckstead JH, Bainton DF: Enzyme histochemistry on bone marrow biopsies: Reactions useful in the differential diagnosis of leukemia and lymphoma applied to 2-micron plastic sections. Blood 55:386, 1980

Breton-Gorius J: The value of cytochemical peroxidase reactions at the ultrastructural level in haematology. Histochem J 12:127, 1980

Cannon MS, Cannon AM et al: Nonspecific esterase activity in plastic-embedded tissues using Meldola blue. Am J Clin Pathol 77:465, 1982

Elias JM: A rapid, sensitive myeloperoxidase stain using 4-chloro-1-naphthol. Am J Clin Pathol 73:797, 1980

Kass L: Kallichrome: A new stain for erythroblasts. Stain Technol 55:31, 1980

Kass L: Niagara sky blue 6B—a new stain for granulocytic cells. Am J Clin Pathol 74:801, 1980

Kass L: Orseillein-aniline blue: A new stain for erythroblasts. Am J Clin Pathol 76:302, 1981

Kass L: Identification of normal and leukemic granulocytic cells with Merocyanine 540. Stain Technol (in press)

Leder LD: Uber die selektive fermentcytochemische Darstellung von neutrophilen myeloischen Zellen und Gewebsmastzellen im Paraffinschnitt. Klin Wochenschr 42:553, 1964

Index

The letter *f* after a page number indicates a figure.

accelerated pyknosis in erythroblasts, 11f, 35, 36f–37f
accessory nuclei in erythroblasts
multiple, small, 26
single, large, 24
acid phosphatase activity
in hairy cells, 153, 361, 363f
method for, 361, 364
in T-cell convoluted lymphoblasts, 143, 361
tartrate resistant, 361
in hairy cells, 153, 363f
acquired immune deficiency
syndrome, plasmacytosis
in, 285, 286f
acute erythremic myelosis, 53,
56f, 60

coarse basophilic stippling in,
41, 41f
cytochemical abnormalities
of erythroblasts in, 53–60
cytoplasmic vacuoles, unusually large, 43, 43f
erythroblastic gigantism in,
22f, 39f, 53, 57f
histiocytoid cells in, 53, 58f
increased proerythroblasts in,
53, 55f
in marrow, 53, 54f
nonspecific esterase activity
in, 59f, 60
PAS stain in, 59f, 60
phosphorylase activity in,
59f, 60
Prussian blue stain in, 60

specific esterase activity in,
59f, 60
acute lymphoblastic leukemia.
See also lymphoblasts,
leukemic
acid phosphatase, unipolar,
150, 361
cytochemical abnormalities
in, 148, 148f–150f, 150
immunological characterization of, 148, 150
L1 variant, 147, 148f
L2 variant, 131f, 147, 148f,
149f
L3 variant, 129f, 146f, 147,
353, 354f
lymphoblasts in, 147–148,
150, 349

423